The International System for Serous Fluid Cytopathology

Ashish Chandra · Barbara Crothers
Daniel Kurtycz · Fernando Schmitt
Editors

The International System for Serous Fluid Cytopathology

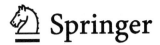 Springer

Editors
Ashish Chandra
Cellular Pathology, Guy's and St. Thomas'
NHS Foundation Trust
London
UK

Barbara Crothers
Gynecology, Breast and Cytopathology
Joint Pathology Center
Silver Spring, MD
USA

Daniel Kurtycz
University of Wisconsin School of Medicine
and Public Health, Department of Pathology
and Laboratory Medicine and
Wisconsin State Laboratory of Hygiene
Madison, WI
USA

Fernando Schmitt
Department of Pathology
Medical Faculty of Porto University and
Unit of Molecular Pathology, Institute of
Molecular Pathology and Immunology
Porto University
Porto
Portugal

ISBN 978-3-030-53907-8   ISBN 978-3-030-53908-5   (eBook)
https://doi.org/10.1007/978-3-030-53908-5

This Springer imprint is published by the registered company Springer Nature Switzerland AG
The registered company address is: Gewerbestrasse 11, 6330 Cham, Switzerland

To my great mentors – Professor Monisha Choudhury, Professor Dulcie Coleman and Dr Amanda Herbert – for their inspiration and encouragement through my early years in cytopathology. AC

To my mother, for giving me freedom to explore, and to the cytopathology community for their cohesion, dedication and unflagging commitment to patients and their health through cytopathology. BC

To my father, Frank Kurtycz, a family man and veteran, who educated three generations of descendants and provided us a model of honor and care. DK

To all who helped, taught and supported me during my scientific career. FS

Foreword

Whilst the pendulum of cytopathology as a diagnostic modality in different organs and systems, through the years, swung both ways, its use in the diagnosis of serous fluids has never been in question. It has stood the test of time as a universally accepted method contributing to clinical management, either in primary diagnosis, staging or follow-up settings. As such, it represents a high proportion of routine specimens in an average diagnostic cytopathology laboratory. Whether a single drop or litres of it, serous fluid is a familiar sample to all cytopathologists and cytotechnologists around the world.

Observing a cytopathologist at work, a fly on the wall might consider our job sedentary and dull. Taking that view, we could compare cytopathology to snorkelling: looking from the shore, a slow moving, breathing tube of a diver on the surface of the water may appear boring, not appreciating that there is a whole underwater planet there to explore. And, drawing a parallel, through the microscope, we are exploring a 'planet body'. There, amongst the cells encountered, those in the serous fluids remind us most vividly of a life submerged under water. Cells float freely, with their tentacle-like processes, unimpeded by the artefacts of other cells obtained by means of brushing, scraping or aspirating. Transporting these delicate cells from the fluid onto a glass slide, in a perfect state of preservation, ready to be observed under a microscope, involves the masterly skill of a cytotechnologist. Excelling in and developing various preparatory techniques should not be underestimated and ultimately can make a major difference between success and failure in their recognition and interpretation.

The interpretation of microscopic findings in serous fluid is challenging. It is often the most difficult part of a trainee cytopathologists' preparation for the final specialist examination/board certification. Unfortunately, it does not end there. It gets worse later when, as a specialist, the interpretation is equally difficult except one's opinion, confirmed by the signature at the bottom of the report, now makes a real life difference to clinical management. This can be a frightening experience if you have no language of communication or coding to convey areas of concern. It is estimated that around one third of serous fluids are difficult to assess by morphology alone, but it takes time to accept one's shortcomings. In the past, the main mode of clinical communication was interpreting cells as 'malignant' or 'not malignant', to the extent that many laboratories had a rubber stamp stating these crude options. This approach reduced cytopathology to issuing machine-like results that were lacking detail and did not allow for grey areas. The use of immunocytochemistry and other ancillary techniques has helped confirm and refine the diagnosis and is now commonplace. Its use is an expected gold standard for the reporting of serous fluids. Laboratories that do not have these facilities available should consider sharing with a larger laboratory rather than giving up on the opportunity of reaching the correct answer.

The International System of Reporting of Serous Fluids (TIS), described in this book, is a new language of communicating the result between the cytopathologist and the clinical team. It should help in all, including the most difficult cases, by stratifying the diagnostic certainty. TIS defines a spectrum of diagnostic categories to be used in daily clinical practice, allowing for doubt and recognising diagnostic dilemmas which sometimes, despite our best efforts, cannot be avoided. Although, for ease of communication, it is a numerical system, partly a nod to our elders who used it in other areas of cytopathology, it is not intended as a substitute for a full diagnostic description, only making the interpretation easier in terms of clinical management. TIS also incorporates the concept of 'risk of malignancy' (ROM) for different diagnostic categories, which has thus far been used successfully elsewhere in cytopathology and adds an important lever to a clinical dialogue which is required more and more frequently.

Communication between the laboratory and the clinic has several aspects, all of which are important. One of the key ones is *clarity*. Nowadays, when formal meetings between the laboratory and clinical teams are held via digital media, communication has to be particularly streamlined to avoid any misunderstanding. TIS addresses the diagnostic part of this communication, serving as a template to aid in patient management. It lends itself to clearer Clinical Management Guidelines. When issuing a TIS report, cytopathologists should be aware of the clinical management protocols and the role their diagnosis plays in it. Ideally, the findings should be discussed with the multidisciplinary clinical team regularly.

In addition to the advantages to direct patient care, the widespread use of TIS will have other benefits, such as a role in collaborative research by making data between laboratories comparable, contributing to easier evaluation of outcomes/audit/follow-up protocols and elucidating teaching conundrums, amongst others.

Looking at cells with our diving mask/microscope, they will still not be labelled with numbers or ROM percentages. In daily practice, the final result will still depend on *expert preparation, careful interpretation* using all available ancillary techniques and a *clear*, if sometimes not definitive, *conclusion*, communicated via the new TIS language including a numerical category. With this triumvirate, serous fluid cytopathology should remain one of the most used diagnostic investigations to make a substantial contribution to clinical management.

Cavtat, Croatia   Gabrijela Kocjan

Preface

This project was a collaborative effort between the International Academy of Cytology (IAC) and the American Society for Cytopathology (ASC) and called upon participation of the international cytopathology and oncology communities to contribute to the development of a truly international system for reporting serous fluid cytology. The project was conceptualized when the authors recognized that cytopathology reporting terminology had been developed and highly adopted for nearly all body sites with the glaring exception of serous fluids. Moreover, the expanding global medical environment necessitated a common language for pathology reporting to ensure appropriate patient management.

The authors organized task forces around each of the book chapters comprised of international experts in those areas, which included 41 individuals from 18 countries. An initial current practices survey was released on the Internet to members of the IAC and ASC, which was used to formulate initial consensus nomenclature and recommendations. A second Internet-based survey of gynecologic oncologists was released through the Society of Gynecologic Oncology to investigate clinical preferences for reporting and uses of peritoneal cytopathology in practice. Among the many challenges faced by the task forces was the lack of evidence-based data to support current practices and proposed changes, but implementation of a baseline standard serous fluid terminology should potentiate further studies and allow for future alterations. The authors also recognized special challenges in serous fluid cytopathology, such as reporting the presence of Mullerian epithelium in peritoneal fluids. What is an appropriate serous fluid volume to ensure adequacy? How should mesothelial proliferations be reported and is it appropriate to make an interpretation of malignant mesothelioma? How specific should a report be regarding the origin and subtyping of tumors found in serous fluids? What are the appropriate quality monitors for this specimen type? Special chapters on considerations for peritoneal washings, cytopreparatory techniques, mesothelioma, and quality management are included to address these issues. Lead authors for each chapter performed literature reviews to eludidate existing evidence in support of current practices and recommendations. Where evidence was lacking, the most common practices were adopted by consensus, and where there was no commonality, expert opinion was employed.

This terminology uses a 5-tier framework of categories that is familiar and popularized by preceding cytopathology terminology systems: nondiagnostic (ND), negative for malignancy (NFM), atypia of undetermined significance (AUS), suspicious for malignancy (SFM), and malignant (MAL). Because the majority of tumors involving serous fluids are metastatic adenocarcinoma, further qualification of tumor cell differentiation and/or primary site are important clinically and the chapter on ancillary studies addresses the importance of additional evaluation. The appropriate clinical management for findings is not specifically addressed in most chapters due to the diversity of possible tumor types recovered.

In an ideal situation, consensus terminology would be widely implemented, supported, and evidence-based, but there must be a starting point, and we hope that this effort will serve as a baseline for international comparative research on outcomes based on its use.

London, UK   Ashish Chandra
Silver Spring, MD, USA   Barbara Crothers

Disclaimer

Contents

1   **The International System for Reporting Serous Fluid Cytopathology: Introduction and Overview of Diagnostic Terminology and Reporting** 1
    Barbara Crothers, Zubair Baloch, Ashish Chandra,
    Sahar Farahani, Daniel Kurtycz, and Fernando Schmitt

2   **Non-diagnostic (ND) and Adequacy** 9
    Mauro Saieg, Kaitlin Sundling, and Daniel Kurtycz

3   **Negative for Malignancy (NFM)** 17
    Eva M. Wojcik, Xiaoyin Sara Jing, Safa Alshaikh,
    and Claudia Lobo

4   **Atypia of Undetermined Significance** 41
    Philippe Vielh, Renê Gerhard, Maria Lozano,
    and Voichita Suciu

5   **Suspicious for Malignancy (SFM)** 53
    Panagiota Mikou, Marianne Engels, Sinchita Roy-Chowdhuri,
    and George Santis

6   **Malignant-Primary (MAL-P) (Mesothelioma)** 63
    Claire Michael, Kenzo Hiroshima, Anders Hjerpe,
    Pam Michelow, Binnur Önal, and Amanda Segal

7   **Malignant-Secondary (MAL-S)** 99
    Yurina Miki, Z. Laura Tabatabai, and Ben Davidson

8   **Ancillary Studies for Serous Fluids** 129
    Lukas Bubendorf, Pinar Firat, Ibrahim Kulac, Pasquale Pisapia,
    Spasenija Savic-Prince, Gilda Santos, and Giancarlo Troncone

9   **Special Considerations for Peritoneal Washings** 167
    Christopher VandenBussche, Barbara Crothers, Amanda Fader,
    Amanda Jackson, Zaibo Li, and Chengquan Zhao

Contents

10 Cytopreparatory Techniques 239
Donna K. Russell and Deepali Jain

11 Quality Management 267
Barbara Centeno, Paul Cross, Marilin Rosa,
and Rosario Granados

12 Serous Effusion Anatomy, Biology, and Pathophysiology 279
Stefan E. Pambuccian and Miguel Perez-Machado

Index 293

Editors

Ashish Chandra, MD, FRCPath, DipRCPath (Cytol) Cellular Pathology, Guy's and St. Thomas' NHS Foundation Trust, London, UK

Barbara Crothers, DO Gynecology, Breast and Cytopathology, Joint Pathology Center, Silver Spring, MD, USA

Daniel Kurtycz, MD University of Wisconsin School of Medicine and Public Health, Department of Pathology and Laboratory Medicine and Wisconsin State Laboratory of Hygiene, Madison, WI, USA

Fernando Schmitt, MD, PhD, FIAC Department of Pathology, Medical Faculty of Porto University and Unit of Molecular Pathology, Institute of Molecular Pathology and Immunology, Porto University, Porto, Portugal

Contributors

Safa Alshaikh, MD Anatomic Pathology and Cytology, Salmaniya Medical Complex, Manama, Kingdom of Bahrain

Zubair Baloch, MD, PhD Department of Pathology & Laboratory Medicine, University of Pennsylvania Medical Center, Perelman School of Medicine, Philadelphia, PA, USA

Lukas Bubendorf, MD, PhD Institute of Pathology, University Hospital Basel, Basel, Switzerland

Barbara Centeno, MD Department of Pathology, H. Lee Moffitt Cancer Center and Research Institute, Tampa, FL, USA

Paul Cross, MD Department of Pathology, Queen Elizabeth Hospital, Gateshead, Tyne and Wear, UK

Gilda Santos, MD, PhD Department of Cellular Pathology, Royal Victoria Hospital, Belfast Health and Social Care Trust, Belfast, UK

Ben Davidson, MD Department of Pathology, Norwegian Radium Hospital, Oslo University Hospital, Oslo, Norway

University of Oslo, Faculty of Medicine, Institute of Clinical Medicine, Oslo, Norway

Marianne Engels, MD Department of Pathology, University of Cologne, Cologne, Germany

Amanda Fader, MD Department of Obstetrics and Gynecology, The Johns Hopkins Hospital, The Johns Hopkins University, Baltimore, MD, USA

Sahar Farahani, MD, PhD Renaissance School of Medicine, Stony Brook University, Department of Pathology, Stony Brook, NY, USA

Pinar Firat, MD Department of Pathology, School of Medicine, Koç University, Istanbul, Turkey

Renê Gerhard, MD Department of Morphologic and Molecular Pathology, Laboratoire National de Santé, Dudelange, Luxembourg

Rosario Granados, MD Pathology Department, Hospital Universitario Getafe, Madrid, Spain

Kenzo Hiroshima, MD Department of Pathology, Tokyo Women's Medical University, Yachiyo, Japan

Anders Hjerpe, MD, PhD Department of Laboratory Medicine, Division of Clinical Pathology/ Cytology, Karolinska Institutet, Karolinska University Hospital Huddinge, Huddinge, Sweden

Amanda Jackson, MD Department of Obstetrics and Gynecology, Walter Reed National Military Medical Center, Bethesda, MD, USA

Deepali Jain, MD Department of Pathology, All India Institute of Medical Sciences, New Delhi, India

Xiaoyin Sara Jing, MD Department of Pathology, Duke University, Durham, NC, USA

Ibrahim Kulac, MD Koc University Schoold of Medicine, Istanbul, Turkey

Zaibo Li, MD, PhD Department of Pathology, The Ohio State University, Columbus, OH, USA

Claudia Lobo, MD Department of Pathology – Cytopathology Division, Portuguese Oncology Institute of Porto, Porto, Portugal

Maria Lozano, MD Department of Pathology, University of Navarra, Pamplona, Navarra, Spain

Claire Michael, MD, PhD Department of Pathology, Case Western Reserve University, University Hospitals Case Medical Center, Cleveland, OH, USA

Pam Michelow, MD Cytology Unit, National Health Laboratory Service, University of the Witwatersrand, Johannesburg, South Africa

Yurina Miki, MBBS, BSc, FRCPath Department of Cellular Pathology, St Thomas' Hospital, Guy's and St Thomas' NHS Foundation Trust, London, UK

Panagiota Mikou, MD Laiko Hospital, Athens, Greece

Binnur Önal, MD Department of Pathology & Cytology, Ankara Diskapi Teaching and Research Hospital, Cankaya, Turkey

Stefan E. Pambuccian, MD Department of Pathology, Loyola University Health Systems, Loyola University, Maywood, IL, USA

Miguel Perez-Machado, MD, PhD, FRCPath Royal Free London NHS Foundation Trust, London, UK

Pasquale Pisapia, MD University of Naples Federico II, Public Health, Naples, Italy

Marilin Rosa, MD Department of Pathology, H. Lee Moffitt Cancer Center and Research Institute, Tampa, FL, USA

Sinchita Roy-Chowdhuri, MD MD Anderson Cancer Center, Houston, TX, USA

Donna K. Russell, MEd, CT(ASCP), HT(ASCP) University of Rochester, Rochester, NY, USA

Mauro Saieg, MD Department of Pathology, AC Camargo Cancer Center, Sao Paulo, SP, Brazil

George Santis, MD Professor of Thoracic Oncology & Interventional Bronchoscopy School of Immunology & Microbial Sciences. King's College London, Guy's & St Thomas' NHS Foundation Trust, London, UK

Spasenija Savic-Prince, MD Institute of Pathology, University Hospital Basel, Basel, Switzerland

Amanda Segal, MBBS Department of Anatomical Pathology, PathWest, QEII Medical Centre, Perth, WA, Australia

Voichita Suciu, MD Department of Medical Biology and Pathology, Gustave Roussy, Villejuif, France

Kaitlin Sundling, MD, PhD Department of Pathology and Laboratory Medicine, Wisconsin State Laboratory of Hygiene, University of Wisconsin Hospitals and Clinics, Madison, WI, USA

Z. Laura Tabatabai, MD Department of Pathology, University of California San Francisco, San Francisco, CA, USA

Giancarlo Troncone, MD, PhD Department of Public Health, University of Naples "Federico II", Naples, Italy

Christopher VandenBussche, MD, PhD Departments of Pathology and Oncology, The John Hopkins University of School of Medicine, Baltimore, MD, USA

Philippe Vielh, MD, PhD Medipath & American Hospital of Paris, Paris, France

Eva M. Wojcik, MD Department of Pathology and Laboratory Medicine, Loyola University Medical Center, Maywood, IL, USA

Chengquan Zhao, MD Magee Women's Hospital, University of Pittsburgh Medical Center, Pittsburgh, PA, USA

Abbreviations

ADASP	Association of Directors of Anatomic and Surgical Pathology
ADC	Adenocarcinoma
ADx-ARMS	ADx amplification refractory mutation system
AEC	3-amino-9-ethylcarbazole
AFB	Acid fast bacillus
AFP	Alpha fetoprotein
AGCT	Adult granulosa cell tumor
AJCC	American Joint Committee on Cancer
ALCL	Anaplastic large cell lymphoma
ALK	Anaplastic lymphoma kinase
ALL	Acute lymphoblastic leukemia
AMP	Association for Molecular Pathology
AP	Anatomic pathology
APC	Allophycocyanin
ARID1A	AT-rich interaction domain 1A
ASC	American Society of Cytopathology
ASCO	American Society of Clinical Oncology
AUS	Atypia of undetermined significance
BAP1	BRCA1 associated protein 1
BCL2/6	B cell lymphoma 2/6
bFGF	Basic fibroblast growth factor
BRCA	Breast cancer (type 1 or 2) gene susceptibility protein
CAIX	Carbonic anhydrase IX
CAF	Cancer-associated fibroblasts
CAP	College of American Pathologists
CAPP-Seq	Cancer Personalized Profiling by Deep Sequencing
CB	Cell block
CCC	Clear cell carcinoma
CD	Cluster designation
CDKN2A	Cyclin-dependent kinase inhibitor 2A protein
CEA	Carcinoembryonic antigen
CEP	Chromosome enumeration probes
CF	Cytocentrifugation
cfDNA	Cell free DNA

CHC	Cytology-histology correlation
CK	Cytokeratin
CLIA	Clinical Laboratory Improvement Amendments of 1988
CLL	Chronic lymphocytic leukemia
CMS	Centers for Medicare and Medicaid Services
CALT	Coelom-associated lymphoid tissue
CS	Cytospin™
CT	Computed tomography
DAB	Diaminobenzidine
DAPI	4,6-diamidino, 2-phenylindole dihydrochloride
DLBCL	Diffuse large B-cell lymphoma
DMM	Diffuse malignant mesothelioma
DNA	Deoxyribonucleic acid
DPAM	Disseminated peritoneal adenomucinosis
dPCR	Digital polymerase chain reaction
DS	Direct smear
DQ	Diff-Quik stain
EBER	Epstein-Barr virus-encoded small RNAs
EBT	Endometrioid borderline tumor
ECA	Endocervical adenocarcinoma
ECCC	Endometrial clear cell carcinoma
EGFR	Epidermal growth factor receptor
EGR	Early growth response factor
EMA	Epithelial membrane antigen
EPP	Extrapleural pneumonectomy
EQA	External quality assurance, European Quality Assurance
ER	Estrogen receptor
FDA	Food and Drug Administration
FC	Flow cytometry
FFPE	Formalin fixed, paraffin embedded
Fig.	Figure
FIGO	Federation International of Gynecologists and Obstetricians
FISH	Fluorescent in situ hybridization
FNA	Fine needle aspiration
FTA	Flinders Technology Associate
GATA3	GATA binding protein 3
GCDFP15	Gross cystic disease fluid protein 15
GMS	Grocott's methenamine silver stain
HCG	Human chorionic gonadotropin
H&E	Hematoxylin and eosin stain
HER2	Human epidermal growth factor receptor 2
HG	HistoGel
HLA	Human leukocyte antigen
HGEC	High grade endometrioid carcinoma
HGMC	High grade mucinous carcinoma

HGSC	High grade serous carcinoma
HGSOC	High grade serous ovarian carcinoma
HHV8	Human Herpes virus 8
HIV	Human immunodeficiency virus
HL	Hodgkin's lymphoma
HMB45	Human Melanoma Black 45
HMWK	High molecular weight keratin
HNF1	Hepatocyte nuclear factor 1
H/RS	Hodgkin/Reed Sternberg cell
IAC	International Academy of Cytology
IASLC	International Association for the Study of Lung Cancer
IC	Immunochemistry
ISH	In situ hybridization
ISO	International Organization of Standardization
JGCT	Juvenile granulosa cell tumor
kD	Kilodalton
LAP	Laboratory Accreditation Program
LBC	Liquid based cytology
LBL	Lymphoblastic lymphoma
LBP	Liquid based preparation
LCM	Laser capture microdissection
LE	Lupus erythematosus
LGEC	Low grade endometrioid carcinoma
LGSC	Low grade serous carcinoma
LIS	Laboratory information system
LM	Localized mesothelioma
LMWK	Low molecular weight keratin
MAL	Malignant
MAL-P	Malignant (Primary)
MAL-S	Malignant (Secondary)
MALT	Mucosa-associated lymphoid tissue
ME	Malignant effusion
MET	Mesenchymal-epithelial-transition
MBT	Mucinous borderline tumor
MGB	Mammaglobin
MGG	May-Grünwald Giemsa
mL	Milliliter
MM	Malignant mesothelioma
MMMT	Malignant Müllerian mixed tumor
MMR	Mismatch repair
MMT	Mesothelial-mesenchymal transition
MPSC	Micropapillary serous carcinoma
MSI	Microsatellite instability
MSS	Microsatellite stable
MT	Molecular testing

MTAP	Methylthioadenosine phosphorylase
MUC	Mucin protein
MUM1	Multiple myeloma 1
MZL	Marginal zone lymphoma
N:C	Nuclear to cytoplasmic ratio
NCB	Needle core biopsy
NCCN	National Comprehensive Cancer Network
ND	Nondiagnostic
NE	Neuroendocrine
NEC	Neuroendocrine carcinoma
NHL	Non-Hodgkin lymphoma
NFM	Negative for malignancy
NGS	Next generation sequencing
NOS	Not otherwise specified
NSCLC	Non-small cell carcinoma lung
NTRK	Neutrotrophic receptor tyrosine kinase
OCCC	Ovarian clear cell carcinoma
OCT3/4	Octamer binding transcription factor 3/4
PanK	Pancytokeratin
Pap	Papanicolaou stain
PAS	Periodic acid Schiff
PASD	Periodic acid Schiff with diastase
PAX	Paired box gene protein
PCR	Polymerase chain reaction
PD-L1	Programmed cell death ligand 1
PEL	Primary effusion lymphoma
PET	Positron emission tomography
PIC	Peritoneal inclusion cyst
PLAP	Placental alkaline phosphatase
PMP	Pseudomyxoma peritonei
PR	Progesterone receptor
PSA	Prostate specific antigen
PSAP	Prostate specific acid phosphatase
PT	Plasma thrombin
QA	Quality assurance
QC	Quality control
QI	Quality improvement
QM	Quality management
RCC	Renal cell carcinoma
RET	Rearranged during transfection
RM	Reactive mesothelium
RNA	Ribonucleic acid
ROM	Risk of malignancy
ROSE	Rapid on site evaluation
RPM	Revolutions per minute

RPMI	Roswell Park Memorial Institute medium
RS	Reed Sternberg cell
RT-PCR	Reverse transcriptase polymerase chain reaction
SALC	Serosa-associated lymphoid clusters
SALL4	Sal-like protein 4
SATB2	Special AT-rich sequence-binding protein 2
SBT	Serous borderline tumor
SCC	Squamous cell carcinoma
SEC	Serous endometrial carcinoma
SLE	Systemic lupus erythematosus
SLL	Small lymphocytic lymphoma
SFM	Suspicious for malignancy
SMA	Smooth muscle actin
SMRP	Soluble mesothelin related peptides
SmCC	Small cell carcinoma
SP	SurePath™ liquid based preparation
STAMP	Sequence tag-based analysis of microbial population dynamics
STIC	Serous tubal intraepithelial carcinomas
TAG	Tumor associated glycoprotein
TAT	Turnaround time
TBS	The Bethesda system
TIS	The International System for Reporting Serous Fluid Cytopathology
TJC	The Joint Commission
TKI	Tyrosine kinase inhibitor
TP	ThinPrep® liquid based preparation
TPS	Tumor proportion score
TTF1	Thyroid transcription factor-1
UK NEQAS	United Kingdom National External Quality Assessment Service
US	United States
VEGF	Vascular endothelial growth factor
WDPM	Well differentiated papillary mesothelioma
WHO	World Health Organization
WT1	Wilms' tumor 1
YST	Yolk sac tumor

The International System for Reporting Serous Fluid Cytopathology: Introduction and Overview of Diagnostic Terminology and Reporting

Barbara Crothers, Zubair Baloch, Ashish Chandra, Sahar Farahani, Daniel Kurtycz, and Fernando Schmitt

Introduction

Cytopathology has always been on the forefront of standardizing terminology, perhaps because many early cytology interpretative reports consisted of a litany of descriptive terms that clinicians found difficult to decipher. Leading this revolution was The Bethesda System (TBS) for Reporting Cervicovaginal Cytology [1–3], the model adopted by all future systems [4–7]. The International System (TIS) for Reporting Serous Fluid Cytopathology is no exception. Foremost among the goals of serous fluid terminology is to enhance consensus on the meanings assigned to diagnostic terminology in order to prevent clinical misunderstanding that might

B. Crothers (✉)
Gynecologic, Breast and Cytopathology, Joint Pathology Center, Silver Spring, MD, USA
e-mail: barbara.a.crothers.civ@mail.mil

Z. Baloch
Department of Pathology & Laboratory Medicine, University of Pennsylvania Medical Center, Perelman School of Medicine, Philadelphia, PA, USA

A. Chandra
Cellular Pathology, Guy's and St. Thomas' NHS Foundation Trust, London, UK

S. Farahani
Renaissance School of Medicine, Stony Brook University, Department of Pathology, Stony Brook, NY, USA

D. Kurtycz
University of Wisconsin School of Medicine and Public Health, Department of Pathology and Laboratory Medicine and Wisconsin State Laboratory of Hygiene, Madison, WI, USA

F. Schmitt
Department of Pathology, Medical Faculty of Porto University and Unit of Molecular Pathology, Institute of Molecular Pathology and Immunology, Porto University, Porto, Portugal

© Springer Nature Switzerland AG 2020
A. Chandra et al. (eds.), *The International System for Serous Fluid Cytopathology*, https://doi.org/10.1007/978-3-030-53908-5_1

undermine therapeutic decisions. The International System serves as a template for improving communication of serous fluid cytology results that strives to reduce reporting variability. Secondary goals include promoting comparison of research results, improving efficiency of electronic record data capture, promoting a common language for teaching, and providing meaningful correlation with follow-up cytology and surgical pathology specimens. In addition, it produces a language that lends itself to clinical practice guidelines. Ultimately, this effort is intended to improve patient management and quality of clinical care.

The International System (TIS) consists of the five diagnostic categories outlined in Table 1.1. These mirror categories adopted by other cytology reporting systems and terminologies are harmonized wherever possible. Diagnostic categories may

Table 1.1 The International System (TIS) for reporting serous effusion cytopathology: diagnostic categories, definitions, and explanatory notes

Diagnostic categories and definitions	Explanatory notes
I. **Nondiagnostic (ND)** *Specimens with insufficient cellular elements for a cytologic interpretation*	This diagnostic category should only be used after an adequate and representative amount of fluid has been processed and examined
II. **Negative for malignancy (NFM)** *Specimens with cellular changes completely lacking evidence of mesothelial or non-mesothelial malignancy*	Specimens classified in this category will include those cellular changes completely lacking evidence of mesothelial and non-mesothelial malignancy The risk of malignancy (ROM) for this category is expected to be low Includes inflammatory, reactive, and metaplastic cells and cellular changes due to infectious agents Includes specimens with a reactive lymphoid infiltrate (flow cytometry and/or immunochemical studies on cell block may be necessary to exclude the possibility of a low-grade lymphoproliferative disorder)
III. **Atypia of undetermined significance (AUS)** *Specimens showing limited cellular (nuclear) and/or architectural atypia (e.g., papillary clusters or pseudo-glandular formations)*	This diagnostic category is for specimens which are indeterminate for mesothelial or non-mesothelial malignancy, and for benign or borderline tumor cells in fluids It represents a true gray zone in effusion cytology This will include cases showing extremes of reactive atypia or specimens containing few or degenerated tumor cells Includes specimens with procurement, processing, and preparation artifacts that obscure cytologic features
IV. **Suspicious for malignancy (SFM)** *Specimens showing features suspicious but not definitively diagnostic for malignancy*	The report may elude to the type of malignancy by providing a differential diagnosis Report comments should direct clinicians to appropriate next steps to procure a diagnosis
V. **Malignant (MAL)** *Specimens include those with definitive findings and/or supportive studies indicating mesothelial or non-mesothelial malignancies*	Further subclassification of all malignant cases using ancillary studies (immunohistochemistry, FISH, molecular and flow cytometry) to determine primary site and tumor differentiation is recommended

stand alone as a diagnosis if further explanation is deemed unnecessary. Categories are to be reported as text (e.g., malignant), not as numerical values alone (e.g., category V). Where uncertainty remains, descriptive diagnoses are preferred along with the diagnostic category. A definitive interpretation should be reported whenever possible. Categorization of cases lends itself to laboratory statistical analysis and can be useful for comparing diagnostic rates between individuals and for documenting laboratory diagnostic trends. Report examples are provided in each chapter.

Particular challenges that the editors strove to address involve how to define specimen adequacy, determining what constitutes a negative sample, the appropriate use of atypical and suspicious categories, and the value of cytology in the primary diagnosis of malignant mesothelioma. Additionally, we recognized that the intraoperative collection of serous fluid, primarily peritoneal fluid, leads to special diagnostic dilemmas, including benign entities that may mimic malignant tumor. Therefore, a chapter is included specifically to address these contingencies.

Although studies supporting the use of a particular terminology for serous fluid cytology are currently scant or nonexistent, we anticipate that with implementation of TIS, subsequent studies (both retrospective and prospective) on its use will direct future terminology modifications. Given the paucity of supportive studies, many final decisions regarding terminology were based on practice surveys illuminating common existing practices, expert consensus, and outcomes resulting from adoption of uniform cytology terminology in other systems. TIS will serve as a baseline model for implementation so that studies on its effectiveness can be initiated. Finally, it is important to recognize that not all cases will fit the model and modification may be necessary for a particular patient.

Format of the Report

The terminology applies to serous fluid collected from the pleura, peritoneal, and pericardial cavities. A primary focus of cytology reporting systems is to minimize the use of "uncertain" diagnoses, which includes atypical and suspicious categories. This may be particularly challenging in serous fluid reporting when clinical information or imaging studies are unavailable. A major principle of this system is that indeterminate categories should be an option of last resort, after all investigative attempts to definitively categorize a lesion have been exhausted. Less definitive preliminary reports may be necessary while awaiting confirmatory data, including receipt of or correlation with surgical specimens. One should emphasize the need for additional information or studies to clarify the diagnosis in a comment when employing atypical and suspicious categories.

One of the challenges of serous fluid cytology is the wide array of disorders that may manifest in fluids, particularly metastases. Unlike other cytology systems, morphology is not limited to a particular body site, and most tumors will produce three-dimensional configurations in fluid, which creates monumental morphologic challenges. Background cellular products that can narrow diagnostic possibilities in fine needle aspiration are largely eliminated when cells metastasize. The architecture of cellular configurations (papillary formation, sheetlike growth, dispersion, and cohesion) are more difficult to assess. There is considerable morphologic overlap among adenocarcinomas of various body sites, and adenocarcinoma is the most common metastatic tumor in fluids. Consequently, ancillary tests (special stains, immunochemistry, and molecular tests) may be paramount to arriving at the correct interpretation. Some of these tests have published standardized reporting templates, such as ER, PR, HER2 [8], and molecular tests in lung cancer [9, 10]. Adoption of these templates is encouraged but not discussed in this publication.

Another principle of cytologic diagnostic terminology is that for malignancies, the cytology report should strive to be as definitive as possible by identifying the primary site or the most likely primary site, as well as defining the precise category of tumor. The ease of this step is significantly aided by comparison with concordant surgical specimens. Because it is impractical to include all possible tumor types in the atypical, suspicious, and malignant chapters, the authors focused on the most common or unusual but perplexing examples. Although there are published manuscripts outlining diagnostic criteria for some of these entities, some of the lesions are represented by images of fine needle aspiration, touch imprint, and scrape preparations or other specimen types, which may not reflect their actual appearance in fluids.

The serous effusion cytology report format is depicted in Table 1.2.

Table 1.2 Reporting format for serous effusion cytopathology specimens

Cytology report headings	Explanatory notes
Specimen Type, Location, Procedure:	For some body cavities (e.g., pericardial), a specific location is not important, whereas for pleural and intraoperative peritoneal washings, the location further clarifies the pattern of tumor spread The procedure type may be included on the requisition, intuited, or unknown
Statement of Adequacy	The adequacy statement usually reflects cellular preservation or processing rather than collection challenges Following TBS example, "Satisfactory for evaluation," "Evaluation limited by (with qualifying limitation stated)," and "Unsatisfactory" are the proposed terms
TIS Diagnostic Category	We do not recommend reporting categories as numerical values (I, II, III, etc.); similar systems were decried prior to the introduction of standardized terminology for being inconsistently applied and diminishing understanding of a report's meaning
Notes and Comments	Reports should also include pertinent notes and all necessary regulatory requirements A brief description of the cytologic features present may be included in the notes, along with the differential diagnosis in cases of uncertainty Summarizing the findings of ancillary tests can provide evidence supporting the interpretation If conclusive evidence is lacking in support of an interpretation, it is helpful to provide direction to the clinical staff on subsequent tests necessary to confirm a diagnosis

Rate and Risk of Malignancy

Farahani and Baloch (2019) [11] have compiled the most comprehensive statistics to date on the accuracy of and risk of malignancy (ROM) for each diagnostic category through a meta-analysis of the literature and assignment of study outcomes using TIS categories (Table 1.3). This study serves as a framework for future investigation and evaluation of evolving risks. Due to the diversity of malignant possibilities in fluid specimens, the editors chose not to address the clinical management for all tumor types.

Mean risk of malignancy (ROM) in this study was calculated using a univariate random effect model by performing meta-analysis of reported 11,799 pleural fluid, 3978 peritoneal fluid, 8540 peritoneal washing, and 941 pericardial fluid specimens in the English literature. The following ranges for mean ROM with standard error for diagnostic categories have been cited in the literature: ND 0–100%, NFM 0–81%, AUS 13–100%, SFM 0–100%, and MAL 87–100% [11]. The results of this systematic review show that when a definite diagnosis of absence or presence of malignancy is considered, serous fluid cytology has a sensitivity and specificity of 72.1% and 99.9%, respectively. This literature analysis also showed that cytology was more sensitive in confirming the diagnosis of malignancy in pleural fluid and peritoneal washing specimens when compared to peritoneal fluid and pericardial fluid specimens. Interestingly, Baloch and Farahani [11] found that the diagnostic accuracy of serous effusion cytology was greater in studies that interpreted serous effusion cytology specimens using diagnostic categories of "NFM," "AUS (atypical)," "SFM," and "MAL" compared to those using a two-tiered system reporting the cases as either "NFM" or "MAL." This finding strongly suggests that a multitiered classification system for reporting serous effusion cytopathology would likely improve the diagnostic performance of malignancy detection in cytology specimens.

Table 1.3 The International System (TIS) for reporting serous fluid cytopathology: implied risk of malignancy (ROM)

Diagnostic category[a]	% ROM[b] (SE)[c]
Nondiagnostic (ND)	17% (± 8.9%)
Negative for malignancy (NFM)	21% (± 0.3%)
Atypia of undetermined significance (AUS)	66% (± 10.6%)
Suspicious for malignancy (SFM)	82% (± 4.8%)
Malignant (MAL)	99% (± 0.1%)[d–g]

[a]Chandra [12]
[b]*ROM* risk of malignancy; from Farahani and Baloch [11]
[c]*SE* standard error
[d]Psallidas et al. [13]
[e]Kremer et al. [14]
[f]Loveland et al. [15]
[g]Rossi et al. [16]

The diagnostic categories of TIS could provide useful inherent information for appropriate clinical management and follow-up. It is important to understand that calculating the risk of malignancy (ROM) by traditional methods, i.e., on tissue follow-up, is most likely flawed. It overestimates ROM due to selection bias, as not all serous effusion cytology specimens classified as nondiagnostic, benign, and atypical will have tissue follow-up. Therefore, the best estimates based on literature review are iterated in Table 1.3. Including the ROM (as shown in Table 1.3) along with the general diagnostic category in the cytology report is optional and left to the discretion of the individual pathologist or laboratory. Ideally, each laboratory would perform its own ROM based on annual statistics and follow-up clinical information and/or surgical resection.

The International System for Reporting Serous Fluid Cytopathology will always be a project in evolution with refinement in the face of new technology and new evidence. The authors welcome new research, criticism, and approaches to better serve the field of cytopathology and the care of patients.

References

1. Kurman RJ, Solomon D, editors. The Bethesda system for reporting cervical/vaginal cytologic diagnoses. Definitions, criteria, and explanatory notes for terminology and specimen adequacy. New York: Springer; 1994.
2. Solomon D, Nayar R. The Bethesda system for reporting cervical cytology. Definitions, criteria, and explanatory notes. 2nd ed. New York: Springer; 2004.
3. Nayar R, Wilbur DC. The Bethesda system for reporting cervical cytology. Definitions, criteria, and explanatory notes. 3rd ed. New York: Springer; 2015.
4. Pittman MB, Layfield LJ, editors. The Papanicolaou Society of Cytopathology system for reporting pancreaticobiliary cytology. Definitions, criteria, and explanatory notes. New York: Springer; 2015.
5. Rosenthal DL, Wojcik EM, Kurtycz DFI, editors. The Paris system for reporting urinary cytology. Switzerland: Springer; 2016.
6. Ali SZ, Cibas ES, editors. The Bethesda system for reporting thyroid cytopathology. Definitions, criteria, and explanatory notes. 2nd ed. Switzerland: Springer; 2018.
7. Faquin WC, Rossi ED, editors. The Milan system for reporting salivary gland cytopathology. Switzerland: Springer; 2018.
8. Fitzgibbons PL, Dillon DA, Berman AR, et al. Template for reporting results of biomarker testing of specimens from patients with carcinoma of the breast. Arch Pathol Lab Med. 2014;138(5):595–601.
9. Lindeman NI, Cagle PT, Beasley MB, et al. Molecular testing guideline for selection of lung cancer patients for EGFR and ALK tyrosine kinase inhibitors: guideline from the College of American Pathologists, International Association for the Study of Lung Cancer, and Association for Molecular Pathology. Arch Pathol Lab Med. 2013;137(6):828–1174.
10. Cree IA, Deans Z, Ligtenberg MJ, for the European Society of Pathology Task Force on Quality Assurance in Molecular Pathology and Royal College of Pathologists, et al. Guidance for laboratories performing molecular pathology for cancer patients. J Clin Pathol. 2014;67(11):923–31.
11. Farahani SJ, Baloch Z. Are we ready to develop a tiered scheme for the effusion cytology? A comprehensive review and analysis of the literature. Diag Cytopathol. 2019;47(11):1145–59.
12. Chandra A. Announcement: the international system for reporting serous fluid cytopathology. Acta Cytol. 2019;63(5):349–51.

13. Psallidas I, et al. Malignant pleural effusion: from bench to bedside. Europ Respir Rev. 2016;25:189–98.
14. Kremer R, et al. Pleural fluid analysis of lung cancer vs. benign inflammatory disease patients. Br J Cancer. 2010;102:1180–4.
15. Loveland P, et al. Diagnostic yield of pleural fluid cytology in malignant effusions: an Australian tertiary center experience. Intern Med J. 2018;48:1138–324.
16. Rossi ED, et al. The role of liquid-based cytology and ancillary techniques in pleural and pericardial effusions: an institutional experience. Cancer Cytopathol. 2015;123:258–66.

Non-diagnostic (ND) and Adequacy

2

Mauro Saieg, Kaitlin Sundling, and Daniel Kurtycz

Background

All samples must be interpreted in the context of the clinical and radiologic findings present. Ideally, an adequate sample would be representative of the underlying disease process. Defining adequacy in terms of cellularity is not feasible because it would require different criteria for distinct entities or processes involving the serous cavities. In the context of a fluid containing largely inflammatory cells, the absence of intact mesothelial cells does not make the sample non-diagnostic (ND) (Fig. 2.1). A specimen obtained from pleural tuberculosis containing only lymphocytes, for example, is adequate in the terms of being representative of the disease process involving the pleura. In patients with metastatic malignancy, although malignant cells may not be represented in the specimen itself, excess fluid may be due to lymphatics blocked by tumor emboli. Thus, a minimum cell count of benign mesothelial cells or inflammatory cells is difficult to propose. Additionally, designating a sample as non-diagnostic may imply that a procedure was unsuccessful and should be repeated. This is problematic because in the face of overwhelming inflammation one will only see the same pattern on repeat sampling.

As for a minimal volume threshold, a small number of robust studies indicate that a minimal threshold of around 50–75 mL may be considered adequate in order to diminish potential false negatives and optimize the test sensitivity [1–6]. A study of more than 2500 pleural fluid samples has advocated a threshold volume of at

M. Saieg (✉)
Department of Pathology, AC Camargo Cancer Center, Sao Paulo, SP, Brazil

K. Sundling
Department of Pathology and Laboratory Medicine, Wisconsin State Laboratory of Hygiene, University of Wisconsin Hospitals and Clinics, Madison, WI, USA

D. Kurtycz
University of Wisconsin School of Medicine and Public Health, Department of Pathology and Laboratory Medicine and Wisconsin State Laboratory of Hygiene, Madison, WI, USA

© Springer Nature Switzerland AG 2020
A. Chandra et al. (eds.), *The International System for Serous Fluid Cytopathology*, https://doi.org/10.1007/978-3-030-53908-5_2

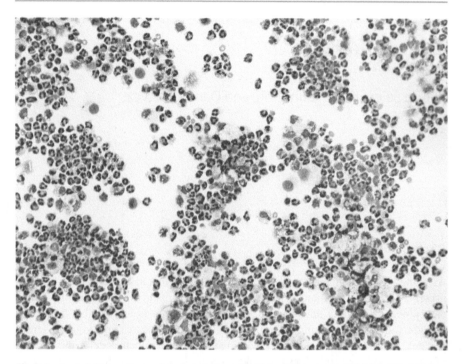

Fig. 2.1 Acute inflammation and degenerated mesothelial cells in a serous fluid (Modified Giemsa stain, high power). The image exhibits neutrophils and degenerated mesothelial cells. Such a pattern does not automatically make the sample non-diagnostic. In TIS, as long as the sample reflects the disease process and provides useful information, it remains helpful to the clinician. In this case acute inflammation can support an existing differential diagnosis, help generate a new differential diagnosis, and/or call for culture of organisms. Designating a sample as non-diagnostic may imply that either the procedure should be repeated or may be useless, when in fact neither supposition is true

least 75 mL, due to a statistically significant increase in the detection of malignancy up to 75 mL [1]. There does not seem to be an upper limit as far as the maximum volume received by the lab. The higher the volume, the smaller the number of samples reported as non-diagnostic or atypical. Clinicians should be encouraged to submit as much of the fluid to the laboratory as reasonable to ensure the greatest possible sensitivity for detection of abnormalities. If specimens are aliquoted for testing in multiple parts of the laboratory (such as for microbiologic culture or cell counts), the fluid should be well-mixed (see Chap. 10, Cytopreparatory Techniques).

Adequate specimens are well-preserved, well-prepared, well-stained, and easily visualized. Poor preservation can result in cellular degeneration and rupture, as well as adversely impact stain penetration (Figs. 2.2 and 2.3). Thick preparations may be uninterpretable. Any factors obscuring the cells from interpretation may limit evaluation, including overlying blood and inflammation. Mechanical factors, such as the sheer forces introduced during smear preparation, can distort or rupture cells. Totally hemolyzed samples are clearly non-diagnostic and show finely granular

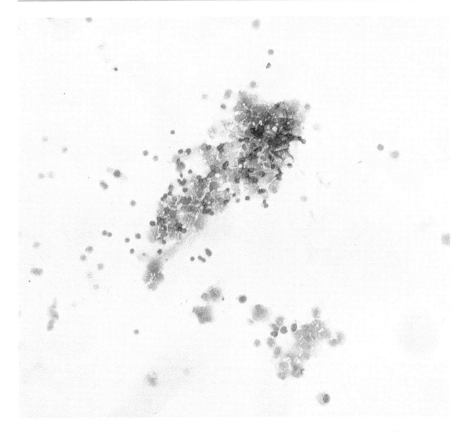

Fig. 2.2 A non-diagnostic (ND) sample (Papanicolaou stain, intermediate power). The specimen is uninterpretable due to the lack of fixation. There are homogenized masses of cytoplasm of unclear origin

debris in different patterns depending on the type of preparation. One cannot even be confident that a hemolyzed sample came from a body cavity unless appropriate cellular elements can be found (Figs. 2.4 and 2.5). Overstaining or incomplete stain penetration can make features uninterpretable. A statement on adequacy should reflect limitations to interpretation. Wholly inadequate specimens are uninterpretable and, hence, non-diagnostic.

Definition

A specimen is considered ND if it provides no diagnostic information in the appropriate clinical context, as in the case of acellular, highly degenerated, or hemorrhagic samples. A specimen that meets the criteria for any other category should be reported as that category and cannot be considered ND, even if the cellularity or specimen volume are low.

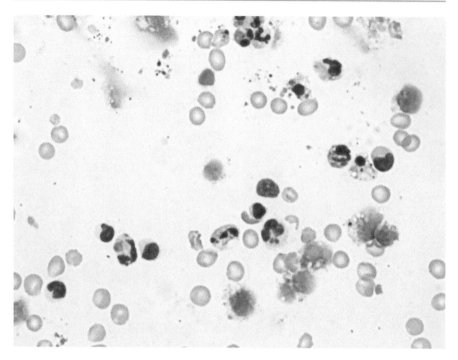

Fig. 2.3 A non-diagnostic (ND) degenerate sample (Modified Giemsa stain, high power). The image displays lysing lymphocytes and neutrophils amid background debris

Explanatory Notes

Paucicellular specimens with a volume less than 50 mL may not be optimal to exclude malignancy. Although no evidence-based minimum number of mesothelial cells has been established to determine adequacy, cases with scant cellularity in which malignancy is suspected could include a brief comment explaining the limited nature of the specimen and the concern for lack of sensitivity. In cases where inflammatory disease is suspected, large numbers of inflammatory cells and few or no mesothelial cells may be considered diagnostic and supportive of an inflammatory disease process.

The adequacy of the sample relies not only on the quantity of cells or volume of the sample but also on the quality of preservation of those cells. This is of pivotal importance in fluids, since badly preserved or poorly processed specimens may compromise cell morphology and degenerated cells should not be considered adequate for evaluation nor interpreted as atypical for the diagnosis of cancer. In addition, talc powder, squamous cells from the skin surface and other external contaminants, as well as extensive hemorrhage/hemolysis, may hamper the sample evaluation and result in a non-adequate specimen.

Fig. 2.4 Generalized hemolysis in a serous fluid (Papanicolaou stain, low power). The sample exhibits fine granular material resulting from hemolysis. Intact cells are not observed at this magnification, and one cannot be confident that the sample actually was derived from a body cavity. It may have come directly from a blood vessel

Clinical Management

Samples reported as ND should be regarded as non-contributory and submission of a repeat aspirate suggested upon reaccumulation of the fluid, if clinically appropriate.

Sample Reports

Example 2.1:
- Ascitic fluid:
- Evaluation limited by scant or absent cellularity.
- Non-diagnostic.

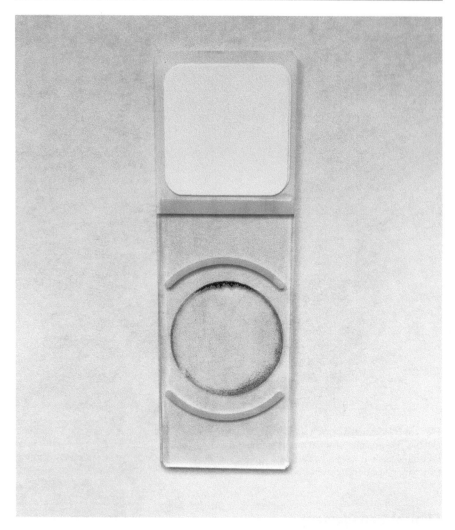

Fig. 2.5 Hemolysis in a liquid based preparation (ThinPrep®, macroscopic image). The image displays the typical pattern of a ThinPrep® preparation in the face of hemolysis. The fine particles of heme and cellular debris clog the ThinPrep® filter during processing and fill all the central pores. A ring of remnant hemolytic debris surrounds the edge of the sample due to unequal pressure forces present during processing of this type of sample

Comment: The specimen is comprised solely of blood. Repeat procedure is advised.

Example 2.2:
- Peritoneal cavity, paracentesis:
- Adequacy: Evaluation limited by external contaminants.
- Diagnosis: Non-diagnostic.

Comment: Evaluation of the present sample is limited or obscured by the presence of external contaminants that are consistent with fecal debris.

Example 2.3:
- Lung, right, thoracentesis:
- Evaluation limited by poor preservation.
- Non-diagnostic.

Comment: Although cells can be visualized, proper morphological evaluation of the present sample is limited due to drying/preservation artifact. Repeat procedure with proper handling and processing of the sample is advised.

References

1. Rooper LM, Ali SZ, Olson MT. A minimum fluid volume of 75 mL is needed to ensure adequacy in a pleural effusion: a retrospective analysis of 2540 cases. Cancer Cytopathol. 2014;122(9):657–65.
2. Rooper LM, Ali SZ, Olson MT. A minimum volume of more than 60 mL is necessary for adequate cytologic diagnosis of malignant pericardial effusions. Am J Clin Pathol. 2016;145(1):101–6.
3. Thomas SC, Davidson LR, McKean ME. An investigation of adequate volume for the diagnosis of malignancy in pleural fluids. Cytopathology. 2011;22(3):179–83.
4. Swiderek J, Morcos S, Donthireddy V, et al. Prospective study to determine the volume of pleural fluid required to diagnose malignancy. Chest. 2010;137(1):68–73.
5. Abouzgheib W, Bartter T, Dagher H, Pratter M, Klump W. A prospective study of the volume of pleural fluid required for accurate diagnosis of malignant pleural effusion. Chest. 2009;135(4):999–1001.
6. Sallach SM, Sallach JA, Vasquez E, Schultz L, Kvale P. Volume of pleural fluid required for diagnosis of pleural malignancy. Chest. 2002;122(6):1913–7.

Negative for Malignancy (NFM)

Eva M. Wojcik, Xiaoyin Sara Jing, Safa Alshaikh, and Claudia Lobo

Background

Pathologic accumulation of excessive fluid in serosal cavities can be associated with systemic or localized disease [1]. Considering how often effusions do occur, fluids are one of the most commonly seen types of non-gynecologic cytology specimens. The list of etiological factors leading to effusions is extensive, and malignancy is only one of them [2]. Nonetheless, the detection of malignant cells in fluid cytology is the main goal of cytologic examination of effusions, even though malignant cells are detected in a small percentage of cases. The great majority (>80%) of effusions are interpreted as "negative for malignancy (NFM)" [3–7].

Definition

A serous effusion specimen obtained from peritoneal, pleural, or pericardial cavities may be considered NFM when the specimen is composed of only benign or reactive cellular components, without malignant tumor cells or cells concerning for

E. M. Wojcik (✉)
Department of Pathology and Laboratory Medicine, Loyola University Medical Center, Maywood, IL, USA
e-mail: ewojcik@lumc.edu

X. S. Jing
Department of Pathology, Duke University, Durham, NC, USA

S. Alshaikh
Anatomic Pathology and Cytology, Salmaniya Medical Complex, Manama, Kingdom of Bahrain

C. Lobo
Department of Pathology – Cytopathology Division, Portuguese Oncology Institute of Porto, Porto, Portugal

© Springer Nature Switzerland AG 2020
A. Chandra et al. (eds.), *The International System for Serous Fluid Cytopathology*, https://doi.org/10.1007/978-3-030-53908-5_3

malignancy. These components include mesothelial cells without apparent neoplastic phenotypic changes, immunohistochemical patterns, or molecular alterations associated with malignancy. Varying ratios and types of inflammatory cells may be present depending on the condition responsible for the effusion, and this category also includes effusions due to infectious causes.

Criteria for Negative for Malignancy

- Mostly mesothelial cells as single cells, small clusters (often with "windows"), or flat sheets
- Rare mesothelial binucleation or multinucleation could be present
- Variable histiocytes, giant cells, lymphocytes, and neutrophils
- No or minimal cellular atypia
- May include other benign components (e.g., psammoma bodies, collagen balls, asbestos bodies, organisms)

Explanatory Notes

Approach to Serous Effusion (Fig. 3.1)

All serous effusions are the result of some kind of pathological process. There is no such state as a "normal effusion." Therefore, all cells within these specimens, and particularly mesothelial cells, can be expected to show some degree of reactive change. The first step in evaluating effusions is deciding if the specimen is adequate for examination. Once considered adequate, one should determine what types of cells are present, overall cellularity (high or low), and architectural composition. Architectural composition refers to whether the cells are arranged singly, in small clusters, or in large, complex cellular formations. The next step is to decide if the cells present are the ones which are expected in serous fluid (mesothelial cells and/ or inflammatory cells, including histiocytes) versus an unexpected cell population (secondary population). In some instances, definitive diagnosis may require additional stains or ancillary studies to confirm cell of origin. In the majority of cases, the diagnosis of NFM can be established on morphology alone.

Expected Cellular Findings

Without Regard to Volume or Distribution

All serous cavities are lined by mesothelial cells. These are usually the predominant cell in serous effusions, with or without various ratios of inflammatory cells. Most mesothelial cells in effusion cytology show some degree of reactive change, so it is not necessary to report reactive mesothelial cells. Among all cells, the mesothelial

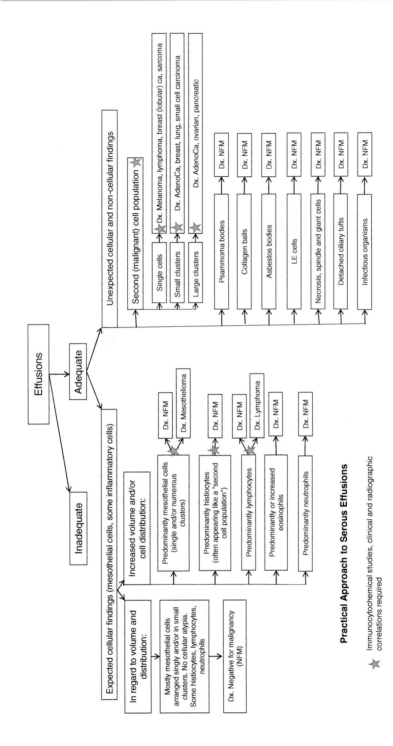

Fig. 3.1 An algorithmic approach to serous effusions

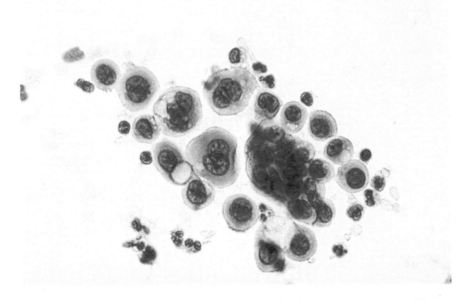

Fig. 3.2 Mesothelial cells. The image demonstrates multinucleation, cytoplasmic vacuolization, and loose clustering. Variability in size and shape is often seen in reactive mesothelial cells. (Pleural fluid, Papanicolaou stain, TP, high magnification)

cell is one of the most malleable, with the greatest plasticity to adapt to environmental changes [8]. Therefore, it is no surprise that reactive changes lead to significant morphologic overlap with malignant cells, which may require additional studies to identify their phenotype. The wide range of cytomorphologic appearances of reactive mesothelial cells are illustrated in Figs. 3.2, 3.3, 3.4, 3.5, 3.6, 3.7, 3.8, 3.9, 3.10, 3.11, and 3.12.

In benign effusions, mesothelial cells appear as round to oval single cells and/ or small cohesive clusters. The cells vary in size, but generally, they exhibit nuclei 1.5–2 times the size of a neutrophil. Nuclei may be centrally or eccentrically located. Binucleated or multinucleated mesothelial cells are not uncommon and these findings usually point to a reactive process. Mesothelial cells usually contain nucleoli, sometimes prominent, but increased numbers of macronucleoli are more characteristic of malignant mesothelioma [9, 10]. It is important to note that in reactive mesothelial cells, both nucleolar profiles and nuclear membranes are usually smooth and very succinctly defined. The nuclear to cytoplasmic ratio may be increased [2, 11]. Cytoplasm may show lace-like edges ("frilly skirt," Fig. 3.3). The frequently described "two-toned" cytoplasm is best appreciated in older Romanowsky-stained preparations and is less apparent in current preparations using thin layer techniques and stained with modified Giemsa or Papanicolaou methods. It is not unusual to see cytoplasmic vacuolization, which may take the form of signet-ring like cells [12] (Fig. 3.7).

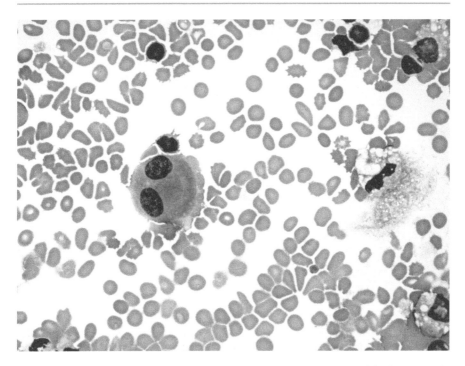

Fig. 3.3 A binucleated mesothelial cell. This binucleate cell demonstrates "frilly" cytoplasmic edges. (Pleural fluid, Modified Giemsa stain, CS, high magnification)

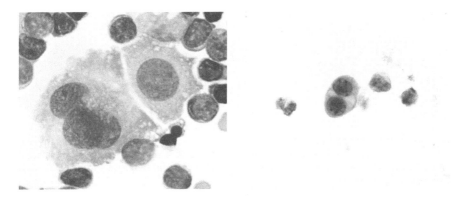

Fig. 3.4 Mesothelial cells with windows. Adjacent mesothelial cells showing a clear gap, or "window" due to microvilli, not visible at the light microscopic level, that exists at the edges of the cells pushing the cytoplasm of the mesothelial cells apart. (Left: Pleural fluid, Modified Giemsa stain, CS, high magnification; Right: Peritoneal fluid, Papanicolaou stain, TP, high magnification)

Mesothelial cells often exfoliate in small clusters with characteristic "windows" or spaces between two cells (Fig. 3.4). These spaces are due to the presence of inter-digitating microvilli on the surface of mesothelial cells not visible to general light microscopy but well visualized on electron micrographs [8]. Peritoneal lavage

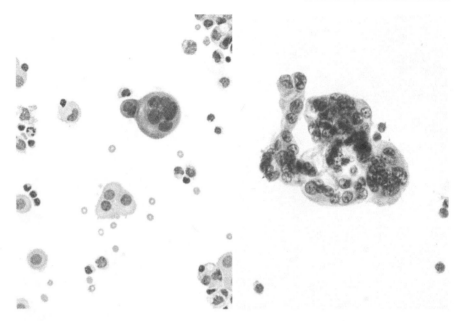

Fig. 3.5 Reactive mesothelial cells. Reactive cells may become multinucleated, with cellular enlargement. Note the small nucleoli and relatively regular nuclear contours. Left: Pleural fluid, Modified Giemsa stain, CS, high magnification. Right: Pleural fluid, Papanicolaou stain, LBP, high magnification

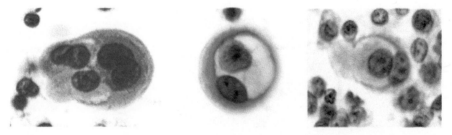

Fig. 3.6 Reactive mesothelial cells. Mesothelial cells showing "cannibalism," clasping, or cell-within-cell appearance. This appearance can be seen in both benign and malignant mesothelial proliferations. (Pleural fluid, Left: Modified Giemsa stain. Middle and right: Papanicolaou stain, LBP, high magnification)

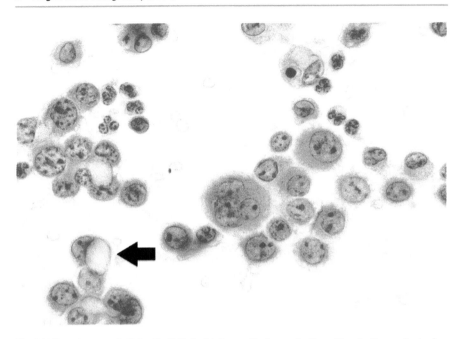

Fig. 3.7 Reactive mesothelial cells. Cells in this image display nucleoli, multinucleation, and cytoplasmic vacuoles with signet ring morphology (arrow). Prominent nucleoli reflect excited cells generating RNA on the pathway to making protein. (Pleural fluid, Papanicolaou stain, TP, high magnification)

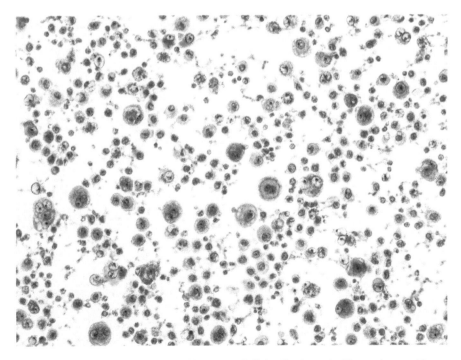

Fig. 3.8 Reactive mesothelial cells. These mesothelial cells show significant pleomorphism – great variation in size, as compared to mesotheliomas, that are often a more uniform ("monomorphic") population. (Pleural fluid, Papanicolaou stain, TP, medium magnification)

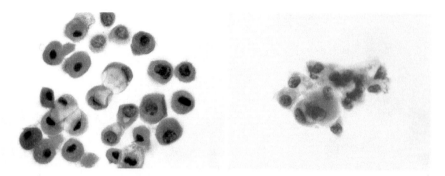

Fig. 3.9 False keratinization and degeneration. Left: "False" keratinization is degenerated dense mesothelial cells that appear orangeophilic due to cytoplasmic collapse with trapping of Orange G stain, mimicking squamous cells. Right: Mesothelial cells with some degenerative change, intracytoplasmic vacuoles, and frayed cytoplasmic borders. (Both images, Pleural fluid, Papanicoloau Stain, TP, high magnification)

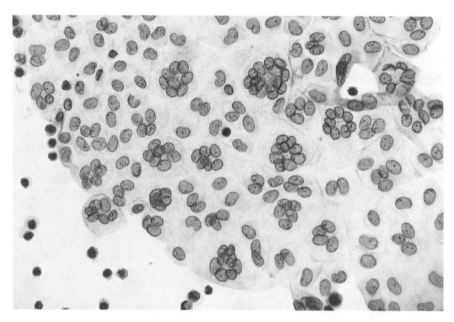

Fig. 3.10 Peritoneal lavage. This image exhibits benign mesothelial cells in a sheet, some with multinucleation and mild nuclear contour lobularity. (Papanicolaou stain, TP, high magnification)

samples may show flat sheets or balls of mesothelial cells. These cells can show lobulated nuclear contours, leading to the term "daisy cells" (Fig. 3.11).

If the specimen contains mostly mesothelial cells arranged singly and/or forming small clusters, and the cells do not express significant cellular atypia, the diagnosis of NFM can be rendered without additional immunochemical (IC) studies. In

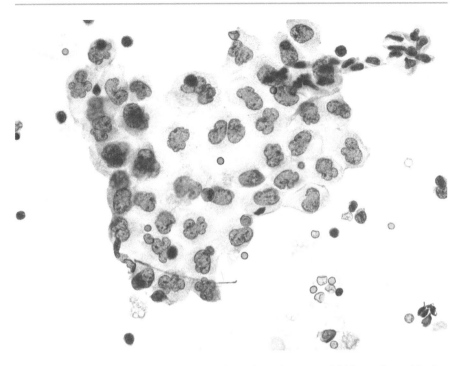

Fig. 3.11 Peritoneal lavage. Sample derived from the peritoneum exhibiting a sheet of benign mesothelial cells with markedly lobular nuclear contours, referred to as "daisy cells." (Papanicolaou stain, TP, high magnification)

general, utilization of IC studies in effusions should be judicious and should not exceed 10–15% of cases [13].

With Increased Volume and/or Distribution of Predominately One Cell Type

Predominantly Mesothelial Cells

Effusion samples can be very cellular and contain abundant single mesothelial cells and/or numerous cohesive clusters, including some with a papillary configuration. Individual cells can show significant reactive changes in the form of nuclear enlargement, binucleation, and multinucleation. Increased phagocytic activity can be present with significant vacuolization in appropriate cell types and even so-called cannibalism (cell within a cell pattern, or cell wrapping) may be seen in non-phagocytic cells [14]. In addition, hyperchromasia and prominent nucleoli may be present. There is significant overlap between the morphologic appearance of reactive mesothelial cells and malignant cells, particularly adenocarcinoma. In these cases, immunohistochemical studies are useful to confirm the mesothelial phenotype of those cells [15, 16]. If atypical cells show a mesothelial phenotype, it could be malignant mesothelioma. Significant cellularity and particularly the number, size, and complexity of cellular clusters should prompt consideration of this diagnosis

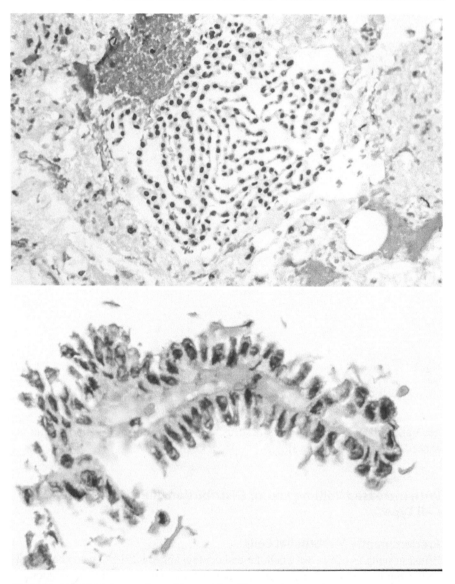

Fig. 3.12 Cell block from peritoneal lavage. Top: The sample shows benign mesothelial cells in a folded-up sheet. Cells are cohesive and low cuboidal without atypia, and do not show any clearing, or "lacunae" around this cell group. Bottom: Reactive mesothelial cells in a folded strip can be a pitfall in peritoneal washings, mimicking a papillary structure. (CB, H&E stain, Top: Low magnification, Bottom: Medium magnification)

[10]. A more detailed discussion of mesothelioma can be found in Chap. 6, Malignant-Primary. If mesothelioma can be excluded based on absence of appropriate clinical history, imaging findings and IC/molecular studies, the diagnosis for a

specimen containing exuberant, predominantly mesothelial cells should be reported as NFM with a comment (see Sample Reports, Example 3.2).

Predominantly Histiocytes

Effusions containing predominantly histiocytes are commonly encountered in daily practice. Differentiating histiocytes from mesothelial cells is very challenging based on morphology alone, and in many cases these cells are misinterpreted as mesothelial in origin [2, 11]. This misinterpretation does not affect the diagnostic category since in both scenarios, NFM would apply. Classically, histiocytes are round with well- to ill-defined borders and are usually single. They may form small, poorly defined clusters with irregular peripheral contours, or cohesive groups, mimicking an epithelial population (Fig. 3.13). In cases where the predominant cell population consists of histiocytes and occasional small clusters of mesothelial cells, this gives the appearance of a two-cell population. In addition, the cytoplasm of histiocytes can be coarsely vacuolated, and single, large vacuoles can push the nucleus to the periphery, giving a signet ring appearance (Fig. 3.14). These features can lead to a false-positive diagnosis of adenocarcinoma. Immunochemistry (e.g., CD68, CD163) is helpful in these challenging cases to confirm the histiocytic nature of these cells [15, 16] (Fig. 3.15).

Predominantly Lymphocytes

Various types of lymphocytes are commonly seen in effusions, with T-cells predominating in reactive processes by approximately 80% [17]. In the majority of cases, they are present as scattered cells with mature morphology. However, there are cases where lymphocytes constitute the predominant population. Patients with tuberculosis present with effusions composed predominantly of T-cells [18] (Fig. 3.16). In general, it is difficult to assess distinctive morphology of lymphoid cells in fluid specimens, particularly those that have been alcohol fixed. The differentiation of a reactive lymphoid proliferation versus lymphoma may be impossible

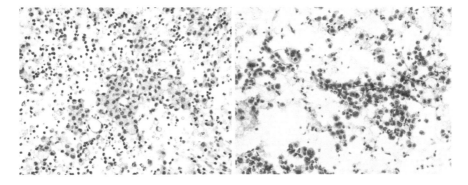

Fig. 3.13 Histiocytes. Histiocytes may aggregate in epithelioid clusters, as shown in both images, mimicking an epithelial malignancy/second population. This obviously is a major pitfall. (Left: Pleural fluid, H&E stain, medium magnification. Right: Pleural fluid, Papanicolaou stain, TP, medium magnification)

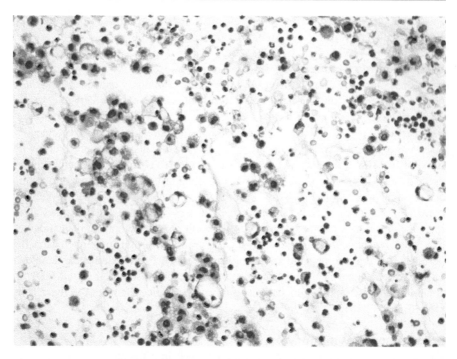

Fig. 3.14 Histiocytes. Degenerating histiocytes may develop a single large cytoplasmic vacuole, pushing the nucleus to the periphery, creating a signet ring-like morphology, which raises the specter of adenocarcinoma. (Pleural fluid, H&E stain, CB, medium magnification)

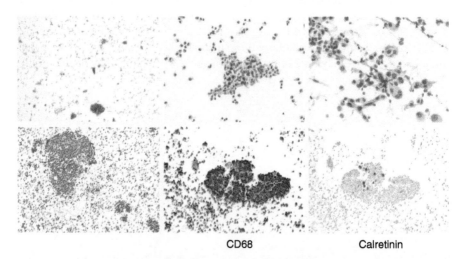

CD68   Calretinin

Fig. 3.15 Histiocytes. Top row: Histiocytes forming epithelioid aggregates may be difficult to distinguish from metastatic carcinoma based on morphology alone. (Pleural fluid, Papanicolaou stain, TP, low, medium, and high magnification). Immunohistochemistry on cell block can be helpful. Bottom row, left: Cell block showing epithelioid aggregates. (Pleural fluid, H&E stain, CB, low magnification). Bottom middle: CD68 immunostain highlights almost all of the cells, confirming that they are histiocytes. (Pleural fluid, CD68 immunostain, CB, low magnification). Bottom right: Calretinin immunostain highlights only scattered mesothelial cells. (Pleural fluid, calretinin immunostain, CB, low magnification)

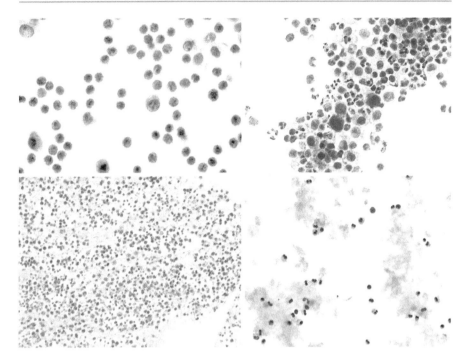

Fig. 3.16 Various inflammatory patterns. Top left: Tuberculous pleuritis, showing lymphocytes (T cells) and very few or no mesothelial cells. (Pleural fluid, Papanicolaou stain, LBP, high magnification). Top right: Mixed acute and chronic inflammation, interspersed with reactive mesothelial cells. (Pleural fluid, Modified Giemsa stain, high magnification). Bottom left and right: Pleural fluid showing a prominent population of eosinophils. Their bilobed nuclei and bright cytoplasmic granules are characteristic. (Bottom left: H&E stain, CB, low magnification; Bottom right: Papanicolaou stain, TP, medium magnification)

based on morphology alone [19, 20]. Therefore, additional studies, including flow cytometry, are necessary in cases with a significant lymphoid population, particularly if there are clinical indications of a lymphoid malignancy.

Predominantly or Increased Eosinophils

It is unusual for an effusion to be composed predominantly of eosinophils. However, there are cases where there is a significant increase in eosinophils (Fig. 3.16). There is no clear definition of what constitutes "significant," but if numerous eosinophils are present, it should be noted in the report and correlated with the clinical history. The presence of eosinophils is most commonly related to the introduction of air into a mesothelial-lined space and may be associated with prior paracentesis/thoracentesis or trauma leading to pneumothorax or hemothorax. However, many cases with serous eosinophilia are idiopathic. Other causes include malignancy, infection, pulmonary infarction, and hypersensitivity reactions [21, 22].

Predominantly Neutrophils
Cases composed predominantly of neutrophils are seen in purulent effusions [23] and should be reported as NFM with a diagnosis of "numerous neutrophils consistent with empyema." Empyema is most commonly caused by infection and rarely by other etiologies such as rheumatoid arthritis [24].

Unexpected Cellular and Noncellular Findings

Unexpected Cell Population (Second Cell Population)

In general, specimens containing a second cell population or unexpected cells are usually malignant. Malignant effusion is discussed in detail in Chaps. 6 and 7. When abnormal populations are present, immunohistochemistry is valuable to further classify these intruders. Correlating cytomorphology with clinical history should result in the prudent selection of appropriate ancillary tests.

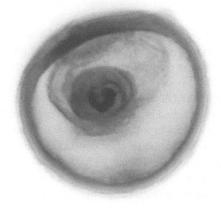

Fig. 3.17 Psamomma body in peritoneal fluid. A psamomma body is a lamellated concentric calcification. Follow-up on this case was benign. (Peritoneal fluid, Papanicolaou stain, TP, high magnification)

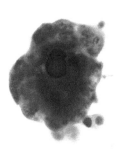
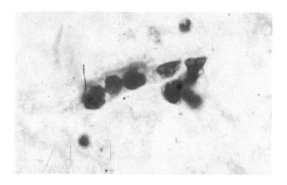

Fig. 3.18 Endosalpingiosis. Left: A psammoma body is surrounded by reactive cells. (Peritoneal fluid, Papanicolaou stain, high magnification) Right: Ciliated epithelial cells suggest endosalpingiosis. (Peritoneal fluid, Papanicolaou stain, TP, high magnification)

Unexpected Benign Cellular and Noncellular Findings

Occasionally an effusion will contain cellular material or benign cells not normally occurring in effusions, as listed below. In these circumstances, the interpretation should be NFM with a comment explaining the findings (see Sample Report 5).

Psammoma Bodies

It is not uncommon to encounter psammoma bodies in effusion fluids. Psammoma bodies are concentrically laminated calcifications (Fig. 3.17). Although psammoma bodies are associated with a variety of malignancies, the presence of psammoma bodies alone (without an accompanying cellular proliferation) is not sufficient to classify a specimen as malignant. In peritoneal fluids in particular, psammoma bodies can be associated with benign processes. Any process that leads to papillary formation, such as papillary mesothelial hyperplasia, endometriosis, and endosalpingiosis can be associated with the formation of psammoma bodies (Fig. 3.18). In addition, benign neoplasms such as ovarian cystadenoma and cystadenofibroma can be associated with psammoma bodies [25–27]. Finding psammoma bodies should lead to a very careful examination of the specimen and correlation with clinical history and imaging studies to exclude a potential neoplasm.

Collagen Balls

Collagen balls are round to oval, small fragments of collagen covered with mesothelial cells. They originate as papillary projections commonly seen on the surface of

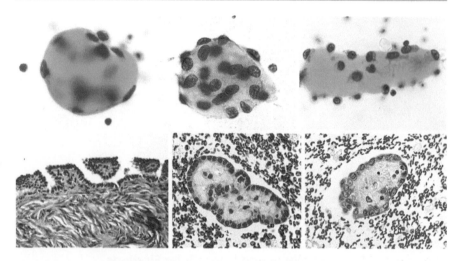

Fig. 3.19 Collagen balls. These structures are a common finding in peritoneal lavage specimens as well as effusion cytology. Three-dimensional balls of collagen wrapped with benign mesothelial cells (Top: Peritoneal fluid, Papanicolaou stain, TP, high magnification; Bottom: Peritoneal fluid, H&E stain, CB, medium magnification)

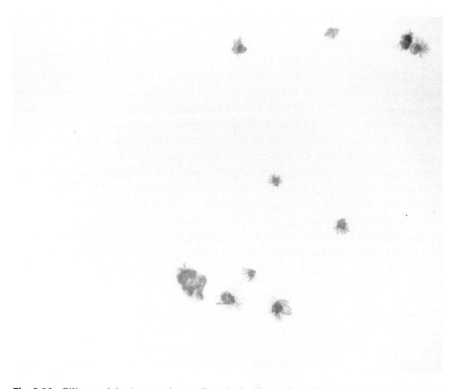

Fig. 3.20 Ciliocytophthoria-type change. Detached ciliary tufts in fluid cytology are sometimes seen in female patients and may be mistaken for a parasite. These have also been noted in dialysis samples. This example is from a case of cyst fluid from a serous cystadenoma; findings in peritoneal fluid would appear similar. (Cyst fluid, Papanicoloau stain, TP, high magnification)

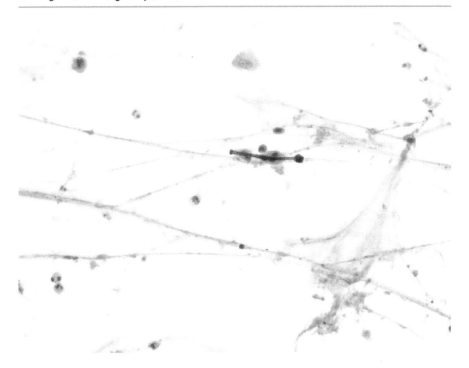

Fig. 3.21 Asbestos (ferruginous) body. These are rarely seen in fluid cytology. A linear structure with rounded ends, usually with a core of asbestos, is covered by brown iron salts. (Pleural fluid, Papanicoloau stain, TP, high magnification)

the ovary. They are relatively often identified in pelvic washings. They are also seen in spontaneous effusions [28] (Fig. 3.19). The most important issue is not to misinterpret them as a malignant process. They are insignificant and incidental findings, so there is no need to report their presence.

Detached Ciliary Tufts

Occasionally, detached ciliary tufts originating from ciliated epithelium lining the fallopian tubes may be seen in peritoneal washings [29] (Fig. 3.20). This finding should not be interpreted as protozoa or parasites [30]. It is not clinically significant and there is no need to include this in the report.

Asbestos (Ferruginous) Bodies

Finding asbestos bodies in a serous fluid is extremely rare. In a pleural fluid, this very rare finding should be regarded as indicative of a heavy asbestos burden in the lung [31] (Fig. 3.21). The diagnosis is NFM; however, considering the serious clinical implications of this finding, the presence of asbestos bodies should be included in the report or comment.

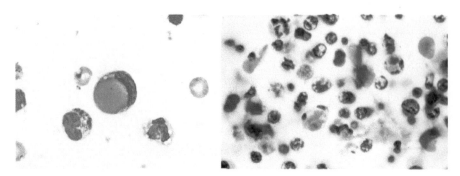

Fig. 3.22 Lupus erythematosus (LE) cells. LE cells are classically seen in effusions related to systemic lupus erythematosus and consist of a cell (neutrophil or macrophage) engulfing a so-called "hematoxylin body." These cells are not always seen in effusions related to SLE. (Left: Pleural fluid, Modified Giemsa stain, CS, high magnification; Right: Pleural fluid, Papanicoloau stain, TP, high magnification)

Curschmann's Spirals

Although extremely rare, Curschmann's spirals may be found in effusions. Presence of these spirals should prompt a close search for cells of a mucin producing adeno-carcinoma, since these are the most common source of Curschmann's spirals in fluids [32, 33]. The presence of Curschmann's spirals alone does not indicate malignancy; the diagnosis would still be NFM.

Lupus Erythematosus (LE) Cells

LE cells are classically described as the characteristic cell found in effusions due to systemic lupus erythematosus (SLE). LE cells are inflammatory cells, usually a neutrophil but sometimes a macrophage, containing a homogenous, smudged hematoxylin body (degraded nuclear material) (Fig. 3.22). Although the presence of LE cells is a characteristic feature of SLE, not all fluids from SLE patients will show LE cells even with close inspection. The LE cell is not entirely pathognomonic and can be seen in other entities [34, 35]. The presence of LE cells should be noted in the report to ensure clinical correlation.

Necrotic Material

The presence of extensive necrosis suggests a malignant process. Necrosis in serous fluid is also characteristic of rheumatoid disease, particularly if the specimen contains round, multinucleated giant cells, spindle cells (resembling spindle squamous cells), necrotic debris, and many degenerated cells [36, 37]. It is important to be familiar with these characteristic changes and not to misinterpret these specimens as malignant to prevent subjecting patients to unnecessary additional investigation to

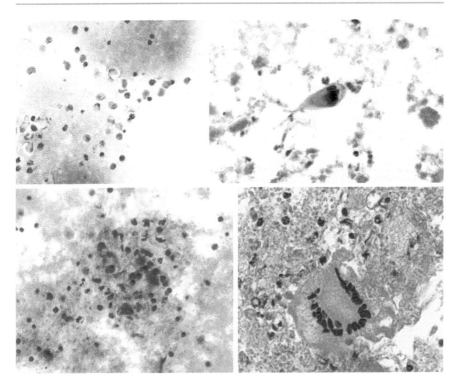

Fig. 3.23 Rheumatoid changes. Samples from an effusion related to rheumatoid serositis. Left top and bottom: Lymphocytes and degenerated neutrophils in a "felt-like" proteinaceous background. (Left top: Pleural fluid, Modified Giemsa stain, CS, medium magnification; Left bottom: Pleural fluid, Papanicolaou stain, direct smear, medium magnification). Right top and bottom: Necrotic material and multinucleated giant cells, which may be elongated and spindle-shaped. (Right top: Pleural fluid, Papanicolaou stain, LBP, medium magnification; Right bottom: Pleural fluid, H&E stain, CB, medium magnification)

confirm malignancy or tuberculosis. Findings in rheumatoid disease such as elongated spindle shaped macrophages, multinucleated giant macrophages, and necrotic granular material should be interpreted as NFM with a comment indicating that these findings are consistent with rheumatoid serositis (Fig. 3.23).

Fistula

Fistulas may arise in various organs and anastomose with serosal cavities, leading to unexpected cellular and other material in fluid samples. The type and quantity of these materials depends on the site of the fistula [38]. For example, a patient with an esophagopleural fistula may show stratified squamous cells and food material in pleural fluid [39]. The presence of foreign material should be noted with a comment indicating that the findings suggest fistula formation.

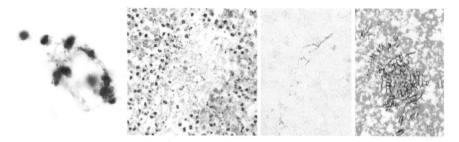

Fig. 3.24 *Nocardia* in fluid. Far left: Pleural fluid showing delicate, rod-shaped bacteria forming branching filaments. (Papanicoloau stain, TP, high magnification) Left middle: The background shows inflammation and debris. (Pleural fluid, H&E stain, CB, medium magnification) Right middle: The bacteria are weakly acid-fast. (Pleural fluid, Acid-Fast Bacillus stain, CB, high magnification) Far right: Bacteria pick up silver staining on a GMS stain. (Pleural fluid, Gomori Methenamine Silver stain, CB, high magnification)

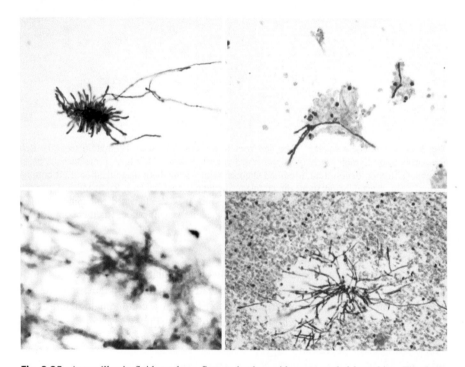

Fig. 3.25 *Aspergillus* in fluid cytology. Septate hyphae with acute-angled branching. The background may show necrotic debris and inflammation. The fungal elements can be identified on routine stains, but special stains for fungus may be helpful in cases where the organisms are scant. (Top left and right: Pleural fluid, Papanicoloau stain, TP, high magnification. Bottom left: Pleural fluid, Papanicoloau stain, direct smear, high magnification. Bottom right: Pleural fluid, H&E stain, CB, medium magnification)

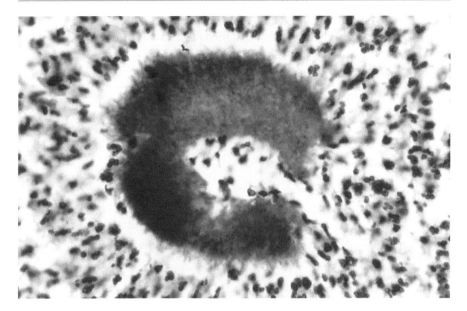

Fig. 3.26 *Actinomyces. Actinomyces* in a fluid appear as "fluffy" ball of bacteria with tangled bacterial filaments surrounded by inflammatory cells. (Pleural fluid, H&E stain, CB, medium magnification)

Infectious Organisms

All types of infectious organisms including parasites, fungi, bacteria, and viruses have been reported in serous effusions, and all are reported in the NFM category. The presence of a specific agent, if identified, should also be reported. Appropriate special stains should be deployed to confirm the diagnosis, if necessary (Figs. 3.24, 3.25, and 3.26).

Rate and Risk of Malignancy

The rate of NFM and risk of malignancy (ROM) for a NFM diagnosis in serous fluids as a whole are not well-studied, but there are numerous publications on the sensitivity, specificity, and positive predictive value of serous fluid cytology for specific body sites or diseases. A recent meta-analysis of 80 English-language studies containing 35 or more cases with results on positive and negative outcomes revealed over 22,000 cases reported as NFM, with a ROM from 0–82%, and a mean ROM of 20.7% [40]. Overall, serous fluid cytology had a sensitivity of 73.1%, specificity of

99.9%, and a negative likelihood ratio of 0.27. Cytology was more sensitive in pleural and peritoneal fluid than in pericardial fluid [40].

Sample Reports

Example 3.1
- Pleural effusion:
- Adequacy: Satisfactory for evaluation
- Diagnosis: Negative for malignancy

Example 3.2
- Abdominal fluid, paracentesis:
- Adequacy: Satisfactory for evaluation
- Diagnosis: Negative for malignancy; reactive mesothelial cells present

Comment: Due to the high cellularity of the specimen, the diagnosis was confirmed with immunohistochemical studies that showed the following results: (appropriate markers are listed with their interpretation and rationale for use).

Example 3.3
- Right lung, pleural fluid:
- Adequacy: Satisfactory for evaluation

Diagnosis: Negative for mlaignancy; Polymorphous lymphoid population consistent with lymphoid hyperplasia
Comment: Please correlate with flow cytometry results.

Example 3.4
- Left pleural fluid:
- Adequacy: Satisfactory for evaluation
- Diagnosis: Negative for malignancy; Increased eosinophils consistent with patient's history of pneumothorax

Example 3.5
- Lung, right, thoracentesis:
- Adequacy: Satisfactory for evaluation
- Diagnosis: Negative for malignancy (see comment)

Comment: Occasional asbestos bodies are identified, indicating significant asbestos exposure.
Comment: Isolated psammoma bodies are present, but there is no evidence of malignancy. Correlation with clinical history and imaging studies is recommended.

Comment: Occasional LE cells are identified. These cells are characteristically seen in SLE. Appropriate clinical correlation is recommended.

References

1. Light RW. Clinical practice: pleural effusion. N Engl J Med. 2002;346:1971–7.
2. Bibbo M, Draganova-Tacheva D, Naylor B. Pleural, peritoneal and pericardial fluids. In: Bibbo M, Wilbur DC, editors. Comprehensive Cytopathology. Philadelphia: Saunders Elsevier; 2014.
3. Dragoescu EA, Liu L. Pericardial fluid cytology: an analysis of 128 specimens over a 6-year period. Cancer Cytopathol. 2013;121(5):242–51.
4. Hsu C. Cytologic detection of malignancy in pleural effusion: a review of 5,255 samples from 3,811 patients. Diagn Cytopathol. 1987;3(1):8–12.
5. Irani DR, Underwood RD, Johnson EH, Greenberg SD. Malignant pleural effusions. A clinical cytopathologic study. Arch Intern Med. 1987;147(6):1133–6.
6. Motherby H, Nadjari B, Friegel P, Kohaus J, Ramp U, Böcking A. Diagnostic accuracy of effusion cytology. Diagn Cytopathol. 1999;20(6):350–7.
7. Rossi ED, Bizzarro T, Schmitt F, Longatto-Filho A. The role of liquid-based cytology and ancillary techniques in pleural and pericardic effusions: an institutional experience. Cancer Cytopathol. 2015;123(4):258–66.
8. Mutsaers SE. The mesothelial cell. Int J Biochem Cell Biol. 2004;36(1):9–16.
9. Hjerpe A, Abd-Own S, Dobra K. Cytopathologic diagnosis of epithelioid and mixed-type malignant mesothelioma: ten years of clinical experience in relation to international guidelines. Arch Pathol Lab Med. 2018;142(8):893–901.
10. Hjerpe A, Ascoli V, Bedrossian C, et al. Guidelines for cytopathologic diagnosis of epithelioid and mixed type malignant mesothelioma. Complementary statement from the International Mesothelioma Interest Group, also endorsed by the International Academy of Cytology and the Papanicolaou Society of Cytopathology. Cytojournal. 2015;12:26.
11. Bedrossian CW. Diagnostic problems in serous effusions. Diagn Cytopathol. 1998;19(2):131–7.
12. Wu JM, Ali SZ. Significance of "signet-ring cells" seen in exfoliative and aspiration cytopathology. Diagn Cytopathol. 2010;38(6):413–8.
13. Alshaikh S, Lapadat R, Atieh MK, et al. The utilization of immunostains in body fluid cytology. Cancer Cytopathol. 2020; https://doi.org/10.1002/cncy.22256.
14. Bansal C, Tiwari V, Singh U, Srivastava A, Misra J. Cell cannibalism: a cytological study in effusion samples. J Cytol. 2011;28(2):57–60.
15. Sundling KE, Cibas ES. Ancillary studies in pleural, pericardial, and peritoneal effusion cytology. Cancer Cytopathol. 2018;126(Suppl8):590–8.
16. Yu GH, Glaser LJ, Gustafson KS. Role of ancillary techniques in fluid cytology. Acta Cytol. 2020;64(1–2):52–62.
17. Spieler P, Kradolfer D, Schmid U. Immunocytochemical characterization of lymphocytes in benign and malignant lymphocyte-rich serous effusions. Virchows Arch A Pathol Anat Histopathol. 1986;409(2):211–21.
18. Spriggs AI, Boddington MM. Absence of mesothelial cells from tuberculous pleural effusions. Thorax. 1960;15(2):169–71.
19. Yu GH, Vergara N, Moore EM, King RL. Use of flow cytometry in the diagnosis of lymphoproliferative disorders in fluid specimens. Diagn Cytopathol. 2014;42(8):664–70.
20. Walts AE, Marchevsky AM. Low cost-effectiveness of CD3/CD20 immunostains for initial triage of lymphoid-rich effusions: an evidence-based review of the utility of these stains in selecting cases for full hematopathologic workup. Diagn Cytopathol. 2012;40(7):565–9.
21. Kalomenidis I, Light RW. Pathogenesis of the eosinophilic pleural effusions. Curr Opin Pulm Med. 2004;10(4):289–93.

22. Oba Y, Abu-Salah T. The prevalence and diagnostic significance of eosinophilic pleural effusions: a meta-analysis and systematic review. Respiration. 2012;83(3):198–208.
23. Davies RJ, Gleeson FV. The diagnosis and management of pleural empyema. Curr Opin Pulm Med. 1998;4(3):185–90.
24. Avnon LS, Abu-Shakra M, Flusser D, Heimer D, Sion-Vardy N. Pleural effusion associated with rheumatoid arthritis: what cell predominance to anticipate? Rheumatol Int. 2007;27:919–25.
25. Covell JL, Carry JB, Feldman PS. Peritoneal washings in ovarian tumors. Potential sources of error in cytologic diagnosis. Acta Cytol. 1985;29(3):310–6.
26. Fanning J, Markuly SN, Hindman TL, et al. False positive malignant peritoneal cytology and psammoma bodies in benign gynecologic disease. J Reprod Med. 1996;41(7):504–8.
27. Parwani AV, Chan TY, Ali SZ. Significance of psammoma bodies in serous cavity fluid: a cytopathologic analysis. Cancer Cytopathol. 2004;102(2):87–91.
28. Wojcik EM, Naylor B. "Collagen balls" in peritoneal washings. Prevalence, morphology, origin and significance. Acta Cytol. 1992;36(4):466–70.
29. Sidawy MK, Chandra P, Oertel YC. Detached ciliary tufts in female peritoneal washings. A common finding. Acta Cytol. 1987;31(6):841–4.
30. Kuritzkes DR, Rein M, Horowitz S, et al. Detached ciliary tufts mistaken for peritoneal parasites: a warning. Rev Infect Dis. 1988;10(5):1044–7.
31. Butler EB, Stanbridge CM. Cytology of body cavity fluids. A colour atlas. London: Chapman and Hall; 1986.
32. Wahl RW. Curschmann's spirals in pleural and peritoneal fluids. Report of 12 cases. Acta Cytol. 1986;30(2):147–51.
33. Naylor B. Curschmann's spirals in pleural and peritoneal effusions. Acta Cytol. 1990;34(4):474–8.
34. Naylor B. Cytological aspects of pleural, peritoneal and pericardial fluids from patients with systemic lupus erythematosus. Cytopathology. 1992;3(1):1–8.
35. Kaplan AI, Zakher F, Sabin S. Drug-induced lupus erythematosus with in vivo lupus erythematosus cells in pleural fluid. Chest. 1978;73(6):875–6.
36. Montes S, Guarda LA. Cytology of pleural effusions in rheumatoid arthritis. Diagn Cytopathol. 1988;4(1):71–3.
37. Boddington MM, Spriggs AI, Morton JA, Mowat AG. Cytodiagnosis of rheumatoid pleural effusions. J Clin Pathol. 1971;24(2):95–106.
38. Weaver KM, Novak PM, Naylor B. Vegetable cell contaminants in cytologic specimens: their resemblance to cells associated with various normal and pathologic states. Acta Cytol. 1981;25(3):210–4.
39. Cherveniakov A, Tzekov C, Grigorov GE, Cherveniakov P. Acquired benign esophago-airway fistulas. Eur J Cardiothorac Surg. 1996;10(9):713–6.
40. Farahani SJ, Baloch Z. Are we ready to develop a tiered scheme for the effusion cytology? A comprehensive review and analysis of the literature. Diag Cytopathol. 2019;47(11):1145–59.

Atypia of Undetermined Significance

4

Philippe Vielh, Renê Gerhard, Maria Lozano,
and Voichita Suciu

Background

Atypia of undetermined significance (AUS) is a diagnostic category associated with a lower outcome of malignancy compared to suspicious for malignancy (SFM) in all reporting systems. The AUS category includes cases with small numbers of cells displaying some features that make it difficult to confidently exclude malignancy but that also overlap with reactive changes. If the features closely approximate malignancy, SFM is the preferred category. If the features are atypical but processing, degeneration or ancillary testing does not confirm their true nature, then AUS is appropriate. Benign epithelial cells in peritoneal fluids that are difficult to definitively identify or are due to benign or borderline tumors may also be categorized as AUS. Clinical data may influence categorization and the decision to perform ancillary tests, but the expectation of malignancy is low. In a recent meta-analysis of 73 studies [1], only 0.6% of effusions were reported as atypical with a reported risk of malignancy (ROM) of 65.9%. It was, however, not clear what features were used to classify specimens as atypical, and a degree of overlap with the suspicious for malignancy (SFM) category is likely. Prospective data using the proposed

P. Vielh (✉)
Medipath & American Hospital of Paris, Paris, France

R. Gerhard
Department of Morphologic and Molecular Pathology, Laboratoire National de Santé,
Dudelange, Luxembourg

M. Lozano
Department of Pathology, University of Navarra, Pamplona, Navarra, Spain

V. Suciu
Department of Medical Biology and Pathology,
Gustave Roussy, Villejuif, France

© Springer Nature Switzerland AG 2020
A. Chandra et al. (eds.), *The International System for Serous Fluid
Cytopathology*, https://doi.org/10.1007/978-3-030-53908-5_4

41

diagnostic criteria may help to modify the ROM of serous fluid atypia of undetermined significance (AUS) and other diagnostic categories.

In our survey of oncologists, only 22% found an AUS diagnosis to be useful, and the majority of respondents would treat AUS as a benign result if the surgical results were benign. However, others indicated that they would follow patients more closely or even treat the patient with hormonal or chemotherapy. Cytologists must guard against using this category as a wastebasket and strive to clarify the differential diagnosis and interpretive difficulties in a note.

Definition

The AUS diagnostic category is reserved for effusion specimens that lack quantitative or qualitative cytological features to be confidently diagnosed as either benign or malignant and exhibit sufficiently clear morphologic features to exclude the possibility of classifying them as nondiagnostic. The atypical morphologic features identified more closely approximate benign, reactive, or degenerative features than malignant features.

Criteria

As compared to normal reference cells of similar derivation, atypical cells may show the following:

- Mild to moderate nuclear enlargement and slightly increased nuclear to cytoplasmic ratio
- Prominent nucleoli or variable nucleoli
- Slight nuclear membrane irregularities
- Altered chromatin
- Altered cytoplasm

The category of AUS can be used in any of the following scenarios:

- Cytological features indefinite for a diagnosis of SFM (Figs. 4.1 and 4.2)
- Low-cellularity specimens with or without pre-analytical artifacts that suggest that the specimen should be included in the negative for malignancy (NFM) category, such as degenerative changes in mesothelial cells or macrophages, but where confidence of benignity remains uncertain (Figs. 4.3 and 4.4)
- Mesothelial proliferations that are indefinite for a diagnosis of SFM (Figs. 4.5, 4.6, and 4.7) (see Chaps. 5 and 6, "Suspicious for Malignancy" and "Malignant Primary")
- Lymphocytosis indefinite for a lymphoproliferative disorder but favoring a reactive process
- Epithelial cells of unknown or indeterminate origin with bland, benign features (see Chap. 9, "Special Considerations for Peritoneal Fluids")

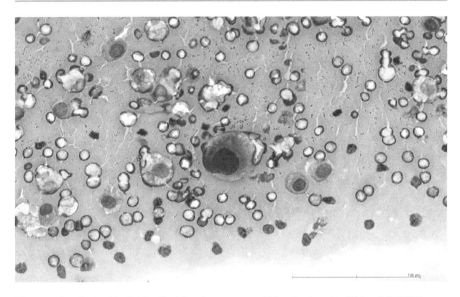

Fig. 4.1 Atypical epithelioid cell with enlargement and binucleation. BerEP4 and MOC31 were negative in this patient with breast carcinoma; this is likely a mesothelial cell (Pleural fluid, smear, Modified Giemsa stain, high magnification)

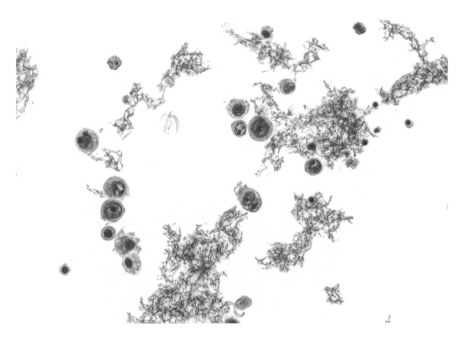

Fig. 4.2 Atypical epithelioid cells. These atypical cells exhibit a high nuclear to cytoplasmic ratio and prominent nucleoli. Clinical follow-up was negative in this patient with prior lung adenocarcinoma (Pleural fluid, TP, Papanicolaou stain, high magnification)

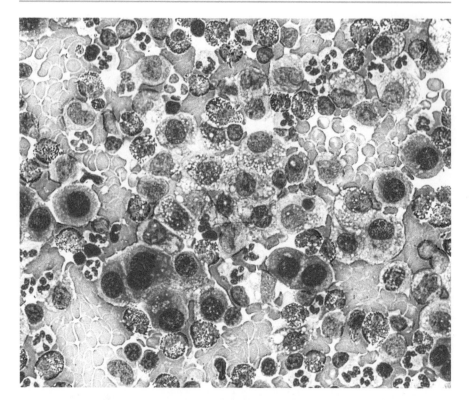

Fig. 4.3 Atypical microvacuolated cells. Atypical microvacuolated (likely mesothelial) cells in an inflammatory background worrisome for carcinoma, but possibly consistent with inflammatory degeneration. The patient had a prior history of breast cancer and current transient pneumonia with negative follow-up (Pleural fluid, smear, Modified Giemsa stain, high magnification)

- Epithelial or other cells from benign or borderline tumors of the ovary or abdominal/pelvic cavities (see Chap. 9, "Special Considerations for Peritoneal Fluids")

Explanatory Notes

One of the challenges of effusion cytology is that the use of "atypia" has proven to be quite variable [2, 3]. What has been deemed AUS in the literature is very heterogeneous. Similar to other diagnostic systems, the domain of atypia resides somewhere between benign reactive change and suspicious for malignancy (SFM). The AUS category should have a higher ROM than benign changes but less than SFM. Problems with degeneration or preparation artifacts can impair morphology such that it is difficult to resolve the malignant and nonmalignant state. Less degeneration and better preparations are more likely to produce a clearer answer. Experience and good quality control can help. Laboratory practices that correlate the histology and the cytology may fine-tune criteria, leading to more secure diagnoses and the avoidance of indeterminate categories.

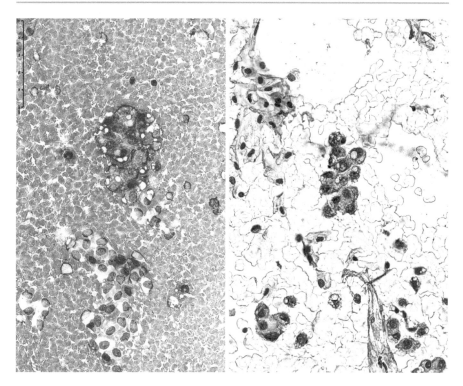

Fig. 4.4 Atypical cell clusters. These cells, that are likely degenerate mesothelial cells, display discrete cytoplasmic vacuoles in a patient with a uterine leiomyoma (Peritoneal fluid, smears, Modified Giemsa stain (left) and Papanicolaou stain (right), medium magnification)

It is difficult to find any medical test that can always separate a "diseased" population from a "normal" population. There is always overlap in the values or features being measured. This concept is valid in clinical chemistry, hematology, and histology. In the morphology of neoplasia, there are patterns that do not allow an observer to resolve tumor versus non-tumor, and this is the domain of atypia (Fig. 4.8). Poor preparations or degenerate material can make the overlap worse. The performance of the test will also change depending on where the observer makes the decision point on the x-axis. The further one goes to the right, the less tendency for false positives and the higher the diagnostic specificity, but with a corresponding lower sensitivity. The more one goes to the left, the higher the tendency for false positives, lowered specificity, and higher sensitivity. The International System proposes to exclude clearly reactive morphology from the AUS category, shift the decision point to the right, and decrease the numbers of atypical diagnoses.

Special attention is required to identify reactive mesothelial cells resulting from conditions such as cirrhosis, ectopic pregnancy, tubo-ovarian abscess, chemotherapy, radiotherapy, and pelvic tumors. Rarely, mesothelial cells may be reported under AUS, but this should be reserved for cases where the clinical picture is not clearly benign or malignant, where there is cytologic mesothelial atypia in low or

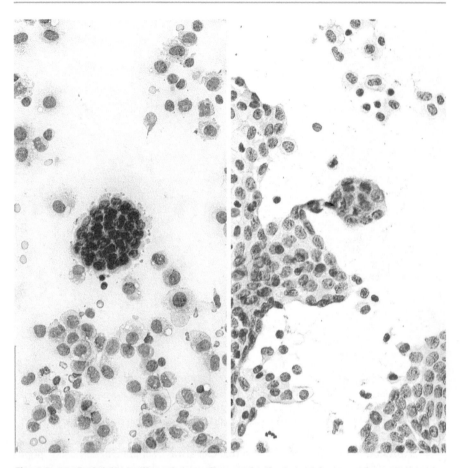

Fig. 4.5 Atypical tight papillary clusters. Groups of cells derived from a young patient with a cystic ovarian mass. Follow-up showed an ovarian serous borderline tumor without extra-ovarian or peritoneal involvement (Peritoneal fluid, smears, Modified Giemsa stain (left) and Papanicolaou stain (right), medium magnification)

moderately cellular effusions, or when ancillary tests to support a definitive malignant or benign mesothelial process are inconclusive.

Pitfalls may occur in cases of endometriosis and endosalpingiosis. In endometriosis, the presence of large aggregates of reactive mesothelial cells (sometimes with calcific concretions) may mimic serous tumors. Endosalpingiosis (Müllerian inclusions) is a potential cause of false positive that may present as tightly cohesive papillary structures with psammoma bodies. Both of these situations are more appropriately reported as negative for malignancy (NFM) whenever possible.

Borderline tumors of the ovary or other tumors of low malignant potential are categorized as AUS, with the diagnostic line stating "consistent with borderline tumor," once the effusion cells have been confirmed as concordant to the surgical specimen with that diagnosis. If the surgical specimen is unavailable or the surgical

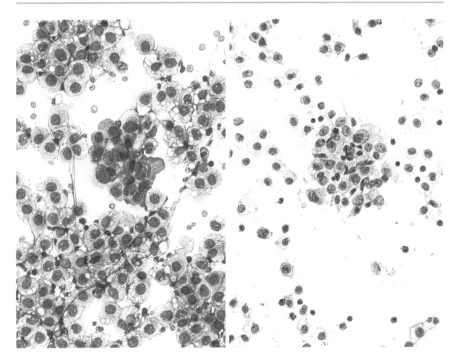

Fig. 4.6 Atypical cells of undetermined origin. Atypical cells associated with chronic inflammation in a woman with a solid and cystic ovarian mass, surgically confirmed endometrioid carcinoma with mesothelial hyperplasia but without peritoneal metastases (Peritoneal fluid, smears, Modified Giemsa stain (left) and Papanicolaou stain (right), medium magnification)

diagnosis unknown, the categorical selection of AUS or SFM is left to the clinical judgment of the pathologist, with the understanding that AUS represents lesions that are likely benign or borderline, whereas SFM represents lesions that are at least borderline and/or suspected to be malignant. It is preferable to qualify the diagnostic line of AUS whenever possible as "favor benign," "favor reactive," "favor borderline tumor," or other appropriate terminology.

As already stressed, a clinically meaningful, standardized diagnostic category of AUS requires a narrow definition of the term atypia, including what is not atypia [4]; preset quantitative criteria; agreed-upon reference images in the form of a well-illustrated atlas or an online collection of benchmark reference images; translatable clinical significance (risk of malignancy); and, ideally, well-defined management options [3]. Consequently, the successful implementation of an AUS diagnostic category in effusion cytology will require continuous education of cytology professionals and quality assurance efforts to monitor its use [3, 5]. Even though most of the previously described criteria are generalized, we believe that this diagnostic category is useful in daily practice. It fills the gap between what is recognizable as normal and unequivocally abnormal and should potentially reduce the number of false-negative and false-positive diagnoses in the "negative for malignancy" and "malignant" diagnostic categories, respectively.

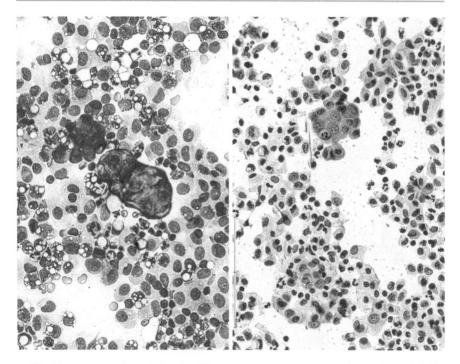

Fig. 4.7 Atypical cellular clusters. The images show tightly packed clusters of cells in a patient with a colorectal mass. Calretinin was positive and CK20 and BerEP4 were negative, confirming mesothelial origin. Surgical specimen showed colorectal adenocarcinoma without peritoneal involvement (Peritoneal fluid, smears, Modified Giemsa stain (left) and Papanicolaou stain (right), high magnification)

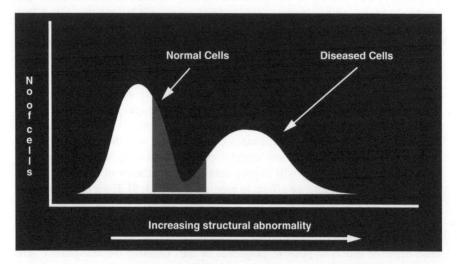

Fig. 4.8 Overlap in morphologic features of normal and diseased cells (see text)

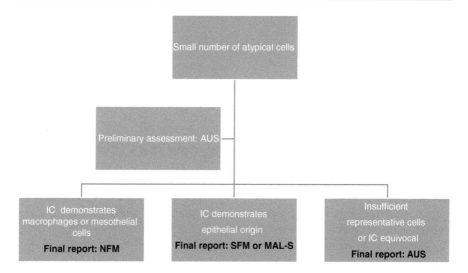

Fig. 4.9 Approach to preliminary reporting of atypia of undetermined significance

The AUS diagnostic category corresponds to cytopathologic findings that are not sufficiently clear-cut to permit a more specific diagnosis after eliminating the morphologic effects on cells due to known or unknown organ (hepatic, cardiac, and renal) diseases, various reactive processes, bacterial or viral infections, and neoplastic or preneoplastic changes [3]. It is difficult to apply a standard set of criteria to all cell types that may present in serous effusions; the comparative reference is a normal cell. AUS should be a *diagnosis of exclusion* and its rate be kept as low as possible in order to increase clinicians' confidence in cytologic reports, reduce patients' anxiety and potential morbidity, and diminish healthcare costs [5].

Our large web-based survey (manuscript in preparation) of current international cytopathology practice favored a two-step reporting approach to AUS: a provisional report (either written or verbal) based on morphology, followed by a more definitive report (either SFM or Malignant, Secondary (MAL-S)) based on the results of ancillary techniques (Fig. 4.9). This survey also indicated that ancillary tests were requested to exclude rather than confirm malignancy when the outcome was expected to be benign. By contrast, the category SFM was preferred when the outcome of ancillary tests was expected to support a malignant process.

Performance of immunostains (IC) on formalin-fixed paraffin-embedded cell blocks, combined with cytomorphology, may help differentiate metastatic epithelial cells from normal, reactive, or malignant mesothelial cells in pleural, peritoneal, and pericardial effusion specimens using panels of antibodies [6]. IC is also useful in lymphocytosis, which is most common in malignant and tuberculous effusions, but can also be attributable to lymphoproliferative diseases or other benign entities such as sarcoidosis, rheumatoid disease, and chylothorax. Immunophenotyping by flow cytometry on fresh effusions is also a useful adjunct when atypical hematologic cells are present.

Sample Reports

Example 4.1:
Provisional report:

- Pleural fluid, right, thoracentesis:
- Atypia of undetermined significance.
- Category: Atypia of undetermined significance.

Note: The preparations are poorly cellular, comprising a mixed population of lymphocytes, macrophages, and mesothelial cells. Very few cells show mild nuclear enlargement but no hyperchromasia or chromatin abnormalities. In view of the clinical history of a 65-year-old male with a unilateral pleural effusion and history of lung adenocarcinoma, a cell block and immunostains are being performed and a supplementary report will follow.

Supplementary report:

- Pleural fluid, right, thoracentesis:
- Atypia of undetermined significance.
- Category: Atypia of undetermined significance.
- Final report: Atypia of undetermined significance.

Note: The cell block consisted only of blood and should be considered as non-representative, so additional ancillary studies were unable to be performed. Consider submission of any further pleural fluid effusion for further evaluation.

Example 4.2:
Provisional report:

- Pleural fluid, left, thoracentesis:
- Atypia of undetermined significance.
- Category: Atypia of undetermined significance.

Note: The preparations are moderately cellular, comprising a mixed population of lymphocytes, macrophages, and mesothelial cells. Scattered cells show mild nuclear enlargement but no hyperchromasia or chromatin abnormalities. In view of the clinical history of a 57-year-old female with a new left pleural effusion and a history of breast adenocarcinoma, a cell block and immunostains are being performed and a supplementary report will follow.

Supplementary report:

- Pleural fluid, left, thoracentesis:
- No malignant cells identified on immunocytochemistry.
- Category: Negative for malignancy.
- Final report: Negative for malignancy.

Note: No epithelial cells are highlighted with immunostains BerEP4 and MOC31 performed on the cell block, indicating that the atypical cells are likely reactive mesothelial cells or macrophages.

Example 4.3:
Peritoneal fluid, paracentesis:
   Atypical epithelioid cells with psammoma bodies, consistent with serous border-line tumor.
   Category: Atypia of undetermined significance.
   (See note)
   Note: The cytology is compared with the patient's surgical specimen, a right ovarian serous borderline tumor, and is morphologically compatible. The category of atypia of undetermined significance (AUS) reflects the uncertain malignant potential of these lesions, although most behave in a benign fashion.

Rate and Risk of Malignancy

As in other cytology reporting systems, the proportion of specimens diagnosed as atypical is anticipated to be low. A benchmark of 5–10% of all effusion specimens seems reasonable for this diagnostic category. However, this benchmark is a work in progress, and it should prompt retrospective and prospective studies.

Since most published series emphasize cases diagnosed as benign or malignant and not those diagnosed as indeterminate (atypical or suspicious), it is difficult to determine the frequency with which atypical cells are seen in fluid specimens, discuss acceptable rates of nondefinitive diagnoses, and evaluate a risk of malignancy (ROM) [7]. In the most recent meta-analysis of Farahani and Baloch [1], the overall ROM was 65.9%. This seems unreasonably high if the AUS category is confined to cases suspected to be benign or behave in a benign fashion. Given the paucity of significant data in the literature on the risk of malignancy (ROM) for the AUS category, it may be expected to fall between the ROMs of the "negative for malignancy" and "suspicious for malignancy" categories. Future studies should help to refine acceptable ROM rates for AUS. In addition, intralaboratory monitoring of the AUS rate, which we recommend, may play a role in avoiding overuse of this diagnostic category [5].

References

1. Farahani SJ, Baloch Z. Are we ready to develop a tiered scheme for the effusion cytology? A comprehensive review and analysis of the literature. Diagn Cytopathol. 2019;47(11): 1145–59.
2. Tabatabai ZL, Nayar R, Souers RJ, Crothers BA, Davey DD. Performance characteristics of body fluid cytology analysis of 344 380 responses from the College of American Pathologists Interlaboratory Comparison Program in Nongynecologic Cytopathology. Arch Pathol Lab Med. 2018;142(1):53–8.

3. Pambuccian SE. What is atypia? Use, misuse, and overuse of the term of atypia in diagnostic cytopathology. J Am Soc Cytopathol. 2015;4(1):44–52.
4. Wojcik EM. What should not be reported as atypia in urine cytology? J Am Soc Cytopathol. 2015;4(1):30–6.
5. Barkan GA, Wojcik EM, Pambuccian SE. A tale of atypia: what can we learn from this? Cancer Cytopathol. 2018;126(6):376–80.
6. Sundling KE, Cibas ES. Ancillary studies in pleural, pericardial, and peritoneal effusion cytology. Cancer Cytopathol. 2018;126(Suppl8):590–8.
7. Raab SS. Significance of atypical cells in cytologic serous fluid specimens. Am J Clin Pathol. 1999;111(1):11–3.

Suspicious for Malignancy (SFM)

5

Panagiota Mikou, Marianne Engels,
Sinchita Roy-Chowdhuri, and George Santis

Literature is sparse on reporting practices in the use of atypical and suspicous categories in serous fluid cytopathology. Most published series with large numbers of cases emphasize cases diagnosed as benign or malignant, not those with inconclusive diagnoses [1–4]. It is difficult to determine the frequency with which suspicious cells are reported in fluid specimens. This may be in part because cytologists interpret these cells differently and only a few interobserver variability stuides in the literature have examined this issue [5–6]. This grey zone may reflect experience as well as the quality of the preparation, the clinical data and the use of ancillary tests. The number of suspicious cells is often small in cases of suspected metastatic carcinoma. However, in suspected lymphoma or mesothelioma, these may be numerous. Also, the number of suspicious cells may be small on routine stains, and many more may be highlighted on immunostains. Therefore, at the present time, a particular number of cells have not been established to distinguish between suspicious for malignancy (SFM) and malignant (MAL) categories. This distinction depends on the confidence in the morphological and ancillary test findings as well as on the clinical data available and the experience of the reporting pathologist.

A survey of current practice [7] revealed that the majority (64.4% respondents) of pathologists already use the suspicious category as a preliminary or provisional category while awaiting immunochemical stains. In cases lacking representative

P. Mikou (✉)
Laiko Hospital, Athens, Greece

M. Engels
Department of Pathology, University of Cologne, Cologne, Germany

S. Roy-Chowdhuri
MD Anderson Cancer Center, Houston, TX, USA

G. Santis
Professor of Thoracic Oncology & Interventional Bronchoscopy School of Immunology & Microbial Sciences. King's College London, Guy's & St Thomas' NHS Foundation Trust, London, UK

© Springer Nature Switzerland AG 2020
A. Chandra et al. (eds.), *The International System for Serous Fluid Cytopathology*, https://doi.org/10.1007/978-3-030-53908-5_5

Table 5.1 Comparison of AUS and SFM categories

	AUS	SFM
Cytological features	Only mild cytological abnormalities such as nuclear enlargement and hyperchromasia present, usually as small numbers of dispersed cells and occasional small groups	Greater degree of cytological abnormalities present, usually as small numbers of cells, including architectural features such as occasional three-dimensional groups
Cell lineage	Benign cell type favored, but epithelial or other benign or low-grade tumor cell of origin not excluded	Epithelial or other malignant cell of origin strongly favored
Immunochemistry	Outcomes may be benign, SFM, malignant, or inconclusive	Outcomes usually malignant or inconclusive
Suggested risk of malignancy [7, 24]	~20%	~80%

material or inconclusive results on immunochemistry (IC), the final report remains SFM. The remaining cases are upgraded from SFM to MAL on the final report following confirmatory studies or downgraded to atypia of undetermined significance (AUS) or negative for malignancy (NFM). Depending on factors such as anticipated time taken for return of immunostains and clinical urgency for results, a provisional SFM report may be issued or communicated verbally on inquiry by the clinical team. However, a single final report may be issued after performing ancillary tests without an interim provisional report. The survey also indicated that the respondents use both atypical and suspicious categories, although there was overlap in their current usage. A comparison of AUS and SFM features is presented in Table 5.1.

Definition

The SFM category is defined as one in which the evidence falls short of confirming malignancy based on cytomorphology and results of any ancillary tests performed.

Cytologic Criteria

- Cells occurring in small or occasionally in large numbers but limited by artifact and raising the suspicion of malignancy
- Monomorphic lymphocytic population or atypical lymphoid cells in varying numbers, suspicious for lymphoma
- Presence of mucinous material alone or with small numbers of bland epithelial cells (pseudomyxoma peritonei) requiring confirmation of malignancy and of the primary site
- Mesothelial proliferation suspicious for mesothelioma (see Chap. 6, "Malignant-Primary")

- Presence of epithelial cells in peritoneal washings (see Chap. 10, "Special Considerations for Peritoneal Fluids")

Explanatory Notes

Definitive cytological diagnosis of serous effusions is sometimes challenging on cytomorphologic grounds alone, and ancillary studies are necessary. Techniques such as DNA ploidy, image analysis, and even artificial intelligence have so far failed to provide anything more than modest results in equivocal cases. Over the last decade, it has become clear that of all the available methods, immunochemical (IC) stains are superior to the above alternatives in the diagnostic workup of effusion cytology [8–19]. In addition to morphology, immunochemistry and clinical data assist in arriving at a decisive diagnosis, thereby reducing the rates of SFM as a final report.

If malignancy has been confirmed on IC on a recent prior sample, repeating immunostains is unnecessary, since the sample may have been obtained for symptomatic relief, for performing genetic studies (next-generation sequencing [NGS], fluorescence in situ hybridization [FISH], etc.), or for theranostic markers such as HER2 (breast and gastric primaries) or PD-L1 (lung, urothelial, and other primaries). Ideally, this information should be supplied by the requesting clinical team, but often comes to light when the pathologist investigates the patient's medical record. Even in the presence of a past medical history of malignancy, a new malignancy should be considered and appropriate IC performed if there are sufficient clinical grounds to suspect a new primary.

A number of clinical scenarios apply to cases suspicious for metastatic malignancy. A common scenario is a patient with no previous history of malignancy and with scant numbers of suspicious cells present in an effusion (see Fig. 5.1). These cells display malignant characteristics such as a high nucleocytoplasmic ratio, deep

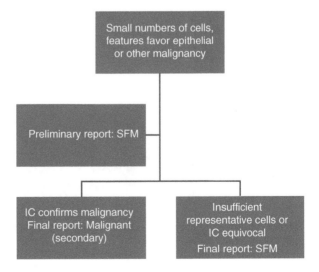

Fig. 5.1 Algorithm for SFM. For suspicious cells seen on routine stains, if residual material available for IC confirms a malignant infiltrate, the case may be assigned to the malignant category. If not, SFM remains the final diagnostic category

hyperchromasia and may have occasional groups with a three-dimensional architecture, suspicious for metastatic carcinoma. The most common culprit is metastatic adenocarcinoma, but others include poorly differentiated squamous cell carcinoma, neuroendocrine carcinoma, melanoma, and sarcoma. These cases may be provisionally labeled SFM until IC demonstrates them to be epithelial, neuroendocrine, melanoma, or sarcoma cells, whereby they may be reassigned to the MAL-S (secondary, metastatic) category. However, cellular preparations with the diagnostic features of malignancy should be reported as MAL regardless of supporting clinical data. In these cases, IC is performed to ascertain the cell of origin rather than confirm malignancy.

Another scenario is a case with small numbers of suspicious cells and insufficient residual material for performing immunostains such that these cannot be upgraded to the MAL category.

A third scenario is a patient with a history of malignancy and an effusion comprised of small numbers of suspicious cells but with IC equivocal for malignancy, either due to technical reasons or due to a non-classic or altered immunoprofile of the tumor (Fig. 5.2).

A fourth scenario is a cellular specimen with large numbers of relatively bland-appearing epithelial cells with some similarity to macrophages and only occasional or absent mesothelial cells. The epithelial cells may appear so bland that a diagnosis

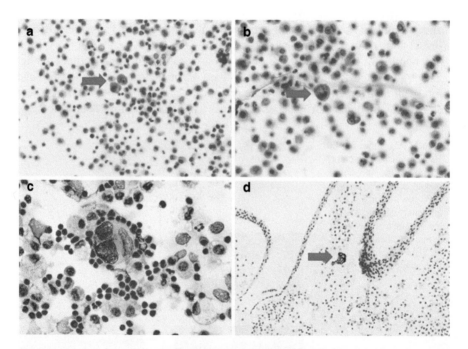

Fig. 5.2 Suspicious for malignancy (SFM). Ascitic fluid with small numbers of suspicious cells on cytospins (**a** and **b**. Papanicolaou stain and **c**. MGG). BerEP4 immunostain on the clot section (**d**) confirms these to be epithelial in origin, hence upgraded to metastatic adenocarcinoma (MAL-S) on the final report. Further immunostains ascertained the primary to be the ovary

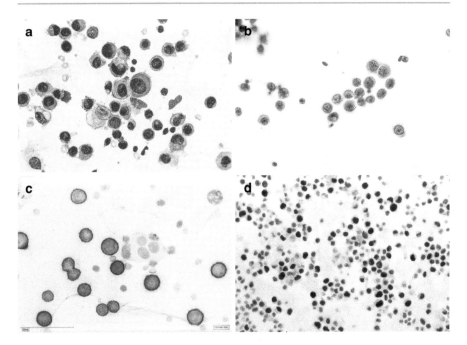

Fig. 5.3 Suspicious for malignancy (SFM). Numerous suspicious cells are present on the sediment smears (**a**. MGG and **b**. Papanicolaou stain). These, however, lack significant nuclear pleomorphism and ancillary testing was performed to confirm the diagnosis. Immunocytochemistry: The suspect cells are positive for BerEP4 (**c**) and GATA3 (**d**), hence upgraded to metastatic adenocarcinoma (MAL-S) on the final report. Primary most likely is breast carcinoma

of malignancy is not made without IC in spite of the large number of suspicious cells. This pattern is not uncommon in breast carcinoma and lung carcinoma and is a potential diagnostic pitfall (Fig. 5.3).

An important group in SFM is lymphocytic effusion. The presence of lymphocytes in large numbers may be a concern, even though there are several causes of benign lymphocytosis, most frequently due to infectious processes (such as tuberculosis). Chronic lymphocytic leukemia (CLL) associated with serosal involvement may be suspected on cytomorphology by virtue of a monotonous population of small, round lymphocytes with very scant cytoplasm, "turtle shell"-like clumped chromatin, and no nucleoli. IC staining for B- and T-cell markers can be helpful in these cases, but flow cytometry provides an accurate phenotypic analysis and is regarded as the gold standard for lymphoma diagnosis in effusions [20, 21] (Fig. 5.4).

Some lymphomas harbor genetic aberrations that support a definitive malignant category, such as t(11;14) in mantle cell lymphoma or t(14;18) in follicular lymphoma. Fluorescence in situ hybridization (FISH) may provide an accurate analysis of these genetic changes and allow a definite diagnosis. Polymerase chain reaction (PCR) for B- or T-cell clonality analysis is helpful in cases of indolent lymphoma. With a suspicious lymphocytic effusion, correlation with the complete blood cell count and a peripheral blood smear is recommended.

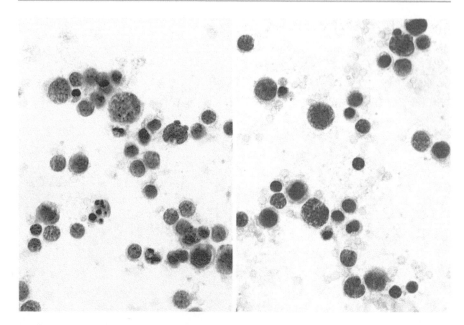

Fig. 5.4 Suspicious for malignancy (SFM). The cytospins contain an increased number of larger lymphoid cells admixed with mature lymphocytes suspicious for lymphoma. Mesothelial cells and macrophages are not conspicuous. Flow cytometry confirmed mantle cell lymphoma

The diagnostic value of some findings may differ depending on demographics. For example, the fact that reactive lymphocytes in effusions are usually of T-cell origin is very helpful in western or northern Europe where most of the indolent lymphomas are of B-cell origin. A lymphocytic effusion with small and medium-sized lymphocytes and strong expression of CD3 proves to be a reactive condition with benign lymphocytosis in most cases. This finding, however, does not help in populations with a high incidence of T-cell lymphomas.

A final critical finding for SFM is the presence of mucin in the peritoneal fluid. Pseudomyxoma peritonei represents spread from a mucin-secreting adenocarcinoma that may be located in the gastrointestinal tract (usually appendix) or gynecological tract (usually ovary). The mucin may be accompanied by epithelial cells which show only mild nuclear pleomorphism and require confirmation of their epithelial nature and site of origin. Rarely, mucin may be present in the peritoneum from rupture of a benign cystic mucinous neoplasm. Clinical correlation is essential in all these scenarios.

Rate and Risk of Malignancy/Clinical Management

There is not much data in the literature about the outcome of suspicious cases or the clinical impact of this diagnosis [22]. Most studies imply that clinicians usually manage patients with suspicious effusions the same way as those with proven malignant ones, taking clinical data into account. Therefore, use of SFM should be reserved for cases where malignancy is highly probable. In a recent meta-analysis of 73 studies [23], 2.3% of all reported effusions (34,941 samples) were reported as suspicious with a reported risk of malignancy (ROM) of 81.8%. Another recent study from a single institution [24] reported an ROM of 83.3% for the suspicious category. These values provide a baseline for further studies that should clarify criteria and appropriate clinical management for this category.

Sample Reports

Example 5.1:
Clinical data: 64-year-old female with ascites. Awaiting scans to exclude malignancy.
   Macroscopic findings: 28 mL of hemorrhagic fluid with a clot measuring 10 × 5 × 3 mm.
   Provisional report:

- Ascitic fluid, paracentesis:
- Satisfactory for evaluation.
- Suspicious for malignancy (adenocarcinoma).

   Note: The cytospins contain lymphocytes, macrophages, and mesothelial cells. A few dispersed cells and an occasional group of cells show large nuclei and hyperchromasia suspicious for malignancy. Clot section and immunostains to follow.
   Supplementary report:

- Ascitic fluid, paracentesis:
- Satisfactory for evaluation.
- Metastatic adenocarcinoma, consistent with serous carcinoma of ovarian origin.
- Category: Malignant.

   Note: A subsequent clot section contains similar groups of cells with vacuolated cytoplasm, high nuclear to cytoplasmic ratio, and chromatin clumping consistent with metastatic adenocarcinoma. Immunostains PAX8, WT1, and BerEP4 are positive in the malignant cells, most likely indicating serous ovarian carcinoma. Correlation with clinical and radiological findings is advised.

Example 5.2:
Clinical data: 73-year-old male with left-sided pleural effusion; uncertain if infectious or malignant.
   Macroscopic findings: 10 mL of straw-colored fluid with no clot.
   Provisional report:

- Lung, left pleura, thoracentesis:
- Satisfactory for evaluation.

- Suspicious for adenocarcinoma.
- Category: Suspicious for malignancy.

Note: The cytospins contain macrophages, a few mesothelial cells, and lymphocytes. Occasional cells show large nuclei and hyperchromasia suspicious for adenocarcinoma. A cell block is being prepared to perform ancillary tests. Cell block and immunostains to follow.
Supplementary report:

- Lung, left pleura, thoracentesis:
- Satisfactory for evaluation.
- Suspicious for adenocarcinoma.
- Category: Suspicious for malignancy.

Note: The cell block and immunostains do not demonstrate any epithelial cells with immunostains BerEP4 and TTF1. WT1 demonstrates mesothelial cells. In view of the cytomorphologic findings, this case is still regarded to be suspicious for malignancy. A repeat sample (ideally 75 mL or greater) is advised for confirmation.

Example 5.3:
Clinical data: 52-year-old male with bilateral pleural effusions, larger on the right.
   Macroscopic findings: 30 mL of cloudy fluid with no clot.
   Provisional report:

- Pleural effusion:
- Satisfactory for evaluation.
- Suspicious for high-grade lymphoma.
- Category: Suspicious for malignancy.

Note: Cytomorphology shows a monotonous population of large lymphoid cells suspicious for high-grade lymphoma. Very few macrophages and mesothelial cells are present. Residual samples are sent for flow cytometry. Results of flow cytometry to follow.
   Supplementary report:

- Pleural effusion:
- Satisfactory for evaluation.
- High-grade lymphoma, consistent with large B-cell lymphoma.
- Category: Malignant.

Note: Flow cytometry confirms the immunoprofile of a large B-cell lymphoma.

References

1. Davidson B, Firat P, Michael CW. Serous effusions: etiology, diagnosis, prognosis and therapy. 2nd ed. New York: Springer; 2018.
2. Chandra A, Cross P, Denton K, et al. The BSCC code of practice–exfoliative cytopathology (excluding gynecological cytopathology). Cytopathology. 2009;20(4):211–23.
3. Johnston WW. The malignant pleural effusion. A review of cytopathologic diagnoses of 584 specimens from 472 consecutive patients. Cancer. 1985;56(4):905–9.
4. Hsu C. Cytologic detection of malignancy in pleural effusion: a review of 5,255 samples from 3,811 patients. Diagn Cytopathol. 1987;3(1):8–12.
5. Raab SS. Significance of atypical cells in cytologic serous fluid specimens. Am J Clin Pathol. 1999;111(1):11–3.
6. Tabatabai ZL, Nayar R, Souers RJ, Crothers BA, Davey DD. Performance characteristics of body fluid cytology: analysis of 344,380 responses from the College of American Pathologists Interlaboratory Comparison Program in Nongynecologic Cytopathology. Arch Pathol Lab Med. 2018;142(1):53–8.
7. Kurtycz DFI, Crothers BA, Schmitt F, Chandra A. International system for reporting serous fluid cytopathology: initial project survey. Acta Cytol. 2019;63(Suppl1):13. https://doi.org/10.1159/000500433.
8. Gupta S, Sodhani P, Jain S. Cytomorphological profile of neoplastic effusions: an audit of 10 years with emphasis on uncommonly encountered malignancies. J Cancer Res Ther. 2012;8:602–9.
9. Esteban JM, Yokota S, Husain S, Battifora H. Immunocytochemical profile of benign and carcinomatous effusions. A practical approach to difficult diagnosis. Am J Clin Path. 1990;94(6):698–705.
10. Tickman RJ, Cohen C, Varna VA, Fekete PS, DeRose PB. Distinction of carcinoma cells and mesothelial cells in serous effusions. Usefulness of immunohistochemistry. Acta Cytol. 1990;34(4):491–6.
11. Athanassiadou P, Kavantzas N, Davaris P, et al. Diagnostic approach of effusion cytology using computerized image analysis. J Exp Clin Cancer Res. 2002;21(1):49–56.
12. Bassen D, Nayak S, Li XC, et al. Clinical decision support system (CDSS) for the classification of atypical cells in pleural effusions. Procedia Computer Sci. 2013;20:379–84.
13. Antonangelo L, Rosolen D, Bottura G, et al. Cytology and DNA ploidy techniques in the diagnosis of malignant pleural effusion. Eur Resp J. 2012;40:4625.
14. Kayser K, Blum S, Beyer M, Haroske G, Kunze KD, Meyer W. Routine DNA cytometry of benign and malignant pleural effusions by means of the remote quantitation server Euroquant: a prospective study. J Clin Pathol. 2000;53(10):760–4.
15. Illei PB, Ladanyi M, Rusch VW, Zakowski MF. The use of CDKN2A deletion as a diagnostic marker for malignant mesothelioma in body cavity effusions. Cancer Cytopathol. 2003;99(1):51–6.
16. Sundling KE, Cibas ES. Ancillary studies in pleural, pericardial, and peritoneal effusion cytology. Cancer Cytopathol. 2018;126(Suppl 8):590–8.
17. Das DK. Serous effusions in malignant lymphomas: a review. Diagn Cytopathol. 2006;34(5):335–47.
18. Czader M, Ali SZ. Flow cytometry as an adjunct to cytomorphologic analysis of serous effusions. Diagn Cytopathol. 2003;29(2):74–8.
19. Savvidou K, Dimitrakopoulou A, Kafasi N, et al. Diagnostic role of cytology in serous effusions of patients with hematologic malignancies. Diagn Cytopathol. 2019;47(5):404–11.

20. Bangerter M, Hildebrand A, Griesshammer M. Combined cytomorphologic and immu-
    nophenotypic analysis in the diagnostic workup of lymphomatous effusions. Acta Cytol.
    2001;45(3):307–12.
21. Bode-Lesniewska B. Flow cytometry and effusions in lymphoproliferative processes and other
    hematologic neoplasias. Acta Cytol. 2016;60(4):354–64.
22. Mårtensson G, Pettersson K, Thiringer G. Differentiation between malignant and non-
    malignant pleural effusion. Eur J Respir Dis. 1985;67(5):326–34.
23. Farahani S, Baloch Z. Are we ready to develop a tiered scheme for the effusion cytology? A
    comprehensive review and analysis of the literature. Diagn Cytopathol. 2019;47(11):1145–59.
24. Valerio E, Nunes W, Cardoso J, et al. A 2-year retrospective study on pleural effusions: a can-
    cer Centre experience. Cytopathology. 2019;30(6):607–13.

Malignant-Primary (MAL-P) (Mesothelioma)

6

Claire Michael, Kenzo Hiroshima, Anders Hjerpe, Pam Michelow, Binnur Önal, and Amanda Segal

Introduction

Primary malignancies occurring in serous fluids generally imply malignant mesothelioma, although other malignancies of mesenchymal and lymphoproliferative origin may also occur in fluids. This chapter is focused on malignancy of mesothelial origin (i.e., mesothelioma) which frequently exfoliates into the serosal cavities. The ability to diagnose malignant mesothelioma by cytology has been well established and guidelines for the diagnosis published [1, 2]. Although the cytologic diagnosis of malignant mesothelioma has been controversial in the past, experts have been successfully diagnosing it for years [3, 4]. This approach represents the consensus view of the authors and contributors, many of whom make definitive diagnoses of malignant mesothelioma by effusion cytology on a regular basis.

C. Michael (✉)
Department of Pathology, Case Western Reserve University, University Hospitals Case Medical Center, Cleveland, OH, USA
e-mail: claire.michael@uhhospitals.org

K. Hiroshima
Department of Pathology, Tokyo Women's Medical University, Yachiyo, Japan

A. Hjerpe
Department of Laboratory Medicine, Division of Clinical Pathology/ Cytology, Karolinska Institutet, Karolinska University Hospital Huddinge, Huddinge, Sweden

P. Michelow
Cytology Unit, National Health Laboratory Service, University of the Witwatersrand, Johannesburg, South Africa

B. Önal
Department of Pathology & Cytology, Ankara Diskapi Teaching and Research Hospital, Istanbul, Turkey

A. Segal
Department of Anatomical Pathology, PathWest, QEII Medical Centre, Perth, WA, Australia

© Springer Nature Switzerland AG 2020
A. Chandra et al. (eds.), *The International System for Serous Fluid Cytopathology*, https://doi.org/10.1007/978-3-030-53908-5_6

Fluids with atypical mesothelial cells can be cytologically categorized as malignant (MAL), suspicious for malignancy (SFM), or atypia of undetermined significance (AUS). The cytologic diagnosis depends primarily upon the cytologic findings and/ or ancillary tests. The preponderance of findings will determine the final category. The constellation of morphologic findings, appropriate clinical history, and radiographic findings drives further steps in patient management.

Background

The incidence of malignant mesothelioma is reported as 2500 cases in the United States and up to 5000 in Western Europe annually. In 2018, it was estimated that over 30,000 patients were diagnosed globally with mesothelioma of which 26,000 succumbed to the disease [5]. In endemic areas such as in Turkey, where the rural population has a high exposure to asbestos, malignant mesothelioma incidence rate in the general population was determined to be 20/100,000 person/year. In a cohort composed of villagers who were above 30 years of age and with known asbestos exposure, the average annual malignant mesothelioma incidence rate was estimated to be 114.8/100,000 person/year for men and 159.8/100,000 person/year for women [6].

It is well established that asbestos exposure and/or erionite fiber exposure can be documented in over 80% of patients with a thorough history and appropriate questions. Other rare causes of malignant mesothelioma have been reported such as history of radiation or exposure to fiberglass, nickel, beryllium, and silica dust [7]. However, it is important to recognize that some patients may genuinely have no known underlying exposures.

As above, the disease is highly associated with asbestos exposure, with a latent period that may exceed 20 years. Patients often present with nonspecific symptoms such as chest pain, shortness of breath, weight loss, and frequently a unilateral, bloody effusion. It is generally more common in males than females. The majority of cases occur in the pleura, far fewer in the peritoneum, and rarely in the pericardium. In the pleura, it characteristically presents as diffuse pleural fibrous thickening known as a "pleural rind" that encases the lung, but it can occasionally present as subpleural nodules. In the peritoneum, it presents as nodular studding or "carcinomatosis."

Malignant mesothelioma is histologically subclassified into epithelioid, sarcomatoid, or mixed (biphasic) variants. While the epithelioid component tends to exfoliate in large numbers, the sarcomatoid component rarely does, and consequently the vast majority of cases diagnosed by cytology reflect the epithelioid and mixed variants.

Mesothelial tumors are classified into diffuse malignant mesothelioma (DMM), localized mesothelioma (LM), well-differentiated papillary mesothelioma (WDPM), and adenomatoid tumor. DMM and LM are further classified into epithelioid, sarcomatoid, and biphasic mesothelioma. DMM and LM are considered malignant with poor outcomes, while WDPM has a more indolent clinical course and behaves as benign when completely resected, although those with stalk invasion tend to recur. Although DMM is the most commonly encountered type, it is important to be familiar with LM and WDPM, since they occasionally exfoliate and their cytological features have been reported. This chapter will focus on the diagnosis of the commonly presenting morphological variants of DMM (e.g., trabecular, tubulopapillary and solid). Other morphologic types such as

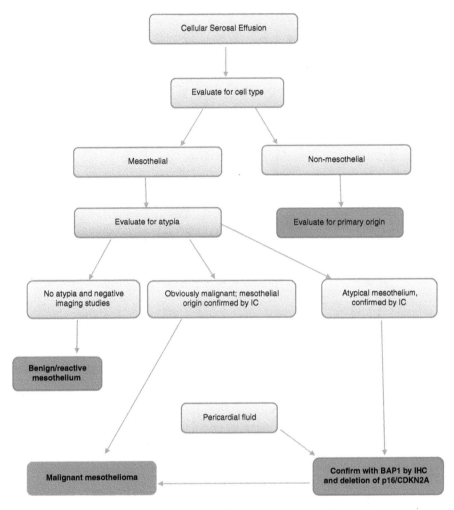

Fig. 6.1 Evaluation of a cellular effusion algorithm

deciduoid, small cell, clear cell, and signet ring are rare, require more experience, and have not been adequately described in the cytology literature.

Cytological Approach to Fluids

The reviewer assesses the fluid for the following features to establish a differential diagnosis (Fig. 6.1). A detailed discussion of this approach follows in the explanatory notes. A cellular sample comprised of mesothelial cells warrants further evaluation for malignant mesothelioma and should be reported as suggested in this chapter.

- Cellularity: Super-cellular, high, moderate, or low cellularity
- Cell type: Mesothelial, non-mesothelial, or both
- Cellular atypia: Obviously malignant, suspicious, atypical, or benign

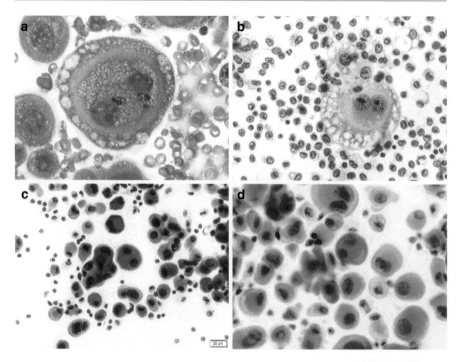

Fig. 6.2 Mesothelial cell. Mesothelial cells with two tone cytoplasm, submembranous and peri-nuclear vacuoles. (**a**) Modified Giemsa stain and (**b**) Papanicolaou stain. (**c** and **d**) Mesothelioma cells with submembranous glycogen detected as yellow droplets; Papanicolaou stain

Since identification of the mesothelial origin of cells is pivotal in initiating the differential and work-up for malignant mesothelioma, the following is a short review of mesothelial cell morphology. More detailed review [8, 9] is beyond the scope of this chapter.

The following features apply to both benign and malignant mesothelium; however, they tend to become more pronounced in reactive cells and are best seen in malignant cells. Mesothelial cells are round cells with central nuclei and moderate amounts of cytoplasm. The cytoplasm is characterized by a two-tone appearance due to endo-ectoplasmic demarcation. Glycogen is present at the periphery and seen as submembranous vacuoles that frequently coalesce and mimic sausage links (Fig. 6.2). Glycogen is demonstrated by periodic acid-Schiff (PAS) stain and should be digested with diastase (PASD) (Fig. 6.3). The long microvilli seen by electron microscopy are frequently noted as a brush-like, vague cellular border, or as peripheral blebs best seen with May-Grünewald-Giemsa (MGG) stain (Fig. 6.4). Perinuclear fat droplets, best recognized by oil red O stain on fresh fluid, are particularly seen in malignant mesothelioma (Fig. 6.5). The nuclei are round and vesicular and may contain a conspicuous nucleolus. Binucleated and multinucleated cells are more common in reactive and malignant effusions (Fig. 6.6). Mesothelial cells have a very characteristic articulation: they tend to have intercellular windows that can be discerned between cells (Fig. 6.7), even in clusters. The cells frequently wrap

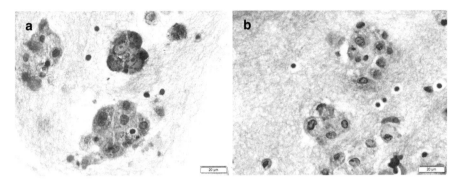

Fig. 6.3 Mesothelial cell glycogen expression. (**a**) Periodic acid-Schiff (PAS) stain illustrates the submembranous glycogen vacuoles. (**b**) The glycogen droplets are digested by diastase (PASD)

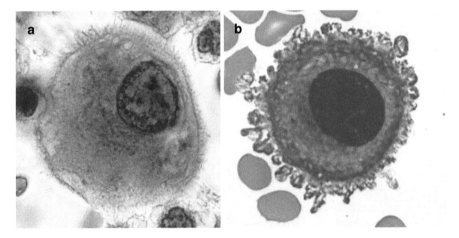

Fig. 6.4 Mesothelial cell brush border. (**a**) Brush border surrounds the cell membrane; Papanicolaou stain. (**b**) Peripheral blebs surrounding the brush border; May-Grünewald-Giemsa stain

around each other in a pattern known as cellular clasping and appear as cell-in-cell (Fig. 6.8), sometimes with cytoplasmic pinching resulting in peripheral cytoplasmic humps (Fig. 6.9). This articulation results in frequent doublets, short cords, and rows of cells.

Malignant Mesothelioma

Definition

Mesothelioma is a malignant proliferation of the mesodermally derived serosal cells lining the pleura, peritoneum, pericardium, and tunica vaginalis.

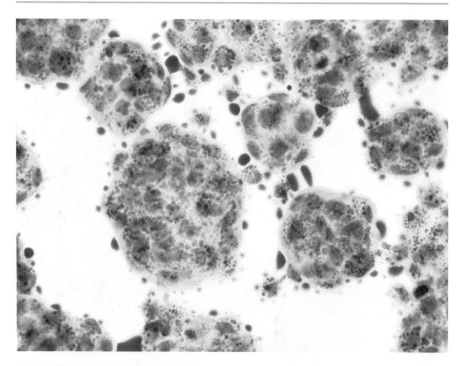

Fig. 6.5 Mesothelioma with lipid. Numerous perinuclear fat droplets; Oil Red O stain

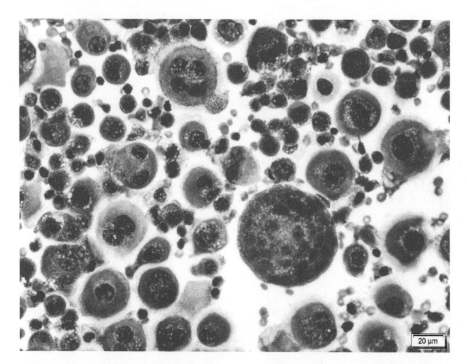

Fig. 6.6 Mesothelioma. A small cellular sphere in a background of numerous binucleated and multinucleated cells with prominent nucleoli; Modified Giemsa stain

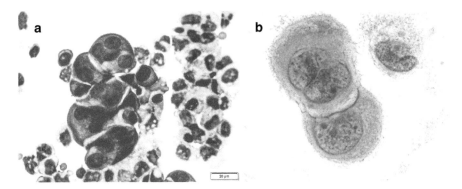

Fig. 6.7 Benign mesothelial cells. (**a**) Cluster of mesothelial cells with intercellular windows; Modified Giemsa stain. (**b**) Intercellular windows between two cells; Papanicolaou stain

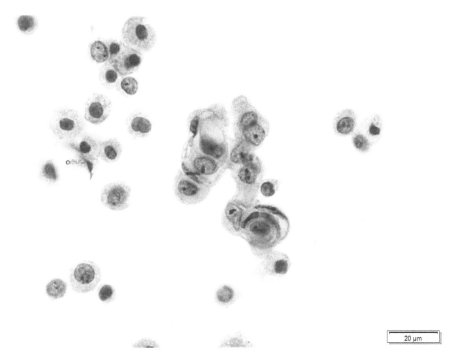

Fig. 6.8 Benign mesothelial cells. "Cellular clasping" is formed when cytoplasmic extensions from one cell wraps around the adjacent cell, or when cells lay on top of one another. Exaggerated clasping may give the appearance of a cell-within-a-cell; Papanicolaou stain

Gross Findings of Serous Effusion

- Frequently manifests as large volumes of effusion that tend to rapidly recur.
- Usually amber in color but can be red due to blood.
- Very viscous with a "tar-like" or "honey-like" consistency, correlating with high hyaluronan concentrations.

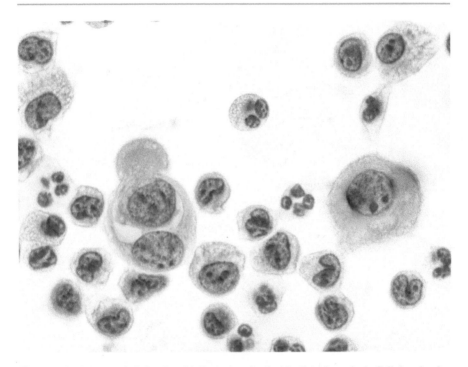

Fig. 6.9 Benign mesothelial cells with "cytoplasmic pinching" (or humping). Cellular clasping may cause pinching of the cytoplasm, giving the appearance of a hump at the cell periphery; Papanicolaou stain

Cytologic Criteria

Definitive Criteria of Malignancy [10–18] (Fig. 6.10)
- Super-cellularity (bird's eye view at low magnification reveals millions of cells)
- Numerous cellular spheres, papillary tissue fragments, berry-like morules, single cells or a mixture of these
- Malignant features identified by either:
  - Overt nuclear abnormalities diagnostic of malignancy (nuclear enlargement, irregular nuclear membranes, macronucleoli, frequent binucleation and multinucleation, cellular pleomorphism, atypical mitoses)
  - Presence of numerous large tissue fragments and cellular clusters

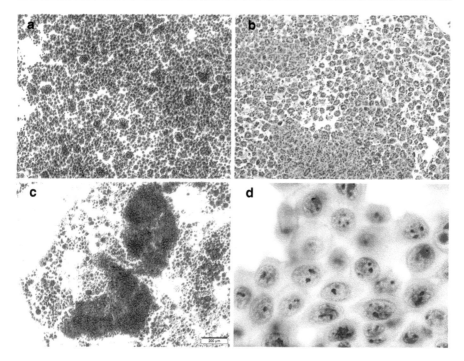

Fig. 6.10 Mesothelioma. (**a**) A bird's-eye view reveals a super-cellular smear with innumerable morules and spheres in a background of many single cells; Papanicolaou stain. (**b**) Highly cellular cell block with innumerable spheres; H&E stain. (**c**) Smear with large tissue fragments in a background of numerous clusters and single cells; Papanicolaou stain. (**d**) Marked nuclear enlargement and cherry red macronucleoli; Papanicolaou stain

Supportive Criteria of Malignancy (Figs. 6.11, 6.12, 6.13 and 6.14)

- Significantly enlarged mesothelial cells with abundant (metachromatic or two-tone) cytoplasm
- Large nuclei with subtle atypia
- Prominent nucleoli often variable in size and number
- Wide variation in cellular size, from normal-appearing mesothelial cell to gigantic
- Numerous multinucleated cells
- Tissue fragments or papillary groups with collagen or basement membrane cores
- Pyknotic, eosinophilic, or orangeophilic cells (pseudokeratotic cells)
- Numerous perinuclear lipid vacuoles on MGG, confirmed by oil-red O stain on fresh fluid
- Pink or red granular background on MGG (representing high hyaluronan concentrations)

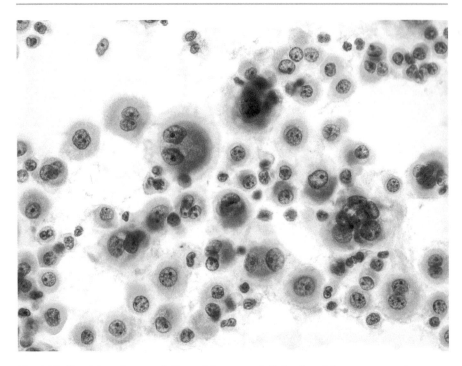

Fig. 6.11 Suspicious for mesothelioma. These mesothelial cells, while monotonous in appearance, have wide variation in cell size, from small to gigantic. Several multinucleated cells are present. The cells have abundant cytoplasm and vesicular nuclei with prominent nucleoli; Papanicolaou stain

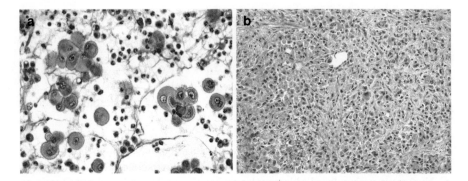

Fig. 6.12 Mesothelioma. (**a**) Moderately cellular specimen with significantly enlarged mesothelial cells containing nuclei with macronucleoli and subtle membrane irregularity; Papanicolaou stain. (**b**) Correlating core biopsy showing diffuse malignant mesothelioma, epithelioid type; H&E stain

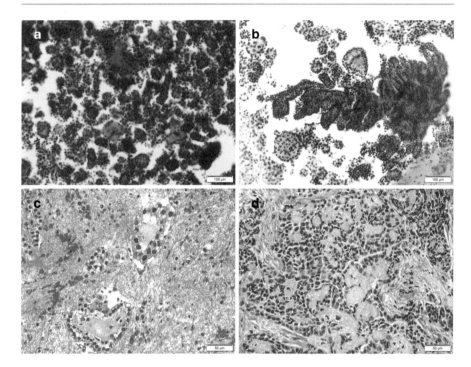

Fig. 6.13 Mesothelioma. (**a**) Cellular smear with numerous clusters, tubules and collagen cores; Papanicolaou stain. (**b**) Focus showing large papillary tissue fragment; Papanicolaou stain. (**c**) Corresponding cell block showing similar hollow clusters with central collagen cores; H&E stain. (**d**) Correlating biopsy with a tubulopapillary pattern and many collagen cores; H&E stain

Explanatory Notes

Malignant mesothelioma may manifest cytologically as a highly cellular effusion with obvious nuclear atypia (frankly malignant), super-cellular fluid with numerous large tissue fragments and clusters (frankly abnormal), or as cellular fluid with mesothelial cells and clusters showing subtle atypia. While the former two presentations can be easily recognized as malignant mesothelioma once mesothelial origin is confirmed, the latter is more challenging, requires experience, and should be confirmed by additional ancillary tests. Similar to any other cytology sample, clinical and radiological correlation is performed during the evaluation of the specimen, but it is important to emphasis that the cytologic diagnosis in a mesothelial proliferative effusion depends primarily on the morphologic findings. Although the medical history and radiological findings can greatly support the diagnosis of mesothelioma, some patients may not have known asbestos and/or erionite exposure. Also, it is not unusual that the malignant effusion is the first manifestation of the disease and is the trigger for further clinical evaluation. A malignant effusion may represent an early mesothelioma (EM) or mesothelioma in situ (MIS). MIS was first introduced in the early 1990s by Whitaker et al. as an abnormal surface mesothelial proliferation that may present as a malignant effusion but lacks the radiological findings classically

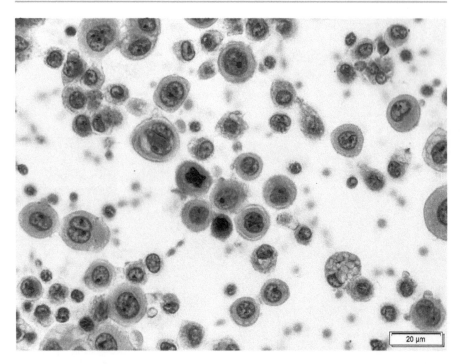

Fig. 6.14 Mesothelioma. Scattered eosinophilic cells with pyknotic nuclei ("pseudokeratotic cells"); Papanicolaou stain

associated with the diagnosis and is subsequently proven to be malignant mesothelioma [19]. While rare, the diagnosis of MIS is becoming more accepted by mesothelioma experts. MIS is stage T0. EM is stage T1 or greater based upon histologic evidence of invasion, although it may be limited in size and have subtle radiological findings [20]. Recent literature suggests that patients with EM and malignant effusion have better survival than cytology-negative patients [21]. This underscores the significance of an early definitive diagnosis and management of disease.

The diagnosis of malignant mesothelioma (MAL-P) can be issued in cases where overtly malignant features are identified. Cases presenting with subtle atypia and many of the additional supportive criteria of malignancy can be diagnosed as malignant mesothelioma (MAL-P) if confirmed by ancillary tests such as loss of BAP1 expression and/or deletion of p16/CDKN2A by fluorescence in situ hybridization (FISH). Cases concerning for malignant mesothelioma but not supported by ancillary tests can be reported as suspicious for malignancy (SFM). Recent literature confirms that malignant mesothelioma can be diagnosed with accuracy in cytologic samples when the above criteria are followed, with sensitivity from 55% to 82% and up to 86% (when suspicious and atypical cases were included). In these cases, predictive value of a malignant mesothelioma diagnosis is 100% [4, 22, 23].

The diagnosis of atypical mesothelial cells (AUS) should be used judiciously and avoided whenever possible. Mesothelial AUS should be reserved for cases where the clinical picture is not supportive of a reactive etiology, where there is concerning atypia in a low or moderately cellular effusion, and/or where ancillary tests are inconclusive.

Table 6.1 Differential diagnosis between reactive mesothelium and malignant mesothelioma

Feature	Reactive mesothelium	Malignant mesothelioma
Cellularity	Moderate to high cellularity	Strikingly high cellularity
Background	Serosanguinous or bloody	Serosanguinous or bloody Thick matrix representing hyaluronan
Cell population	Monotonous population of mesothelial cells with minimal variation in size	Monotonous population of mesothelial cells with wide variation in size
Features at low magnification	Predominantly single cells with relatively increased number of clusters	Super-cellular with innumerable clusters, single cells or a mixture of both
Inflammatory cells	May be prominent as part of the etiology	Varies. Acute inflammation increases significantly post- tube insertion
Cellular features		
Size	Slightly enlarged	Significantly enlarged
Size variation	Minimal variation	Vary from benign to gigantic
Atypia	Mild to moderate	Vary from mild to severe
Nuclei	Slightly enlarged	Markedly enlarged
Nucleoli	May be prominent	Macronuclei in many cases, vary from 2 to innumerable nucleoli
Multinucleation	Cells may contain 2–3 nuclei, rarely more	Vary from 2 to innumerable nuclei
Cytoplasm	Moderate	Abundant
Perinuclear fat droplets	Rare	Numerous
Pseudokeratotic cells	Rare	Common
Cluster features		
Shape	Predominantly two-dimensional with scalloped borders	Predominantly three-dimensional and may be raspberry-like morules with scalloped borders or spheres with smooth borders
Complexity	Mostly simple small clusters	Vary from small to large, very complex and sometimes branching papillae
Collagenous cores	Rare	Occasionally present and may be conspicuous
Hollow clusters	Not seen	Occasionally seen
Ancillary tests		
Desmin	Positive	Negative
EMA (E29 clone)	Negative	Positive
BAP1	Positive	Lost in 60% of cases
p16/CDKN2A (FISH) deletion	Not deleted	Homozygous deletion in up to 80%.
Hyaluronan	<150 μg/mL	>150 μg/mL
Mesothelin	Absent[a]	Present[b]

[a]May be present in cases with renal failure
[b]Better considered a marker of malignancy since it is also present in ovarian and pancreatic adenocarcinoma

The main differential diagnoses for malignant mesothelioma presenting with cellular morules or clusters include reactive mesothelium (RM) and carcinomas, particularly adenocarcinoma (Tables 6.1 and 6.2). For mesotheliomas presenting predominantly as single cells, the differential also includes other malignancies such as melanoma, single-cell patterned adenocarcinomas, and large cell lymphoma.

Table 6.2 Differential diagnosis between malignant mesothelioma and carcinoma

Feature	Malignant mesothelioma	Metastatic carcinoma
Cellularity	Highly cellular	Variable
Background	Serosanguinous or bloody Thick matrix (hyaluronan)	Frequently bloody Mucin in mucinous carcinomas
Cell population	Monotonous population	Two cell population ("alien" cells)
Features at low magnification	Numerous clusters, single cells or a combination of both	Varies depending on the primary origin
Cellular features		
Shape and size	Round large cells	Varies by cell origin
Size variation	Wide variation	Minimal variation
Atypia	Monotonous atypia	Heterogeneous
Nuclei	Enlarged	Enlarged
Nuclear/cytoplasmic ratio	Minimally increased	High
Nucleoli	Prominent	Prominent
Multinucleation	Common	Not common
Cytoplasm	Abundant	Scant to moderate at best
Perinuclear fat droplets	Numerous	Not characteristic
Cluster features		
Shape	Either scalloped borders or perfect spheres	Three-dimensional with common cell borders
Complexity	Variable	Varies depending on primary
Collagenous cores	Common	Uncommon. Fibro-vascular cores may be seen in papillary tumors
Hollow clusters	May be present	Not characteristic
Immunochemistry		
Calretinin	Positive	Negative (most cases)
D2–40	Positive	Negative
WT-1	Positive	Variable
CK5/6	Positive	Negative (most cases)
Claudin 4	Negative	Positive
GATA-3	Positive (50%)	Positive in breast, urothelial and some squamous carcinoma
MOC-31 and BerEp4	Negative (may react with up to 15% of cases)	Positive
Broad spectrum epithelial markers	Positive	Positive
p40 and p63	Negative	Positive in squamous and urothelial carcinoma

Reactive mesothelium (RM) bears a morphologic kinship to malignant mesothelioma and is currently the most common cause of an underdiagnosed mesothelioma on cytology [24]. However, the cellularity is usually far more striking in malignant mesothelioma, exhibiting more and larger cells and cell clusters [16]. Both contain a monotonous population of mesothelial cells. Cells in RM show little variation in size, while malignant mesothelioma shows a wide variation in size, from that of resting mesothelium to gigantic cells. Multinucleated cells may be seen in both but are more numerous in mesothelioma and contain more nuclei. They may attain the

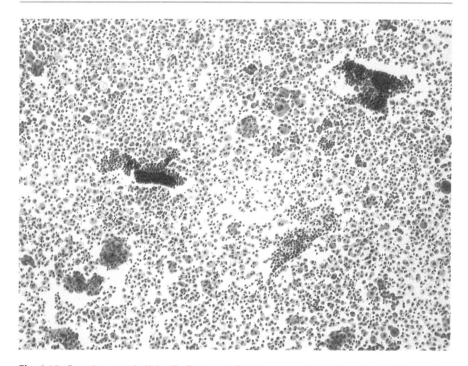

Fig. 6.15 Reactive mesothelial cells. Peritoneal fluid from a renal dialysis patient with hyperplastic mesothelium. The smear is highly cellular with some two-dimensional clusters and large flat sheets. Cells appear monotonous, similar in size and show no nuclear atypia; Papanicolaou stain

size of small neighboring cell morules. Both exhibit conspicuous nucleoli, but RM rarely exhibit macronucleoli such as those seen in malignant mesothelioma. Clusters of mesothelium may be increased in RM, but they tend to remain as two-dimensional groups and rarely form spheres (Fig. 6.15). In contrast, clusters in malignant mesothelioma tend to be large, have scalloped "raspberry-like" borders, or form three-dimensional cellular spheres. In some mesotheliomas, these spheres contain collagen, seen best on cell block sections, reflecting their papillary nature. Rarely, RM in the setting of cirrhosis and renal dialysis will exhibit clusters of mesothelium surrounding metachromatic cores, which probably represent fibrinous material (Fig. 6.16). Other features of malignant mesothelioma are usually lacking in those cases. RM in patients with liver cirrhosis and peritoneal dialysis may present with many of the atypical features described above but with less cellularity than malignant mesothelioma. The pathologist should exercise caution in this context. Similarly, reactive pericardial effusions can present with a pronounced degree of atypia in comparison with other effusion sites due to the friction produced on mesothelium from heart contractions (Fig. 6.17). A diagnosis of malignant mesothelioma should be issued with great care in a pericardial fluid and only if supported by the clinical history, presentation, and ancillary tests.

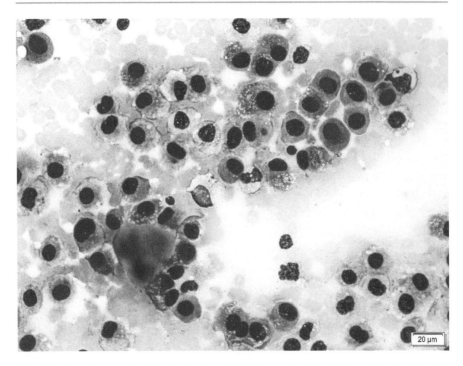

Fig. 6.16 Reactive mesothelial cells. Peritoneal fluid from a patient with liver cirrhosis. The cells are similar in size; a few foci contain fibrin-like material surrounded by scant mesothelial cells; Modified Giemsa stain

Squamous and urothelial carcinoma are great mimickers of malignant mesothelioma [25, 26]. They share some common cellular features, such as two-tone cytoplasm and cellular articulation. Luckily, these malignancies rarely present as a malignant effusion and are traditionally concurrent with known metastatic disease. The differential diagnosis of a malignant effusion can be easily resolved in the majority of cases using immunochemistry (IC). Adenocarcinoma (ADC) may also mimic malignant mesothelioma and in the past was considered the biggest challenge in the differential diagnosis. This is no longer true, due to recent advancements in IC. Effusions with metastatic carcinoma may vary in cellularity and contain two cell populations, namely, the malignant cells and background benign mesothelial cells. Morphology varies widely depending on the type of carcinoma. ADC clusters predominantly exhibit common cell borders, with nuclei bordering the periphery, in contrast to the scalloped borders of malignant mesothelioma with central nuclei and cytoplasm at the periphery. Carcinomas manifest with overtly malignant features, and the cells tend to be very pleomorphic. Despite their pleomorphism, cell size in ADC remains within a limited range, in contrast to malignant mesothelioma.

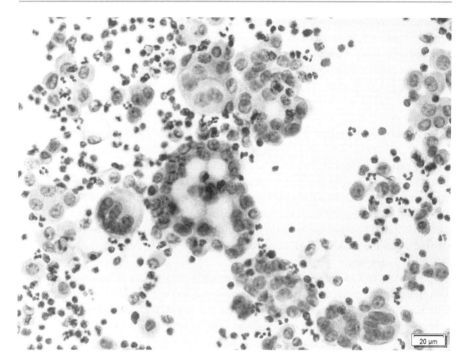

Fig. 6.17 Reactive mesothelial cells. Pericardial effusion in a patient with pericarditis. Mesothelial cells show slight variation in size, multinucleation and prominent nucleoli; Papanicolaou stain

Role of Immunochemistry (IC) in the Work-Up of Mesothelioma

There are various controversies associated with how IC is employed in effusion diagnosis of malignant mesothelioma. There is debate regarding whether cell block or smear preparations are more suitable for IC; whether IC can distinguish benign from malignant mesothelial proliferations; which are the best IC panels; and how many IC stains should be performed to distinguish malignant mesothelioma from ADC? Pathologists use different approaches, and there is no consensus on the best approach. Each laboratory must determine, through validation studies, which IC panel works best for that laboratory, and pathologists must decide the appropriate IC panels for each individual case.

Immunochemistry on Cell Block Versus Smears

IC can be performed on smears or cell block material. Cell blocks have the advantage of having the same processing as formalin-fixed paraffin-embedded surgical pathology specimens, and so do not require special validation procedures. They are suitable for molecular testing and are a robust way to preserve tissue for future requirements. For these reasons, cell block preparations are the preferred option and can be prepared in various ways [27]. Laboratories that have validated IC on cytospins or smears should feel reassured that this is also a reliable and well-accepted technique [28, 29].

Determining Benign Versus Malignant Mesothelial Cells

The use of IC in this differential has been highly controversial. Various markers have been examined in this setting, and there has been wide variation in how these stains have performed and been applied. Recently, the combination of BAP1 loss by IC (Fig. 6.18) and CDKN2A deletion by FISH provide a sensitive and highly specific method of proving malignancy [30] and are currently considered the gold standard. Either the loss of BAP1 expression or CDKN2A deletion is sufficient to establish malignancy.

BAP1 loss of expression by IC has become a widely accepted technique to establish mesothelial malignancy both in histological and cytological samples [31, 32]. The BAP1 immunostain is a nuclear marker that highlights the presence of a tumor suppressor, ubiquitin hydrolase. Biallelic *BAP1* mutations result in loss of nuclear

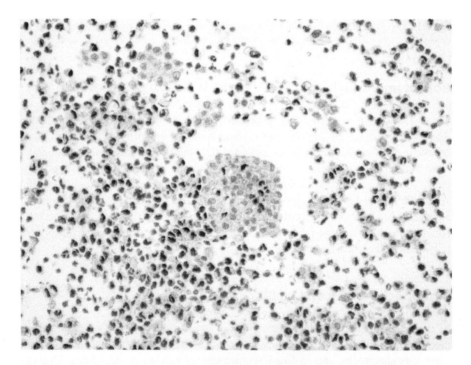

Fig. 6.18 Mesothelioma, loss of BAP1. Notice the negative clusters of mesothelioma cells in a background of reactive lymphocytes, which serve as internal control cells; BAP1 stain

staining, seen in approximately 55–80% of malignant mesothelioma [33].
Background inflammatory cells act as a useful internal positive control (Fig. 6.18).
In effusion samples, careful examination is required to detect negatively stained
mesothelial cell nuclei which may be scattered among and obscured by abundant
positively stained inflammatory cell nuclei. Notably, loss of BAP1 expression is a
rare event in non-small cell lung carcinoma (NSCLC), so BAP1 loss is also potentially useful to distinguish malignant mesothelioma from pleural metastasis of
NSCLC [34, 35].

Methylthioadenosine phosphorylase (MTAP) is a recently described 9p21.3-
related protein which can be used to distinguish reactive from malignant mesothelial cells with 100% specificity, [36, 37] potentially enabling IC assessment instead
of FISH to detect 9p21 deletions (Fig. 6.19). A high degree of concordance was
observed between the results of MTAP IC and 9p21 FISH in cell blocks, [38] providing a potentially useful surrogate for FISH studies, which are more time consum-
ing and expensive and may not be available in some laboratories. Studies have
shown the combination of MTAP and BAP1 IC staining allowed separation of reactive from malignant mesothelial proliferations in 90% of cases [39].

A more controversial but very useful IC marker of malignancy is epithelial membrane antigen (EMA). This IC can be used to establish the presence of a malignant
population and is heavily used in some laboratories, while not accepted in others. When

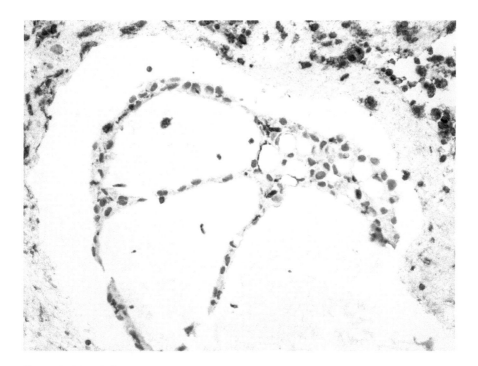

Fig. 6.19 Mesothelioma. Loss of methylthioadenosine phosporylase. The loss of MTAP indicates
a deletion of 9p21; MTAP stain

the appropriate E29 clone is used [40, 41] and there is strong *membranous* staining in the majority of cells (Fig. 6.20), several studies have confirmed that EMA has a sensitivity of approximately 80% in confirming malignancy, with no false positives [40, 42, 43]. However, the following provisos are worth noting: weak cytoplasmic staining or only occasional cells demonstrating weak membranous staining should not be interpreted as a positive result; EMA does not distinguish between mesothelioma and metastatic carcinoma; and plasma cells can demonstrate quite strong EMA staining but should be identifiable on morphological grounds. It also appears that some laboratories experience technical difficulties with this antibody, and this probably explains the differences in how it is applied. EMA can be very useful to identify small populations of malignant cells in the setting of metastatic ADC because the majority of common ADC (lung, breast, gastrointestinal and gynecological tract) are EMA positive.

Desmin demonstrates positive staining in benign mesothelial cells, with loss of staining in approximately 85% of malignant mesotheliomas (Fig. 6.21) [44, 45].

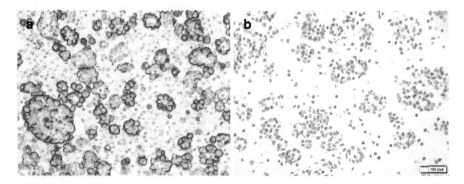

Fig. 6.20 Mesothelioma. (**a**) Malignant cells show strong cytoplasmic membranous staining with epithelial membrane antigen; EMA stain and (**b**) Are negative for cytoplasmic desmin; desmin stain

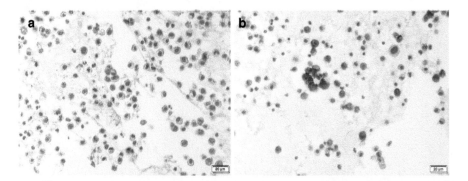

Fig. 6.21 Reactive mesothelial cells. (**a**) Benign mesothelial cells are negative for epithelial membrane antigen; EMA stain and (**b**) Show strong cytoplasmic staining with desmin; desmin stain

Interpretation requires that the appropriate population is assessed, since background benign mesothelial cells in mesothelioma will stain positively.

An IC panel may be useful to confirm a suspected malignancy when morphological features of malignancy are not present. A reasonable panel is BAP1, EMA, desmin, and MTAP, with the addition of FISH for CDKN2A loss, if necessary.

Determining Malignant Mesothelioma Versus Carcinoma

Once it has been determined that an effusion sample contains malignant cells, the next step is accurate phenotyping. The morphological features of malignant mesothelioma, while sometimes very characteristic of mesothelial differentiation, should not be considered enough to establish the diagnosis and confirmatory IC is highly recommended. Generally, two positive mesothelial markers and two negative carcinoma markers are recommended to establish the diagnosis of mesothelioma. With the advent of fairly sensitive and specific mesothelial markers, the distinction between malignant mesothelioma and ADC is less problematic than in the past, and new promising specific mesothelial markers continue to be described [46]. Not all malignant mesothelioma will stain with all mesothelial markers. If a case is positive for calretinin and WT1, but negative for D2–40 and CK5/6, it is probably still malignant mesothelioma; however, had the initial mesothelial panel included only D2–40 and CK5/6, mesothelioma may have been excluded. The fact that mesothelial markers do not have 100% sensitivity means that for each marker, some malignant mesotheliomas will be negative. Similarly, there are mesotheliomas that will stain with one or several carcinoma markers. BerEp4 and MOC31 are positive in approximately 15–25% of malignant mesothelioma (Fig. 6.22), usually in a patchy fashion. Mesothelin has also been found to lack sensitivity and specificity [47]. Be prepared to extend the IC panel of positive and negative mesothelial markers when there are any discordant or unexpected results. A simple periodic acid-Schiff with diastase digestion (PASD) stain, which when positive supports adenocarcinoma, can sometimes be as useful in an IC panel. The importance of thorough morphological assessment, in combination with detailed clinical and imaging information, is exemplified when IC availability is limited or expensive. Very rarely, electron microscopy may be required when there is significant discordance in IC results.

The IC panel is usually directed at distinguishing malignant mesothelioma from metastatic carcinoma when there are tight, cohesive spheres, but other malignancies may also present in this fashion [48]. If the presentation is single cells or loose aggregates, the differential diagnosis is broader and includes melanoma, lymphoma, sarcoma, germ cell, and pediatric tumors as well as malignant mesothelioma and carcinoma.

The many commercially available mesothelial markers vary in sensitivity and specificity. Calretinin is probably the most widely used and has a sensitivity and specificity for mesothelial cells of approximately 90% and 80%. Other commonly used mesothelial markers include WT1, CK5/6, and D2–40 (Figs. 6.23, 6.24, 6.25, and 6.26). Adenocarcinomas can react with all of these markers. WT1 will be

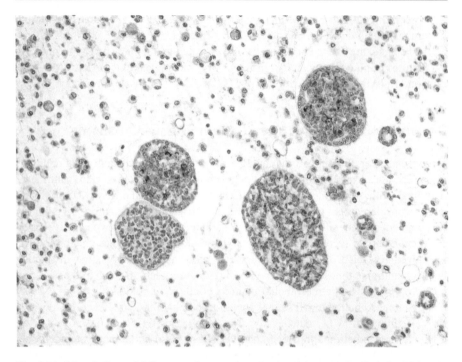

Fig. 6.22 Mesothelioma. Malignant cells may show focal staining with BerEp4; BerEP4 stain. These cells were reactive to calretinin, WT1 and CK 5/6, indicating mesothelial origin

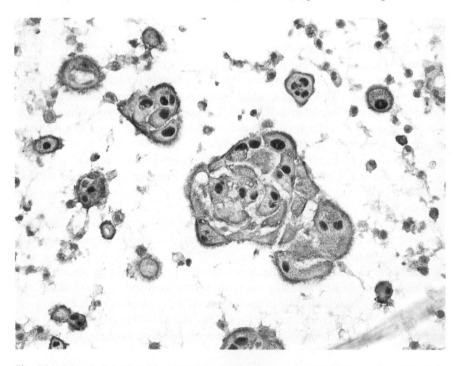

Fig. 6.23 Mesothelial cells with calretinin stain. The image exhibits calretinin stain with nuclear and membranous pattern imparting a "fried egg" appearance; calretinin stain

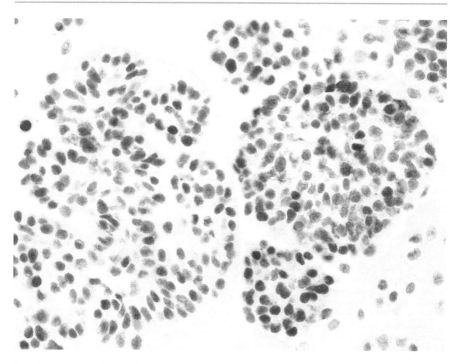

Fig. 6.24 Mesothelioma with WT-1 stain. Wilms Tumor-1 nuclear staining supports mesothelial origin but is also found in some gynecologic tumors, notably serous carcinoma; WT1 stain

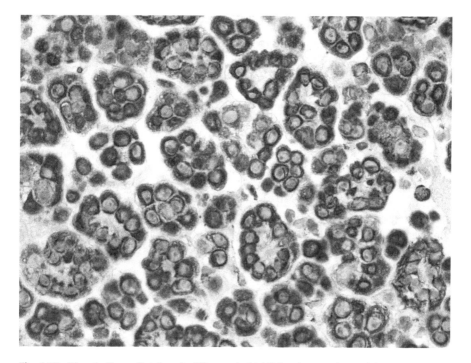

Fig. 6.25 Mesothelioma. Cytokeratin 5/6 strongly highlights the cytoplasm of the mesothelioma cells; CK5/6 stain

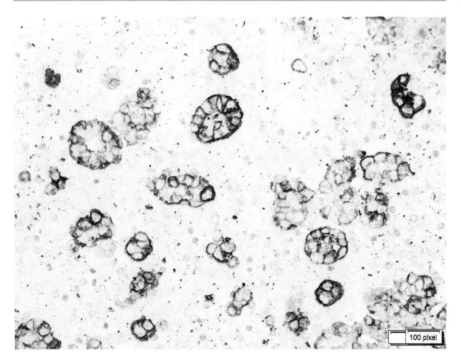

Fig. 6.26 Mesothelioma with D2–40 stain. D2–40 highlights the cellular membrane; D2–40 stain

positive in gynecological tract malignancies, and calretinin is positive in basal phenotype breast cancer and some squamous cell carcinomas. D2–40 has variable specificity, but one study reported positivity in approximately 30% of lung and breast and 60% of ovarian cancers [49].

Broad spectrum carcinoma markers include simple stains (PASD, mucicarmine) for epithelial mucin and IC markers such as CEA, TAG/B72.3, BerEP4, MOC31, MUC4 and the more recently described, seemingly very reliable claudin4. Claudin4 is a tight junction-associated protein that is expressed in most epithelial cells but not in mesothelial cells. It is a relatively new marker but seems to effectively distinguish adenocarcinoma from malignant mesothelioma with high sensitivity and specificity [50, 51].

Site-specific markers may be included in the initial panel if there is a particular clinical history or morphological clue: e.g., TTF1 and napsin for lung; TTF1 and PAX8 for thyroid; GATA3 for breast and urothelium; PAX8 for gynecological tract, renal, and thyroid; CK20, CDX2, and SATB2 for colorectal; and PSA and ERG for prostate. It is beyond the scope of this chapter to discuss all of these markers in detail, but extensive studies and reviews are available [52].

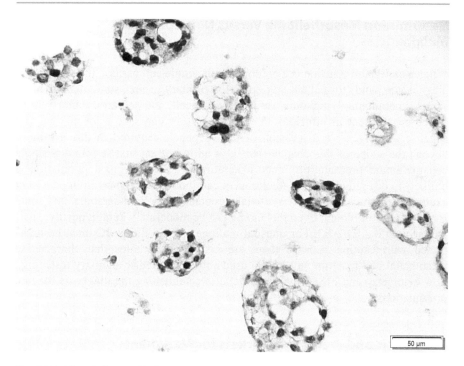

Fig. 6.27 Mesothelioma with GATA-3 stain. GATA-3 nuclear staining may occur in up to half of malignant mesothelioma and is documented to be positive in sarcomatoid mesothelioma; GATA-3 stain

Of the site-specific markers, TTF1 seems to be very valuable and reliable, with only one possible case report of a TTF1-positive malignant mesothelioma [53]. Since the lung is the most common primary to metastasize to pleura, this IC is often routinely included in an initial panel.

Several so-called specific ADC markers can be positive in malignant mesothelioma: GATA3 will stain over 50% of mesothelioma (Fig. 6.27) [54] and is even recommended to distinguish between sarcomatoid lung carcinoma (negative) and sarcomatoid mesothelioma (positive) [37]. CK20 can be positive in mesothelioma [55] and can also stain benign mesothelial cells.

Although metastatic squamous cell carcinoma (SCC) is uncommon in pleural fluid, there can be overlapping morphological and IC features between SCC and malignant mesothelioma. Both are CK5/6 positive, and both can be calretinin and D2–40 positive. Both p63 and p40 are useful since they are strongly positive in SCC and almost invariably negative or very weakly positive in malignant mesothelioma. WT1, usually positive in mesothelioma, is only very rarely positive in SCC.

Determining Mesothelioma Versus Non-epithelial Malignancies

When a malignant effusion is a predominantly single cell pattern, the differential diagnosis expands to include non-epithelial primary or metastatic malignancies such as melanoma, lymphoma, sarcoma, germ cell, and pediatric tumors, all of which can present in effusions. A relevant history can save a lot of time and expense. An extensive discussion of the IC panels required in this setting is beyond the scope of this chapter, but IC is an important first step in any single cell malignant presentation, since a keratin-negative malignant population is unlikely to be epithelioid mesothelioma or carcinoma. Keratin positivity does not exclude sarcoma, particularly synovial sarcoma, epithelioid sarcoma, and some forms of angiosarcoma. Even melanoma can be moderately keratin positive, particularly with AE1/AE3. For unusual malignancies in fluids, IC must be interpreted with caution because there are insufficient studies that characterize mesothelial cell reaction with rarely used antibodies. Other ancillary tests (e.g., flow cytometry and FISH) may be crucial in establishing the diagnosis for rare presentations.

Prognostic and Predictive Markers for Malignant Mesothelioma

In the future, new mesothelioma prognostic and predictive markers will be implemented, highlighting the importance of preserving adequate material in cell blocks. The typical abundant cellularity of malignant mesothelioma effusion renders this material ideal for ancillary studies.

Programmed cell death ligand 1 (PD-L1) is an immune modulator that promotes immunosuppression by binding to programmed cell death 1 (PD-1). PD-L1 is upregulated on the surface of tumor cells, and the PD-1/PD-L1 pathway plays a critical role in tumor immune evasion, providing a target for anti-tumor therapy. Malignant mesothelioma effusions are suitable for IC assessment of PD-L1 expression, and the results are similar to those reported for histological specimens [56]. PD-L1 is expressed in a substantial proportion of malignant mesotheliomas, and a subset of patients may benefit from immunotherapy [57].

Some studies have suggested that loss of BAP1 staining and positive p16 staining by IC is an indicator of prolonged survival in malignant mesothelioma patients, [58] while others report a limitation to the usefulness of BAP1 in this setting [59]. In addition, BAP1 has been associated with prediction of response to chemotherapy [60, 61]. These are all relatively recent studies, and further investigation will be required to confirm the validity of these results.

Role of FISH

Fluorescence in situ hybridization (FISH) of p16/CDKN2A gene is helpful to separate malignant from benign proliferations of mesothelial cells. Studies have reported homozygous deletion (HD) of p16/CDKN2A gene in up to 80% of pleural mesothelioma, but not in reactive mesothelial hyperplasia [62]. Several studies have documented that deletion of the p16/CDKN2A gene could be analyzed on cytology serous effusion specimens from patients with malignant mesothelioma [63–68]. However, the cut-off value of HD of p16/CDKN2A gene ranges from 5% to 48% in these reports. As a result, the sensitivity of p16 FISH in the diagnosis of mesothelioma in effusion cytology is between 48.5% and 92%.

Because FISH analysis on cell blocks can be achieved on archival samples, it may be useful in diagnosing a pleural effusion where the differential diagnosis is between early stage malignant mesothelioma and reactive pleuritis [30, 38, 69, 70] where the HD of p16/CDKN2A gene in cell blocks and in the corresponding tumor tissue was between 73% and 77% for malignant mesothelioma cases (Fig. 6.28). Because there was 100% concordance between the results in the cell blocks and tissue biopsies, p16 FISH results obtained from the cell blocks was as reliable as those from the tissue sections. The cut-off value of HD of p16/CDKN2A gene in these studies was between 12–15% [30, 69]. Each laboratory should calculate its own cut-off value because its staining procedures and types of fluorescent microscope differ.

The main challenge in the assessment of p16/CDKN2A gene deletion by FISH in cell blocks is the presence of admixed reactive mesothelial cells and inflammatory cells that can be indistinguishable from malignant mesothelioma cells by

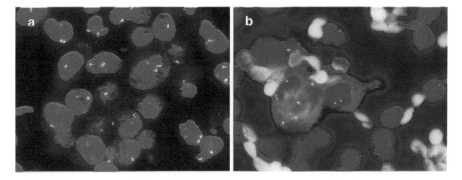

Fig. 6.28 Mesothelioma FISH Study. Homozygous deletion of p16/CDKN2A in malignant mesothelioma is demonstrated by loss of both red signals, but retention of green signals in malignant cell nuclei in cell block "A" and smear "B." Lymphocytes, as the internal control cells, retain both red and green signals; p16 fluorescent in situ hybridization (FISH)

fluorescence microscopy because the cell cytoplasm is digested during the FISH preparation process, leaving only nuclei for evaluation [62]. Since mesothelioma cell blocks often show characteristic three-dimensional clusters, such as papillary or acinar formations, [69] these clusters can be used as targets to analyze the mesothelioma cells by p16/CDKN2A FISH. Minimizing the digestion process to preserve the cytoplasm of mesothelial cells during FISH preparation will help to identify the target cells for recognition by fluorescence microscopy [69].

Role of Soluble Biomarkers

Malignant mesothelioma is a unique form of cancer in many aspects. This is the basis for the diagnostic use of cytochemistry, characterizing cell bound biomarkers. Biomarkers may enter the effusion supernatant, either as a secreted product, indirectly because of paracrine stimulation of the tumor stroma, or as cell decay. The analysis of these soluble compounds in effusions can provide further diagnostic information. In clinical practice, biochemical analyses have been established for diagnostic use, and attempts to predict drug sensitivity using biomarkers are under development. Today three markers – hyaluronan, mesothelin and osteopontin – have been recommended for establishing the diagnosis or as markers to follow effect of treatment when analyzed in serum. In the future, further compounds found in genomic and proteomic screening may add to the battery, although they have not yet been evaluated in clinical practice.

Hyaluronan (previously named hyaluronic acid) was the first diagnostic marker shown to have importance for the diagnosis of a malignant mesothelioma, even before the concept of biomarkers was generally used [71–73]. Hyaluronan is a linear glycosaminoglycan that interacts with various extra- and intracellular components. The chain is synthesized in the cell membrane from where it is released as a water-soluble macromolecule, which is difficult to monitor by IC.

The routine analysis of hyaluronan concentration was first performed using a simple ion suppression HPLC separation [74, 75]. Subsequent techniques based on hyaluronan binding proteins are now commercially available [76]. These reagents may, however, cross react with some bacterial sugars, causing false-positive results, which emphasizes the importance of establishing malignancy by other means. A concentration of hyaluronan exceeding 225 µg polysaccharide per mL (corresponding to 75 µg hyaluronan-derived uronic acid per mL) may indicate a malignant mesothelioma with a sensitivity of 50–60% [77]. In repeated thoracentesis, hyaluronan concentrations tend to be lower, indicating that fluid and polysaccharide enter the pleural cavity at different rates.

Mesothelin/ERC is a protein also presented as a possible marker for malignant mesothelioma [78]. Newly synthesized mesothelin/ERC becomes anchored in the cell membrane, where it sheds a 31 kD fragment (N-ERC, also called megakaryocyte potentiating factor, MPF). The remaining 40 kD C-ERC fragment persists in the cell membrane as the receptor for CA125 [79]. There are also various splice variants, including soluble mesothelin-related protein (SMRP).

Both mesothelin fragments can be used as biomarkers, and they are both commercially available as ELISA tests. Levels exceeding those in benign effusions are seen in 84% of patients with malignant mesothelioma [78]. They are, however, less specific for mesothelioma, since other cancers, such as ovarian and pancreatic carcinomas, also produce mesothelin. Furthermore, elevated effusion values can also be found in patients with renal failure [80, 81]. Thus, mesothelin/ERC can be regarded as a biomarker for malignancy, making this a suitable complement to hyaluronan when diagnosing an effusion as malignant mesothelioma.

Osteopontin is a less established diagnostic biomarker in malignant mesothelioma. It is a phosphoglycoprotein of importance for cell-matrix interactions, binding the hyaluronan binding receptor CD44 and various integrins. Apart from mesothelioma, osteopontin is also associated with cancers of breast, lung, colon, and prostate, and it can be upregulated in other diseases such as psoriasis. The sensitivity for detecting malignant mesothelioma or monitoring tumor burden over time varies in different reports. The diagnostic use of this biomarker is so far limited to following the effects of treatment.

Other suggested biomarkers for the diagnosis of malignant mesothelioma include the 12 kDa redox-enzyme Trx1, which is upregulated in mesothelioma cell lines. The protein is readily stained in sections from this tumor [82, 83]. Broad screening strategies studying gene expression and proteomics patterns can be a way to find new possible markers. Other promising examples are tenascin and high mobility group box 1 (HMGB1), which are over-expressed in malignant mesotheliomas [84, 85]. The diagnostic value of such compounds awaits validation in effusions. Incorporating the information from multiple markers can be a strategy to improve diagnostic sensitivity, but these biomarkers often correlate, and the diagnostic importance of extended biomarker batteries is so far limited.

These analyses can, together with routine cytology and other ancillary studies, contribute to an accurate malignant mesothelioma diagnosis in the first effusion. Measurements of soluble markers must be interpreted together with cell bound biomarkers. Although the positive predictive value of hyaluronan can be higher than most IC reactions, the diagnosis should never be based on hyaluronan analysis alone. However, the analysis of soluble biomarkers can contribute to attaining the diagnosis of a malignant mesothelioma earlier with effusion cytology.

Risk of Malignancy/Clinical Management

As mentioned above, the positive predictive value of a malignant mesothelioma diagnosis can be up to 100% in cases with strong supporting ancillary testing. To our knowledge, the risk of malignancy for malignant mesothelioma as a separate diagnosis has not been evaluated by a meta-analysis and would be a useful addition to the literature.

With proper use of ancillary studies, the diagnosis is sufficient to initiate treatment without further delay or invasive tissue sampling. There are some malignant mesothelioma cases with massive pleural effusion that lack the radiological findings of typical pleural mesothelioma. The definitive diagnosis of malignant mesothelioma can still be made with the use of ancillary studies (IC, analysis of soluble biomarkers, and p16 FISH). Some patients have thoracoscopic biopsies of parietal pleura which are diagnosed as MIS. However, treatment of patients with MIS is not yet established. According to the NCCN guidelines, malignant mesothelioma can be treated with chemotherapy only if inoperable. Operable mesothelioma patients may be treated with pleurectomy/decortication or extrapleural pneumonectomy (EPP). Patients with operable mesothelioma can receive chemotherapy either before or after surgery. In patients who do not receive induction chemotherapy before EPP, postoperative sequential chemotherapy with hemithoracic radiation therapy is recommended [86]. The detection of malignant mesothelioma early enough to improve chances for curative treatment would probably require screening blood samples and the employment of new biomarkers yet to be defined.

Sample Reports

Example 6.1
Frankly malignant with supportive immunochemistry

- Body cavity fluid, right, paracentesis:
- Satisfactory for interpretation
- Malignant mesothelioma (see note)
- Category: Malignant.

Note: The malignant cells are positive for (state mesothelial markers) and negative for (state epithelial markers). This immunochemical pattern corroborates the above diagnosis.

Example 6.2
Frankly malignant with supportive immunochemistry confirmed by additional ancillary tests but no radiological abnormalities

- Body cavity fluid, right, paracentesis:
- Satisfactory for interpretation
- Malignant mesothelioma (see note)
- Category: Malignant.

Note: This specimen is morphologically malignant and the cells are positive for (state mesothelial markers) and negative for (state epithelial markers). Increased soluble biomarkers, loss of BAP1 expression, and deletion of p16/CDKN2 FISH test support the above interpretation. These additional tests corroborate the diagnosis of malignant mesothelioma; however, video-assisted thoracoscopic biopsy is suggested to exclude the possibility of mesothelioma in situ or other mesothelial tumors.

Example 6.3
Frankly malignant with appropriate clinical presentation but inconclusive immunochemistry

- Body cavity fluid, left, paracentesis:
- Satisfactory for interpretation
- Malignant cells most consistent with mesothelioma (see note)
- Category: Malignant.

Note: The malignant cells are positive for (state markers) and negative for (state markers). While the morphology and the clinical presentation are highly suggestive of mesothelioma, this pattern of staining is inconclusive for a definitive categorization of tumor type.

Example 6.4
Highly cellular mesothelial sample with subtle atypia and supportive ancillary tests

- Body cavity fluid, left, paracentesis:
- Satisfactory for interpretation
- Mesothelioma (see note)
- Category: Malignant.

Note: The atypical cells are positive for (state mesothelial markers) and negative for (state epithelial markers). A cellular mesothelial sample with increased soluble biomarkers, loss of BAP1 expression, and/or deletion of p16/CDKN2 FISH test supports the above interpretation.

Example 6.5
Highly cellular sample with atypia and inconclusive ancillary tests

- Body cavity fluid, left, paracentesis:
- Interpretation limited by processing artifact
- Suspicious for malignant mesothelioma (see note)
- Category: Suspicious for malignancy.

Note: This is a highly cellular sample consisting of numerous mesothelial cells with atypia and (state immunostaining pattern). However, malignancy cannot be confirmed by ancillary tests such as soluble biomarkers, loss of BAP1 expression, and/or deletion of p16/CDKN2A by FISH. A biopsy confirmation is recommended.

Example 6.6
Highly cellular sample with atypia and supportive ancillary tests but no radiological abnormalities

- Pleural fluid, thoracentesis:
- Malignant mesothelioma (see note)
- Category: Malignant

Note: The atypical cells are positive for (state mesothelial markers) and negative for (state epithelial markers). Mesothelioma is suspected because loss of BAP1 expression and /or deletion of p16/CDKN2 FISH have been confirmed. However, video-assisted thoracoscopic biopsy is recommended to exclude the possibility of mesothelioma in situ or other mesothelial tumors.

Example 6.7
Highly atypical mesothelial cells but insufficient material for further work-up

- Body cavity fluid, paracentesis:
- Interpretation limited by insufficient volume submitted for evaluation
- Suspicious for malignant mesothelioma (see note)
- Category: Suspicious for malignancy

Note: Highly atypical cells morphologically consistent with mesothelial origin; however, further evaluation is not possible due to insufficient cellularity. Only (specify volume) was submitted for evaluation. Some studies recommend a minimum of 50–100 mL for optimal evaluation.

Example 6.8
Moderately cellular sample with atypia and inconclusive ancillary tests

- Body cavity fluid, left, thoracentesis:
- Satisfactory for interpretation
- Atypical mesothelial cells (see note)
- Category: Atypia of undetermined significance

Note: The atypical cells are positive for (state markers) and negative for (state markers), confirming mesothelial origin. However, malignancy cannot be confirmed by ancillary tests such as soluble biomarkers, loss of BAP1 expression, and/or deletion of p16/CDKN2A by FISH. It is not possible to distinguish between a reactive and a malignant process based on the present specimen. The differential diagnosis includes reactive mesothelial hyperplasia versus malignant mesothelioma; clinical and radiological correlation are recommended.

References

1. Hjerpe A, Ascoli V, Bedrossian CW, et al. Guidelines for the cytopathologic diagnosis of epithelioid and mixed-type malignant mesothelioma. Complementary statement from the International Mesothelioma Interest Group, also endorsed by the International Academy of Cytology and the Papanicolaou Society of Cytopathology. Acta Cytol. 2015;43(7):563–76.
2. Hjerpe A, Dobra K. Comments on the recently published "guidelines for the cytopathologic diagnosis of epithelioid and mixed-type malignant mesothelioma". Cancer Cytopathol. 2015;123(8):449–53.

3. Paintal A, Raparia K, Zakowski MF, Nayar R. The diagnosis of malignant mesothelioma in effusion cytology: a reappraisal and results of a multi-institution survey. Cancer Cytopathol. 2013;121(12):703–7.
4. Segal A, Sterrett GF, Frost FA, et al. A diagnosis of malignant pleural mesothelioma can be made by effusion cytology: results of a 20 year audit. Pathology. 2013;45(1):44–8.
5. Bray F, Ferlay J, Soerjomataram I, Siegel RL, Torre LA, Jemal A. Global cancer statistics 2018: GLOBOCAN estimates of incidence and mortality worldwide for 36 cancers in 185 countries. CA Cancer J Clin. 2018;68(6):394–424.
6. Turkey Asbestos Control Strategic Plan Final Report. Turk Thorac J. 2015;16(Suppl 2):S27–52.
7. Bedrossian CW. Asbestos-related diseases: a historical and mineralogic perspective. Semin Diagn Pathol. 1992;9(2):91–6.
8. Davidson B, Firat P, Michael CW. Serous effusions. 2nd ed. Cham, Switzerland: Springer; 2018.
9. Michael CW, Chhieng DC, Bedrossian CWM, editors. Cytohistology of the serous membranes. Cambridge, UK: Cambridge University Press; 2015.
10. Boon ME, van Velzen D, Ruinaard C, Veldhuizen RW. Analysis of number, size and distribution patterns of lipid vacuoles in benign and malignant mesothelial cells. Anal Quant Cytol. 1984;6(4):221–6.
11. Naylor B. The exfoliative cytology of diffuse malignant mesothelioma. J Pathol Bacteriol. 1963;86:293–8.
12. Whitaker D. Cell aggregates in malignant mesothelioma. Acta Cytol. 1977;21(2):236–9.
13. Leong AS, Stevens MW, Mukherjee TM. Malignant mesothelioma: cytologic diagnosis with histologic, immunohistochemical, and ultrastructural correlation. Semin Diagn Pathol. 1992;9(2):141–50.
14. Tao LC. The cytopathology of mesothelioma. Acta Cytol. 1979;23(3):209–13.
15. Whitaker D, Shilkin KB. The cytology of malignant mesothelioma in western Australia. Acta Cytol. 1978;22(2):67–70.
16. Nguyen GK. Cytopathology of pleural mesotheliomas. Amer J Clin Pathol. 2000;114(Suppl):S68–81.
17. Kho-Duffin J, Tao LC, Cramer H, Catellier MJ, Irons D, Ng P. Cytologic diagnosis of malignant mesothelioma, with particular emphasis on the epithelial noncohesive cell type. Diagn Cytopathol. 1999;20(2):57–62.
18. Chen L, Caldero SG, Gmitro S, Smith ML, De Petris G, Zarka MA. Small orangeophilic squamous-like cells: an underrecognized and useful morphological feature for the diagnosis of malignant mesothelioma in pleural effusion cytology. Cancer Cytopathol. 2014;122(1):70–5.
19. Whitaker D, Henderson DW, Shilkin KB. The concept of mesothelioma in situ: implications for diagnosis and histogenesis. Semin Diagn Pathol. 1992;9(2):151–61.
20. Churg A, Hwang H, Tan L, et al. Malignant mesothelioma in situ. Histopathology. 2018;72(6):1033–8.
21. Negi Y, Kuribayashi K, Funaguchi N, et al. Early-stage clinical characterization of malignant pleural mesothelioma. In Vivo. 2018;32(5):1169–74.
22. Hjerpe A, Abd-Own S, Dobra K. Cytopathologic diagnosis of epithelioid and mixed-type malignant mesothelioma: ten years of clinical experience in relation to international guidelines. Arch Pathol Lab Med. 2018;142(8):893–901.
23. Rakha EA, Patil S, Abdulla K, Abdulkader M, Chaudry Z, Soomro IN. The sensitivity of cytologic evaluation of pleural fluid in the diagnosis of malignant mesothelioma. Diagn Cytopathol. 2010;38(12):874–9.
24. Henderson DW, Reid G, Kao SC, van Zandwijk N, Klebe S. Challenges and controversies in the diagnosis of mesothelioma: Part 1. Cytology-only diagnosis, biopsies, immunohistochemistry, discrimination between mesothelioma and reactive mesothelial hyperplasia, and biomarkers. J Clin Pathol. 2013;66(10):847–53.
25. Huang CC, Attele A, Michael CW. Cytomorphologic features of metastatic urothelial carcinoma in serous effusions. Diagn Cytopathol. 2013;41(7):569–74.
26. Huang CC, Michael CW. Deciduoid mesothelioma: cytologic presentation and diagnostic pitfalls. Diagn Cytopathol. 2013;41(7):629–35.

27. Jing X, Li QK, Bedrossian U, Michael CW. Morphologic and immunocytochemical per-
    formances of effusion cell blocks prepared using 3 different methods. Am J Clin Pathol.
    2013;139(2):177–82.
28. Fetsch PA, Simsir A, Brosky K, Abati A. Comparison of three commonly used cyto-
    logic preparations in effusion immunocytochemistry. Diag Cytopathol. 2002;26(1):
    61–6.
29. McCroskey Z, Staerkel G, Roy-Chowdhuri S. Utility of BRCA1-associated protein 1 immu-
    noperoxidase stain to differentiate benign versus malignant mesothelial proliferations in cyto-
    logic specimens. Diag Cytopathol. 2017;45(4):312–9.
30. Hwang HC, Sheffield BS, Rodriguez S, et al. Utility of BAP1 immunohistochemistry and p16
    (CDKN2A) FISH in the diagnosis of malignant mesothelioma in effusion cytology specimens.
    Am J Surg Pathol. 2016;40(1):120–6.
31. Cozzi I, Oprescu FA, Rullo E, Ascoli V. Loss of BRCA1-associated protein 1 (BAP1) expres-
    sion is useful in diagnostic cytopathology of malignant mesothelioma in effusions. Diag
    Cytopathol. 2018;46(1):9–14.
32. Cigognetti M, Lonardi S, Fisogni S, et al. BAP1 (BRCA1-associated protein 1) is a highly
    specific marker for differentiating mesothelioma from reactive mesothelial proliferations. Mod
    Pathol. 2015;28(8):1043–57.
33. Hatem L, McIntire PJ, He B, et al. The role of BRCA1-associated protein 1 in the diagnosis
    of malignant mesothelioma in effusion and fine-needle aspiration cytology. Diag Cytopathol.
    2019;47(3):160–5.
34. Carbone M, Shimizu D, Napolitano A, et al. Positive nuclear BAP1 immunostaining helps
    differentiate non-small cell lung carcinomas from malignant mesothelioma. Oncotarget.
    2016;7(37):59314–21.
35. Owen D, Sheffield BS, Ionescu D, Churg A. Loss of BRCA1-associated protein 1 (BAP1)
    expression is rare in non-small cell lung cancer. Hum Pathol. 2017;60:82–5.
36. Hida T, Hamasaki M, Matsumoto S, et al. Immunohistochemical detection of MTAP and
    BAP1 protein loss for mesothelioma diagnosis: comparison with 9p21 FISH and BAP1 immu-
    nohistochemistry. Lung Cancer. 2017;104:98–105.
37. Berg KB, Churg A. GATA3 immunohistochemistry for distinguishing sarcomatoid and
    desmoplastic mesothelioma from sarcomatoid carcinoma of the lung. Am J Surg Pathol.
    2017;41(9):1221–5.
38. Kinoshita Y, Hida T, Hamasaki M, et al. A combination of MTAP and BAP1 immunohisto-
    chemistry in pleural effusion cytology for the diagnosis of mesothelioma. Cancer Cytopathol.
    2018;126(1):54–63.
39. Berg KB, Dacic S, Miller C, Cheung S, Churg A. Utility of methylthioadenosine phosphory-
    lase compared with BAP1 immunohistochemistry, and CDKN2A and NF2 fluorescence in
    situ hybridization in separating reactive mesothelial proliferations from epithelioid malignant
    mesotheliomas. Arch Pathol Lab Med. 2018;142(12):1549–53.
40. Creaney J, Segal A, Sterrett G, et al. Overexpression and altered glycosylation of MUC1 in
    malignant mesothelioma. Br J Cancer. 2008;98(9):1562–9.
41. Saad RS, Cho P, Liu YL, Silverman JF. The value of epithelial membrane antigen expression
    in separating benign mesothelial proliferation from malignant mesothelioma: a comparative
    study. Diag Cytopathol. 2005;32(3):156–9.
42. Attanoos RL, Griffin A, Gibbs AR. The use of immunohistochemistry in distinguishing reac-
    tive from neoplastic mesothelium. A novel use for desmin and comparative evaluation with
    epithelial membrane antigen, p53, platelet-derived growth factor-receptor, P-glycoprotein and
    Bcl-2. Histopathology. 2003;43(3):231–8.
43. Shen J, Pinkus GS, Deshpande V, Cibas ES. Usefulness of EMA, GLUT-1, and XIAP for
    the cytologic diagnosis of malignant mesothelioma in body cavity fluids. Am J Clin Pathol.
    2009;131(4):516–23.
44. Hyun TS, Barnes M, Tabatabai ZL. The diagnostic utility of D2-40, calretinin, CK5/6, desmin
    and MOC-31 in the differentiation of mesothelioma from adenocarcinoma in pleural effusion
    cytology. Acta Cytol. 2012;56(5):527–32.

45. Hasteh F, Lin GY, Weidner N, Michael CW. The use of immunohistochemistry to distinguish reactive mesothelial cells from malignant mesothelioma in cytologic effusions. Cancer Cytopathol. 2010;118(2):90–6.
46. Tsuji S, Washimi K, Kageyama T, et al. HEG1 is a novel mucin-like membrane protein that serves as a diagnostic and therapeutic target for malignant mesothelioma. Sci Rep. 2017;7(3):45768.
47. Pu RT, Pang Y, Michael CW. Utility of WT-1, p63, MOC31, mesothelin, and cytokeratin (K903 and CK5/6) immunostains in differentiating adenocarcinoma, squamous cell carcinoma, and malignant mesothelioma in effusions. Diagn Cytopathol. 2008;36(1):20–5.
48. Hattori Y, Yoshida A, Sasaki N, Shibuki Y, Tamura K, Tsuta K. Desmoplastic small round cell tumor with sphere-like clusters mimicking adenocarcinoma. Diagn Cytopathol. 2015;43(3):214–7.
49. Bassarova AV, Nesland JM, Davidson B. D2-40 is not a specific marker for cells of mesothelial origin in serous effusions. Am J Surg Pathol. 2006;30(7):878–82.
50. Jo VY, Cibas ES, Pinkus GS. Claudin-4 immunohistochemistry is highly effective in distinguishing adenocarcinoma from malignant mesothelioma in effusion cytology. Cancer Cytopathol. 2014;122(4):299–306.
51. Ordonez NG. Value of claudin-4 immunostaining in the diagnosis of mesothelioma. Am J Clin Pathol. 2013;139(5):611–9.
52. Ordonez NG. Application of immunohistochemistry in the diagnosis of epithelioid mesothelioma: a review and update. Hum Pathol. 2013;44(1):1–19.
53. Richter G, Heidersdorf H, Hirschfeld D, Krebbel F. Positive TTF-1 expression in malignant mesothelioma: a case report. Am J Case Rep. 2016;17:133–6.
54. Miettinen M, McCue PA, Sarlomo-Rikala M, et al. GATA3: a multispecific but potentially useful marker in surgical pathology: a systematic analysis of 2500 epithelial and nonepithelial tumors. Am J Surg Pathol. 2014;38(1):13–22.
55. Manur R, Lamzabi I. Aberrant cytokeratin 20 reactivity in epithelioid malignant mesothelioma: a case report. Appl Immunohistochem Mol Morphol. 2017. Feb;28 https://doi.org/10.1097/PAI.0000000000000504.
56. Mansour MSI, Seidal T, Mager U, Baigi A, Dobra K, Dejmek A. Determination of PD-L1 expression in effusions from mesothelioma by immuno-cytochemical staining. Cancer Cytopathol. 2017;125(12):908–17.
57. Chapel DB, Stewart R, Furtado LV, Husain AN, Krausz T, Deftereos G. Tumor PD-L1 expression in malignant pleural and peritoneal mesothelioma by Dako PD-L1 22C3 pharmDx and Dako PD-L1 28-8 pharmDx assays. Hum Pathol. 2019;87:11–7.
58. Chou A, Toon CW, Clarkson A, Sheen A, Sioson L, Gill AJ. The epithelioid BAP1-negative and p16-positive phenotype predicts prolonged survival in pleural mesothelioma. Histopathology. 2018;72(3):509–15.
59. McGregor SM, McElherne J, Minor A, et al. BAP1 immunohistochemistry has limited prognostic utility as a complement of CDKN2A (p16) fluorescence in situ hybridization in malignant pleural mesothelioma. Hum Pathol. 2017;60(2):86–94.
60. Guazzelli A, Meysami P, Bakker E, et al. BAP1 status determines the sensitivity of malignant mesothelioma cells to gemcitabine treatment. Int J Mol Sci. 2019;20(2):pii: E429.
61. Kumar N, Alrifai D, Kolluri KK, et al. Retrospective response analysis of BAP1 expression to predict the clinical activity of systemic cytotoxic chemotherapy in mesothelioma. Lung Cancer. 2019;127(1):164–6.
62. Husain AN, Colby TV, Ordonez NG, et al. Guidelines for pathologic diagnosis of malignant mesothelioma: 2017 update of the consensus statement from the International Mesothelioma Interest Group. Arch Pathol Lab Med. 2018;142(1):89–108.
63. Illei PB, Ladanyi M, Rusch VW, Zakowski MF. The use of CDKN2A deletion as a diagnostic marker for malignant mesothelioma in body cavity effusions. Cancer. 2003;99(1):51–6.
64. Flores-Staino C, Darai-Ramqvist E, Dobra K, Hjerpe A. Adaptation of a commercial fluorescent in situ hybridization test to the diagnosis of malignant cells in effusions. Lung Cancer. 2010;68(1):39–43.

65. Factor RE, Dal Cin P, Fletcher JA, Cibas ES. Cytogenetics and fluorescence in situ hybridization as adjuncts to cytology in the diagnosis of malignant mesothelioma. Cancer. 2009;117(4):247–53.
66. Onofre FB, Onofre AS, Pomjanski N, Buckstegge B, Grote HJ, Bocking A. 9p21 deletion in the diagnosis of malignant mesothelioma in serous effusions additional to immunocytochemistry, DNA-ICM, and AgNOR analysis. Cancer. 2008;114(3):204–15.
67. Savic S, Franco N, Grilli B, et al. Fluorescence in situ hybridization in the definitive diagnosis of malignant mesothelioma in effusion cytology. Chest. 2010;138(1):137–44.
68. Matsumoto S, Nabeshima K, Kamei T, et al. Morphology of 9p21 homozygous deletion-positive pleural mesothelioma cells analyzed using fluorescence in situ hybridization and virtual microscope system in effusion cytology. Cancer Cytopathol. 2013;121(8):415–22.
69. Hiroshima K, Wu D, Hasegawa M, et al. Cytologic differential diagnosis of malignant mesothelioma and reactive mesothelial cells with FISH analysis of p16. Diagn Cytopathol. 2016;44(7):591–8.
70. Walts AE, Hiroshima K, McGregor SM, Wu D, Husain AN, Marchevsky AM. BAP1 immunostain and CDKN2A (p16) FISH analysis: clinical applicability for the diagnosis of malignant mesothelioma in effusions. Diagn Cytopathol. 2016;44(7):599–606.
71. Blix G. Hyaluronic acid in the pleural and peritoneal fluids from a case of mesothelioma. Acta Soc Med Ups. 1951;56(1–2):47–50.
72. Harington JS, Wagner JC, Smith M. The detection of hyaluronic acid in pleural fluids of cases with diffuse pleural mesotheliomas. Br J Exp Pathol. 1963;44:81–3.
73. Friman C, Hellstrom PE, Juvani M, Riska H. Acid glycosaminoglycans (mucopolysaccharides) in the differential diagnosis of pleural effusion. Clin Chim Acta. 1977;76(3):357–61.
74. Hjerpe A. Liquid-chromatographic determination of hyaluronic acid in pleural and ascitic fluids. Clin Chem. 1986;32(6):952–6.
75. Thylen A, Wallin J, Martensson G. Hyaluronan in serum as an indicator of progressive disease in hyaluronan-producing malignant mesothelioma. Cancer. 1999;86(10):2000–5.
76. Chichibu K, Matsuura T, Shichijo S, Yokoyama MM. Assay of serum hyaluronic acid in clinical application. Clin Chim Acta. 1989;181(3):317–23.
77. Nurminen M, Dejmek A, Martensson G, Thylen A, Hjerpe A. Clinical utility of liquid-chromatographic analysis of effusions for hyaluronate content. Clin Chem. 1994;40(5):777–80.
78. Robinson BW, Creaney J, Lake R, et al. Mesothelin-family proteins and diagnosis of mesothelioma. Lancet. 2003;362(9396):1612–6.
79. Rump A, Morikawa Y, Tanaka M, et al. Binding of ovarian cancer antigen CA125/MUC16 to mesothelin mediates cell adhesion. J Biol Chem. 2004;279(10):9190–8.
80. Hollevoet K, Bernard D, De Geeter F, et al. Glomerular filtration rate is a confounder for the measurement of soluble mesothelin in serum. Clin Chem. 2009;55(7):1431–3.
81. Park EK, Thomas PS, Creaney J, Johnson AR, Robinson BW, Yates DH. Factors affecting soluble mesothelin related protein levels in an asbestos-exposed population. Clin Chem Lab Med. 2010;48(6):869–74.
82. Rundlof AK, Fernandes AP, Selenius M. al. Quantification of alternative mRNA species and identification of thioredoxin reductase 1 isoforms in human tumor cells. Differentiation. 2007;75(2):123–32.
83. Kahlos K, Soini Y, Saily M, et al. Up-regulation of thioredoxin and thioredoxin reductase in human malignant pleural mesothelioma. Int J Cancer. 2001;95(3):198–204.
84. Yuan Y, Nymoen DA, Stavnes HT, et al. Tenascin-X is a novel diagnostic marker of malignant mesothelioma. Amer J Surg Pathol. 2009;33(11):1673–82.
85. Chen Z, Gaudino G, Pass HI, Carbone M, Yang H. Diagnostic and prognostic biomarkers for malignant mesothelioma: an update. Transl Lung Cancer Res. 2017;6(3):259–69.
86. Ettinger DS, Wood DE, Aisner DL, et al. National Comprehensive Cancer Network. NCCN Clinical Practice Guidelines in Oncology (NCCN Guidelines): Malignant Pleural Mesothelioma, version 2.2019-April 1, 2019. https://www.nccn.org/professionals/physician_gls/pdf/mpm.pdf

Malignant-Secondary (MAL-S)

7

Yurina Miki, Z. Laura Tabatabai, and Ben Davidson

Background

Cytological evaluation of serous effusion specimens remains an extremely valuable means of diagnosing malignancy, particularly with the growing repertoire of ancillary techniques that are available to help resolve diagnostically challenging cases. Although the reported sensitivity and specificity of serous effusion cytology in the detection of malignancy vary (40–80% and 89–98%, respectively) and depend upon various factors (such as tumor type, preparation technique, and experience of the reporting cytopathologist), these values improve with the appropriate use of ancillary studies [1–3]. Furthermore, in conjunction with clinical and radiological findings, a diagnosis of the specific type of malignancy (including determination of the site of origin) can be made on serous effusion specimens, emphasizing its clinical utility, particularly in cases where the development of a pleural, pericardial, or peritoneal effusion may be the first manifestation of disease in a patient with an occult tumor.

The overall rate of malignancy in serous effusions varies from 10% to 50% [1, 4, 5]. Of these, metastatic disease (primarily metastatic adenocarcinoma) accounts for the majority of malignant effusions [4–6]. This chapter aims to provide an approach in categorizing malignant effusions that are secondary (metastatic) in nature by cell

Y. Miki
Department of Cellular Pathology, St Thomas' Hospital, Guy's and St Thomas' NHS Foundation Trust, London, UK

Z. L. Tabatabai
Department of Pathology, University of California San Francisco, San Francisco, CA, USA

B. Davidson (✉)
Department of Pathology, Norwegian Radium Hospital, Oslo University Hospital, Oslo, Norway

University of Oslo, Faculty of Medicine, Institute of Clinical Medicine, Oslo, Norway
e-mail: ben.davidson@medisin.uio.no

© Springer Nature Switzerland AG 2020
A. Chandra et al. (eds.), *The International System for Serous Fluid Cytopathology*, https://doi.org/10.1007/978-3-030-53908-5_7

of origin and to outline the key cytomorphological criteria of specific entities that belong to this diagnostic category, with the main differential diagnosis and useful ancillary studies highlighted in the explanatory notes.

Definition

Serous effusion specimens classified as malignant-secondary (MAL-S) show cytomorphological features that, either alone or in combination with ancillary studies, are diagnostic of a secondary malignancy (metastatic disease). The cell type of origin should be identified as epithelial, neuroendocrine, hematolymphoid, melanocytic, mesenchymal, or germ cell (bearing in mind that involvement of serous effusions by sarcomas and germ cell tumors is rare).

For serous effusions involved by metastatic adenocarcinoma, an indication of the site of origin should be given, guided initially by the serous cavity involved, clinical data (including age, sex, and previous medical history), and radiological findings. The site can subsequently be confirmed by ancillary studies. In contrast, involvement by squamous cell carcinoma, small cell neuroendocrine carcinoma, lymphoma, melanoma, sarcoma, and germ cell tumors (where confirming the cell of origin is enough to place them in the MAL-S category), the anatomical site of origin is determined by clinical and radiological findings.

Diagnostic Approach

As in the algorithm presented in Chap. 3, Negative for Malignancy, the presence of a second ("foreign") population of cells is a key defining feature of a metastatic malignant effusion [7]. In well-preserved specimens, the cellular morphology and architectural pattern may be sufficient to allow designation into the MAL-S category with identification of the cell of origin (see Sample Reports, Example 7.1). However, ancillary studies, mainly immunochemistry (IC), are invariably required for confirmation. A panel of IC stains can be used to first confirm the non-mesothelial nature of the atypical cells in question, enabling confident designation into the MAL-S category. Subsequently, ancillary studies (e.g., IC or flow cytometry) may be used to determine the cell type of origin and render a specific diagnosis. In cases of metastatic adenocarcinoma, site-specific IC stains can be used in the workup of the primary site of origin. This diagnostic algorithmic approach is summarized in Fig. 7.1.

A judicious selection of IC stains is of particular importance to help reduce costs and conserve material in cell block preparations. This may be facilitated by considering the frequent causes of secondary malignant effusions in adults based on the patient's sex and the serous cavity involved (Table 7.1).

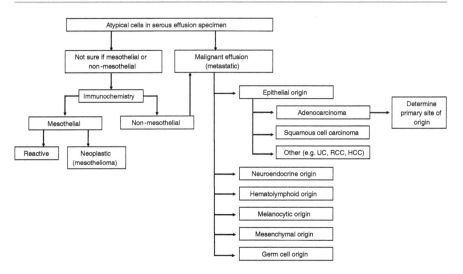

Fig. 7.1 Diagnostic approach for serous effusion specimens suspected to be involved by metastatic malignancy and when designation into MAL-S category confirmed. *(Abbreviations: UC, urothelial carcinoma; RCC, renal cell carcinoma; HCC, hepatocellular carcinoma)*

Table 7.1 Common sources of secondary malignant effusions in adults based on sex and serous cavity involved

	Pleural	Peritoneal	Pericardial
Male	Lung	Gastrointestinal tract	Lung
	Lymphoma	Lymphoma	Lymphoma
	Gastrointestinal tract	Pancreas	Gastrointestinal tract
	Pancreas	Genitourinary	
Female	Breast	Ovary	Breast
	Lung	Uterus	Lung
	Ovary	Breast	Lymphoma
	Lymphoma	Gastrointestinal tract	Gastrointestinal tract
	Gastrointestinal tract	Lymphoma	
	Pancreas		

Reprinted with permission from Davidson et al. [8]

Malignant Effusions of Epithelial Origin

Adenocarcinoma

Metastatic adenocarcinoma accounts for the vast majority of malignant effusions in adults. For pleural effusions involved by metastatic adenocarcinoma, the most common primary site in men is the lung, followed by the gastrointestinal tract, pancreatobiliary tract, and genitourinary tract; in women, the most common primary source is the breast, followed by the lung, gynecological tract, gastrointestinal tract, and pancreatobiliary tract [7]. Similarly, the most common primary site of metastatic adenocarcinoma involving pericardial effusions in men is the lung, followed by the gastrointestinal tract; in women, the breast and lung account for the most common primary sources, followed by the gastrointestinal tract [7]. For peritoneal effusions involved by metastatic adenocarcinoma, the most common primary site in men is the gastrointestinal tract, followed by the pancreatobiliary tract and genitourinary tract; in women, the most common primary source is the gynecological tract (primarily the ovary/fallopian tube and secondarily the uterus), followed by the breast and gastrointestinal tract [7].

The cytomorphological features of metastatic adenocarcinoma in serous effusion specimens can be quite variable depending on various factors, including the primary tumor site and type, the degree of tumor differentiation or tumor grade, the level of tumor cellularity, the presence or absence of associated degenerative and reactive changes, and the previous therapy. In cases of a known primary, a diagnosis of metastatic adenocarcinoma can usually be made based on either cytomorphology alone or in combination with a limited panel of IC stains. In cases of an unknown primary, a more extensive panel of IC stains may be necessary to arrive at the correct diagnosis.

Cytological Criteria

- A "foreign" population of cells arranged in small or large, rounded, three-dimensional clusters with smooth contours, papillary clusters (with or without psammoma bodies), glandular acini, and single or signet ring cells
- Increased nuclear-to-cytoplasmic ratio; enlarged, irregular nuclei with variable pleomorphism, coarse chromatin, and prominent nucleoli (nuclear abnormalities may be more subtle in certain cases – e.g., in gastric carcinoma or lobular breast carcinoma)
- Intracellular mucin demonstrated as single or multiple intracytoplasmic secretory mucin vacuoles and/or extracellular mucin

Explanatory Notes

Analysis of the architectural pattern may be helpful in determining the possible primary sites of metastatic adenocarcinoma, but is not specific. Very large, smooth-bordered cell balls, sometimes referred to as "cannonballs," suggest breast adenocarcinoma (Fig. 7.2). Linear cell patterns may be seen in lobular breast carcinoma. Single or signet ring cells may point to breast or gastric origin (Fig. 7.3). Acinar formation with columnar cells showing elongated, hyperchromatic nuclei and necrosis suggests colorectal origin (Fig. 7.4). Small acinar clusters and single uniform tumor cells showing large, prominent nucleoli may be seen in prostatic adenocarcinoma. Papillary clusters are most commonly associated with ovarian and gastrointestinal tract primaries in peritoneal effusion specimens (Fig. 7.5) and with lung, breast, and thyroid primaries in pleural effusion specimens. Psammoma bodies, when present, may suggest ovarian, lung, breast, or thyroid origin, although mesothelial hyperplasia and neoplasia should also be considered.

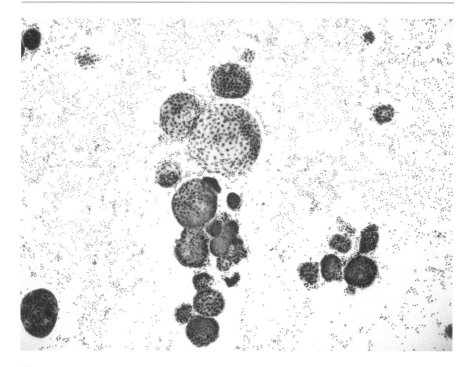

Fig. 7.2 Metastatic breast adenocarcinoma. Large, rounded "cannonball" cell clusters with smooth, community borders. *(Pleural fluid, Papanicolaou stain, low magnification)*

Intracytoplasmic vacuoles, although common in adenocarcinoma, can also be seen in a variety of other settings and are nonspecific unless they contain mucin. Degenerated mesothelial cells, histiocytes, and degenerating tumor cells of various types can all show cytoplasmic vacuoles. Large vacuoles can impart a signet ring-like appearance common to gastric, lobular breast, colonic, or pancreatic adenocarcinomas. Extreme vacuolization may be seen in therapy-related changes and adenocarcinomas of the lung (Fig. 7.6), ovary, pancreatobiliary tract, renal cell carcinomas, and some sarcomas. Conversely, clear spaces ("windows") between tumor cells, a feature commonly associated with mesothelial cells, can occasionally be seen in adenocarcinoma.

In pseudomyxoma peritonei, the serous fluid is characteristically thick due to abundant extracellular mucin. Cellularity is usually very low and may consist of muciphages or bland endocervical-like mucinous tumor cells arranged singly or in small clusters. Other cellular components such as mesothelial cells or leukocytes are usually sparse to absent.

Given the variation and sometimes overlapping features of reactive and malignant mesothelial cells and adenocarcinomas in serous effusion specimens, cell block preparation for confirmatory ancillary studies is recommended to avoid pitfalls in diagnosis. Positive markers for adenocarcinoma include MOC31, Ber-EP4,

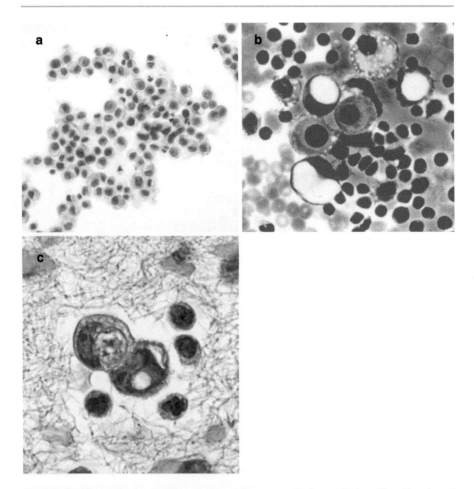

Fig. 7.3 (a) Metastatic gastric adenocarcinoma. Numerous single neoplastic cells with enlarged nuclei, coarse chromatin, prominent nucleoli, and intracytoplasmic vacuoles imparting a "signet ring" appearance. *(Pleural fluid, Papanicolaou stain, medium magnification)*. (b) Metastatic gastric adenocarcinoma. Single neoplastic cells with prominent intracytoplasmic vacuoles and peripherally displaced nuclei, imparting a "signet ring" appearance. *(Ascitic fluid, modified Giemsa stain, high magnification)*. (c) Metastatic gastric adenocarcinoma. Intracytoplasmic mucin vacuole highlighted by mucicarmine stain in a signet ring cell. *(Peritoneal fluid, mucicarmine stain, high magnification)*

claudin 4, B72.3, and CEA. Common malignant mesothelial markers include calretinin, D2-40, and WT1, as well as loss of BAP1; however, some of these IC stains, particularly WT1 and D2-40, should be interpreted with caution in the setting of gynecological adenocarcinomas, as the latter may also show positive staining for these markers.

To determine the primary site of origin of metastatic adenocarcinoma, IC stains for CK7 and CK20 can be used initially to narrow the differential in the setting of

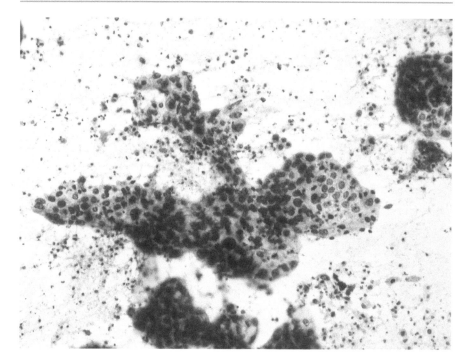

Fig. 7.4 Metastatic colorectal adenocarcinoma. Sheets and clusters of highly atypical epithelial cells with pleomorphic nuclei and coarse chromatin. Note the abundant "dirty" necrosis in the background. *(Pleural fluid, Papanicolaou stain, medium magnification)*

an unknown primary, followed by the use of more site-specific markers. The latter include TTF1 and napsin A for the lung; mammaglobin, GCDFP-15, and GATA3 for the breast; CDX2 and SATB2 for the colorectum or pancreas; PAX8 and ER for the ovary and uterus (with p53 and WT1 as additional markers for serous carcinoma and HNF1β and napsin A as additional markers for clear cell carcinoma); P504S, NKX3, PSA, and PSAP for the prostate; and thyroglobulin and TTF1 for the thyroid gland [8].

Squamous Cell Carcinoma

While squamous cell carcinoma is a common malignancy, it is rarely encountered in serous fluids, comprising only 0.5%–2.7% of malignant effusions [9, 10]. However, when involved, the pleural cavity is the most commonly affected, followed by the peritoneal and pericardial cavities. The most common primary site of origin of metastatic squamous cell carcinoma involving serous effusions is the lung; other less common primary sources include the head and neck, esophagus, and cervix [9, 10].

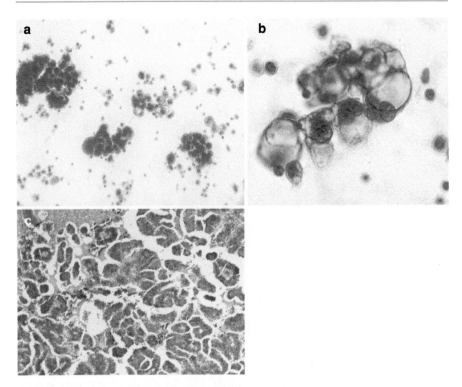

Fig. 7.5 (a) Metastatic high-grade serous carcinoma of the ovary. Cohesive, papillary clusters of atypical epithelial cells with enlarged, hyperchromatic nuclei, coarse chromatin, and focal cytoplasmic vacuolation. *(Peritoneal fluid, Papanicolaou stain, medium magnification)*. (b) Metastatic high-grade serous carcinoma of the ovary. Cluster of atypical epithelial cells with enlarged, hyperchromatic nuclei, coarse chromatin, and large, discrete cytoplasmic vacuoles. *(Peritoneal fluid, Papanicolaou stain, high magnification)*. (c) Metastatic high-grade serous carcinoma of the ovary. Numerous papillary clusters lined by crowded atypical epithelial cells. *(Peritoneal fluid, cell block, H&E stain, low magnification)*

Cytological Criteria
Well-differentiated or keratinizing squamous cell carcinoma (Fig. 7.7)

- Predominantly single-cell pattern or small clusters
- Enlarged, irregular, hyperchromatic nuclei
- Variable amounts of dense, cyanophilic to eosinophilic to dyskeratotic/orangeophilic cytoplasm (on Papanicolaou staining)
- Sharply defined cell borders
- Polygonal cells, tadpole cells, fiber cells, and anucleated cells
- Keratin debris, squamous pearls

Poorly differentiated or non-keratinizing squamous cell carcinoma

- Clusters or syncytial groups of cells
- High nuclear-to-cytoplasmic ratio

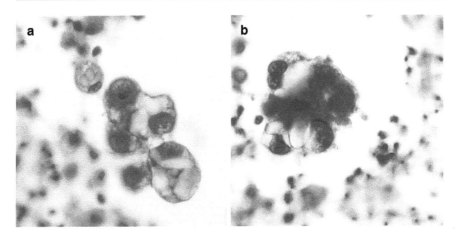

Fig. 7.6 (**a**) Metastatic pulmonary adenocarcinoma. Abundant vacuolization of the cytoplasm, imparting a "soap-bubble" appearance to the neoplastic cells. *(Pleural fluid, Papanicolaou stain, high magnification).* (**b**) Metastatic pulmonary adenocarcinoma. Cluster of malignant glandular epithelial cells with enlarged, pleomorphic, hyperchromatic nuclei and moderate to abundant amounts of vacuolated cytoplasm. *(Pleural fluid, Papanicolaou stain, high magnification)*

- Enlarged, irregular, hyperchromatic nuclei
- Coarse chromatin.
- Thin rim of ill-defined, delicate, granular cytoplasm to focally dense, cyanophilic cytoplasm

Explanatory Notes

When serous effusions are involved by metastatic well-differentiated or keratinizing squamous cell carcinoma, the diagnosis can usually be made without difficulty based on the characteristic cytomorphological features, especially in the context of a known clinical history. However, it has been noted that serous effusions involved by certain non-squamous malignancies (e.g., malignant mesothelioma) may show small degenerated orangeophilic cells, leading to misinterpretation as keratinizing squamous cell carcinoma [11]. Furthermore, the diagnosis becomes more challenging in cases of squamous cell carcinomas that are less differentiated. As tumor cells from a poorly differentiated or non-keratinizing squamous cell carcinoma have a tendency to form cellular clusters, they may be mistaken for those from a poorly differentiated adenocarcinoma or malignant mesothelioma [10]. Certain cytomorphological features of a poorly differentiated or non-keratinizing squamous cell carcinoma may also overlap with those seen in cases of small cell neuroendocrine carcinoma. Benign conditions such as rheumatoid effusions can also mimic squamous cell carcinoma; epithelioid histiocytes in this setting can be slender or elongate with dense, orangeophilic cytoplasm and pyknotic nuclei due to degenerative changes, resembling tadpole cells of squamous cell carcinoma. The orangeophilia in these degenerative histiocytes occurs as a staining artifact and do not reflect true keratinization which has a glassy and refractile quality [12]. A select panel of IC stains, together with the clinical history, will usually help to arrive at the correct

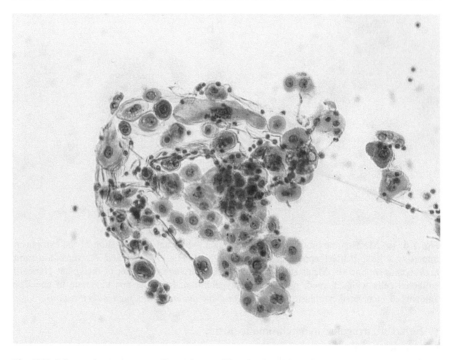

Fig. 7.7 Metastatic squamous cell carcinoma. Neoplastic cells with variable amounts of dense, cyanophilic to eosinophilic to dyskeratotic/orangeophilic cytoplasm and sharply defined cell borders, arranged in loosely cohesive clusters and as single cells. *(Pleural fluid, Papanicolaou stain, high magnification)*

diagnosis. Benign and malignant squamous cells are positive for p40, CK5/6, and p63, and malignant squamous cells often stain for p16 and mCEA. Benign squamous cells can be seen in serous fluids in the setting of fistulas (e.g., esophago-pleural fistula) or contamination but usually lack significant cytological atypia. Correlation with clinical findings is helpful.

Other Carcinomas

Other carcinomas that may involve the serous cavities include high-grade urothelial carcinoma, renal cell carcinoma, and hepatocellular carcinoma.

Cytological Criteria
Urothelial carcinoma (Fig. 7.8)

- Single cells or small clusters
- Increased nuclear-to-cytoplasmic ratio; hyperchromatic nuclei, irregular nuclear membranes, and variably prominent nucleoli

Fig. 7.8 Metastatic urothelial carcinoma. Loosely cohesive neoplastic cells with enlarged, irregular nuclei, coarse chromatin, variably prominent nucleoli, and well-defined, granular to dense cytoplasm. *(Pleural fluid, Papanicolaou stain, high magnification)*

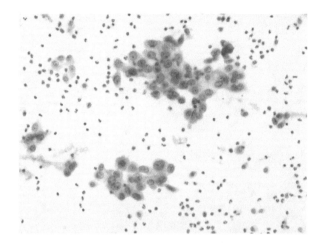

- Well-defined, granular to dense cytoplasm
- May show divergent squamous or glandular differentiation
- Tumor cells express CK7, CK20, uroplakin, p63, and GATA3

Renal cell carcinoma (Fig. 7.9)

- Cohesive clusters or single cells.
- Enlarged nuclei, smooth to irregular nuclear membranes, and prominent nucleoli.
- Moderate to abundant amounts of vacuolated, clear to granular cytoplasm.
- Tumor cells express PAX2, PAX8, EMA, RCC antigen, CAIX, and CD10 but are typically negative for CK7 and CK20 (papillary subtype may express CK7).

Hepatocellular carcinoma

- Clustered or single cells.
- Oval to irregular nuclei with macronucleoli.
- Polygonal, granular, eosinophilic cytoplasm that may contain bile pigment.
- Tumor cells express arginase 1, glypican 3, HepPAR1, α-fetoprotein but are negative for CK7 and CK20.

Malignant Effusions of Neuroendocrine Origin

Small Cell Neuroendocrine Carcinoma

Small cell neuroendocrine carcinoma may arise in the lung, pancreas, gastrointestinal, gynecological or genitourinary tracts, and other anatomic sites (e.g., head and neck). Involvement of serous cavities by metastatic small cell neuroendocrine carcinoma is rare (occurring in less than 3% of cases); nonetheless, as the lung is the

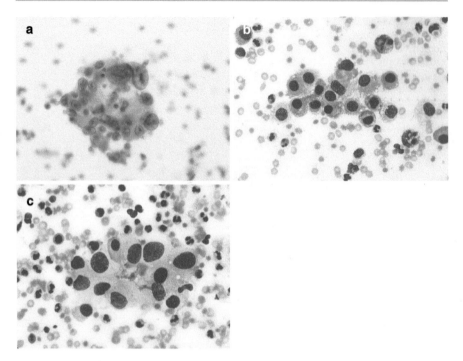

Fig. 7.9 (**a**) Metastatic renal cell carcinoma. Cluster of neoplastic cells with enlarged, pleomorphic nuclei, coarse chromatin, prominent nucleoli, and moderate to abundant amounts of delicate granular cytoplasm. *(Pleural fluid, Papanicolaou stain, high magnification).* (**b**) Metastatic renal cell carcinoma. Neoplastic cells with enlarged, round to oval nuclei, prominent nucleoli, and moderate to abundant amounts of cytoplasm with numerous small vacuoles, imparting a frothy or bubbly appearance. *(Pleural fluid, modified Giemsa stain, high magnification).* (**c**) Metastatic renal cell carcinoma. Neoplastic cells with enlarged, round to oval nuclei, prominent nucleoli, and moderate to abundant amounts of delicate granular cytoplasm. *(Pleural fluid, modified Giemsa stain, high magnification)*

most common primary site affected, the pleural cavity is the most common serous cavity involved [13]. Cytologically, small cell neuroendocrine carcinoma in serous fluids is similar to that in other anatomic sites (Fig. 7.10).

Cytological Criteria
- Single cells, short chains, or moderately cohesive clusters
- Tumor cells approximately two to three times larger than small mature lymphocytes
- High nuclear-to-cytoplasmic ratio
- Scant, delicate cytoplasm
- Oval to irregular nuclei, stippled chromatin, and inconspicuous to absent nucleoli
- Nuclear molding
- Nuclear crush artifact or streaking
- Frequent mitoses, necrosis, and apoptosis

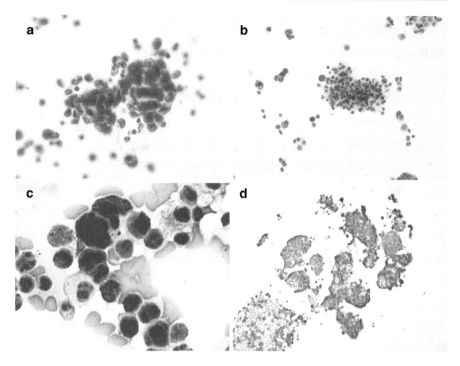

Fig. 7.10 (**a**) Metastatic small cell neuroendocrine carcinoma. Cluster of small- to medium-sized cells with high nuclear-to-cytoplasmic ratios, scant delicate cytoplasm, irregular nuclei, and nuclear molding. *(Pleural fluid, Papanicolaou stain, high magnification).* (**b**) Metastatic small cell neuroendocrine carcinoma. Singly dispersed and clusters of small- to medium-sized cells with high nuclear-to-cytoplasmic ratios, scant delicate cytoplasm, stippled chromatin, and nuclear molding. Note the abundant apoptosis in the cell cluster. *(Pleural fluid, Papanicolaou stain, medium magnification).* (**c**) Metastatic small cell neuroendocrine carcinoma. Neoplastic cells with high nuclear-to-cytoplasmic ratios, scant delicate cytoplasm, and nuclear molding. *(Pleural fluid, modified Giemsa stain, high magnification).* (**d**) Metastatic small cell neuroendocrine carcinoma. Cohesive clusters of neoplastic cells showing cytoplasmic expression of synaptophysin. *(Pleural fluid, cell block, synaptophysin stain, medium magnification)*

Explanatory Notes

Although cytomorphological features of neuroendocrine carcinoma are generally readily recognizable in serous effusion specimens, the use of ancillary studies is recommended to confirm the diagnosis. The differential diagnosis includes neoplastic or non-neoplastic cells of hematolymphoid origin, metastatic Merkel cell carcinoma, other metastatic high-grade carcinomas with basaloid features (such as basaloid squamous cell carcinoma), poorly differentiated carcinomas, and small round blue cell tumors [13]. Small cell and large cell neuroendocrine carcinomas are positive for the neuroendocrine markers synaptophysin and chromogranin A. NSE and CD56 are often positive but are nonspecific markers which cannot be used for diagnosing neuroendocrine differentiation. Those tumors originating from the lung and sometimes from other sites may also be positive for TTF1. Similar to Merkel cell carcinoma, small cell neuroendocrine carcinoma can also show perinuclear dot-like CK20 staining but is negative for Merkel cell polyomavirus. The Ki-67 proliferative index is high (> 70%). Correlation with the clinical and imaging findings, together with IC stains, helps to arrive at the correct diagnosis.

Malignant Effusions of Hematolymphoid Origin

Serous effusions are a common occurrence in patients with hematolymphoid malignancies, often developing during the clinical course of the disease due to a variety of mechanisms, but are rarely the first presentation of disease. Of the serous effusion specimens submitted for cytological analysis which are positive for a hematolymphoid malignancy, lymphomas account for the great majority of cases. Various studies have reported rates of lymphoma in up to 10–15% of malignant effusions, predominantly in pleural effusions and less commonly in peritoneal and pericardial effusions [4, 6, 14–16]. Of note, lymphomas/leukemias represent the most frequent cause of malignant effusions in the pediatric population [17, 18].

Lymphomatous involvement of serous effusions can be attributed to both non-Hodgkin lymphoma (NHL) and Hodgkin lymphoma (HL). The development of pleural effusions in NHL and HL may arise as a result of a variety of mechanisms: obstruction of lymphatic drainage secondary to pulmonary or mediastinal lymph nodes, direct pleural involvement by lymphoma, or thoracic duct obstruction leading to chylothorax (although this mechanism is unusual in HL) [19–21].

Studies have shown that a diagnosis of a specific subtype of NHL (according to the WHO classification) is possible in serous effusion specimens in conjunction with appropriate ancillary techniques [14, 22, 23]. The more common subtypes of NHL diagnosed in serous effusion specimens include chronic lymphocytic leukemia/small lymphocytic lymphoma, follicular lymphoma, mantle cell lymphoma, diffuse large B-cell lymphoma, Burkitt lymphoma, T-cell acute lymphoblastic leukemia/lymphoma, anaplastic large cell lymphoma, and primary effusion lymphoma [14, 22, 23]. With the increasingly complex and ever-evolving WHO classification of lymphoid malignancies, the diagnosis of a particular type of lymphoma ultimately requires specialist hematopathological review and integration of the results of ancillary studies, including flow cytometry, IC staining, and cytogenetic/molecular genetic studies. Nonetheless, some degree of subclassification can be achieved on cytomorphological criteria as outlined below; subsequently, the serous effusion specimen can be appropriately triaged for ancillary studies to reach a more specific diagnosis.

Non-Hodgkin Lymphoma

The general diagnostic principles and approach used in the cytological assessment of lymphoid proliferations in fine-needle aspirations of lymph nodes can equally be applied to serous fluid specimens. However, it is important to note that the lymphoid population in serous fluid specimens may be highly concentrated (due to preparation type) and susceptible to rapid cellular degeneration, making application of such criteria more difficult [24]. Nonetheless, when evaluating lymphocyte-rich serous effusions, the following features should be assessed: (1) the homogeneity of the lymphoid population (i.e., whether there is a polymorphic or monomorphic lymphoid population) and (2) the size of the lymphoid cells (i.e., whether there is a predominance of small-, medium-, or large-sized lymphoid cells) [25]. Small lymphoid cells are equal to or smaller than a resting (naïve) lymphocyte or double the size of an erythrocyte, while large lymphoid cells are two to three times the size of a resting (naïve) lymphocyte; medium-sized lymphoid cells are those in between small and large lymphoid cells [25]. Based on whether the lymphoid proliferation is composed of predominantly small- to medium-sized lymphoid cells or medium-sized to large-sized lymphoid cells, NHL can be broadly classified into low-grade or high-grade, in turn narrowing the differential diagnosis. The general cytomorphological features of low-grade and high-grade NHL are summarized below, highlighting key characteristics of some of the more commonly encountered subtypes of NHL in serous effusion specimens. The precursor lymphoid neoplasm of T-cell acute lymphoblastic leukemia/lymphoma (T-cell ALL/LBL) will be addressed in the high-grade NHL section as it often poses differential diagnostic problems with other entities in this category.

Cytological Criteria: Low-Grade Non-Hodgkin Lymphoma

- Highly cellular preparation.
- At low magnification: predominant population of discohesive small- to medium-sized lymphoid cells, usually with minimal cytological atypia.
- At high magnification: certain cytomorphological (e.g., nuclear) features may be appreciated, providing clues to the specific subtype of low-grade NHL.
  - Chronic lymphocytic leukemia/small lymphocytic lymphoma (CLL/SLL) (Fig. 7.11): predominance of small lymphoid cells with relatively uniform nuclei and coarse clumped chromatin, may be admixed with slightly larger lymphoid cells (prolymphocytes and paraimmunoblasts) with more dispersed nuclear chromatin and distinct nucleoli
  - Follicular lymphoma (low-grade): predominance of centrocytes with cleaved or angulated nuclei, with fewer numbers of admixed centroblasts with vesicular nuclei and one to three nucleoli often apposed to the nuclear membrane
  - Mantle cell lymphoma (classic variant): predominance of small- to medium-sized lymphoid cells with irregular nuclei, condensed chromatin, and inconspicuous nucleoli
  - Marginal zone lymphoma: heterogeneous appearance with small- to medium-sized lymphoid cells with monocytoid, centrocyte-like, and/or plasmacytoid morphology, with variable numbers of admixed larger transformed lymphoid cells reminiscent of centroblasts or immunoblasts
- *Triage sample for immunophenotyping by flow cytometry or IC staining on cell block preparation.*

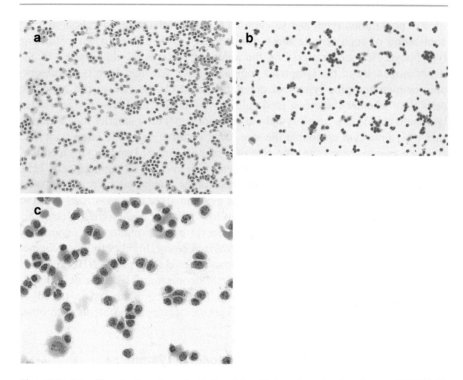

Fig. 7.11 (**a**) Chronic lymphocytic leukemia/small lymphocytic lymphoma (CLL/SLL). Monomorphic population of discohesive small lymphoid cells, highly suspicious for involvement by a low-grade NHL. Ancillary studies are required for diagnostic confirmation and accurate subtyping. *(Pleural fluid, Papanicolaou stain, medium magnification).* (**b**) Chronic lymphocytic leukemia/small lymphocytic lymphoma (CLL/SLL). Monomorphic population of discohesive small lymphoid cells, highly suspicious for involvement by a low-grade NHL. Ancillary studies are required for diagnostic confirmation and accurate subtyping. *(Pleural fluid, modified Giemsa stain, medium magnification).* (**c**) Chronic lymphocytic leukemia/small lymphocytic lymphoma (CLL/SLL). Monomorphic population of discohesive small lymphoid cells with relatively uniform nuclei and coarse clumped chromatin, highly suspicious for involvement by a low-grade NHL. Ancillary studies are required for diagnostic confirmation and accurate subtyping. *(Pleural fluid, Papanicolaou stain, high magnification)*

- – *Fluorochrome-conjugated antibodies used in flow cytometry will vary based on institutional practices but may include CD2, CD3, CD4, CD5, CD7, CD8, CD10, CD19, CD20, CD22, CD23, CD200, CD45, FMC7, and kappa, lambda.*
- – *Suggested IC panel on cell block preparation: CD20, CD79a, CD3, CD5, CD23, CD10, BCL6, BCL2, Cyclin D1, kappa, lambda, MIB1.*

Cytological Criteria: High-Grade Non-Hodgkin Lymphoma
- Highly cellular preparation.
- At low magnification: predominant population of discohesive medium- to large-sized atypical lymphoid cells (the malignant nature of the neoplastic lymphoid cells is usually obvious).

- At high magnification: certain cytomorphological (e.g., nuclear) features may be appreciated in cases of Burkitt lymphoma and T-cell ALL/LBL.
  - Burkitt lymphoma (Fig. 7.12): medium-sized lymphoid cells with often vacuolated cytoplasm, round or slightly irregular nuclei, finely granular to coarse chromatin, and multiple nucleoli
  - T-cell ALL/LBL (Fig. 7.13): lymphoblasts range from small, round blasts with a high nuclear-to-cytoplasmic ratio, relatively condensed chromatin, and inconspicuous nucleoli to larger cells with slightly more cytoplasm, irregular nuclei, dispersed chromatin, and variable numbers of distinct nucleoli
- *Triage sample for IC staining on cell block preparation (examples of suggested panels below).*
  - *Suggested IC panel for medium-/large-sized B-cell lymphomas: CD20, CD79a, CD3, CD10, BCL6, MUM1, CD5, CD23, CD30, BCL2, MIB1, EBER*
  - *Suggested IC panel for B-cell/T-cell ALL/LBL: CD34, TdT, CD117, CD99, CD1a, CD2, CD3, CD4, CD5, CD7, CD8, CD10, CD19, CD20, CD79a, MIB1*

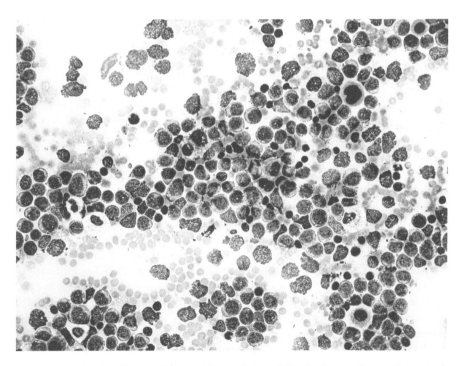

Fig. 7.12 Burkitt lymphoma. Monomorphic population of discohesive, medium- to large-sized, atypical lymphoid cells with round nuclei, coarse chromatin, and multiple nucleoli, indicating involvement by a high-grade NHL. Note the small vacuoles in the cytoplasm of some of these atypical lymphoid cells. Ancillary studies are required for accurate subtyping. *(Pleural fluid, modified Giemsa stain, medium magnification)*

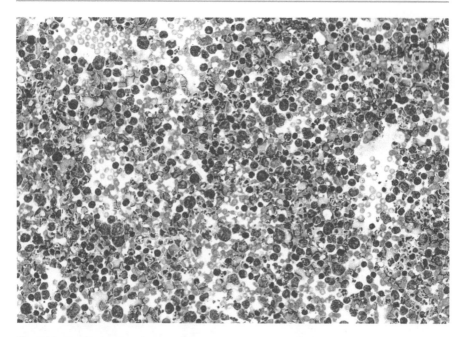

Fig. 7.13 T-cell acute lymphoblastic leukemia/lymphoma (T-cell ALL/LBL). Monomorphic population of discohesive, medium- to large-sized, atypical lymphoid cells with round to irregular nuclei, interspersed by numerous apoptotic bodies. T-cell ALL/LBL often poses diagnostic problems with entities in the high-grade NHL category. *(Pleural fluid, Modified Giemsa stain, medium magnification)*

Explanatory Notes

In routine clinical practice, "lymphocyte-rich" serous fluid specimens are commonly encountered, and one of the main difficulties is distinguishing between a reactive lymphoid population and an indolent low-grade NHL based on cytomorphological features alone. Although the presence of a monomorphic lymphoid population is highly suspicious of lymphoma morphologically (and can be designated as such – i.e., placed in the suspicious for malignancy (SFM) diagnostic category), some low-grade NHL (e.g., follicular lymphoma and marginal zone lymphoma) can show a more heterogeneous cytomorphology, thereby mimicking a reactive pattern. As a result, immunophenotyping (either by flow cytometry or IC) is required for diagnostic confirmation. Indeed, the value of flow cytometry as an adjunct to cytomorphological analysis of serous fluid specimens in the diagnosis of lymphoproliferative diseases is well-established and is helpful both in patients with and without a previous history of lymphoma [15, 22–24, 26–30]. In the former setting, sending "lymphocyte-rich" serous fluid specimens for flow cytometry is generally recommended because lymphomatous malignant effusions occur in greater frequency in patients with a known history of lymphoma than those without. Furthermore, in these settings, the adjunct use of flow cytometry invariably allows a definitive diagnosis of lymphoma in serous effusions since typically the patient's original lymphoma diagnosis has been fully evaluated and classified on a separate tissue specimen. In patients without a prior history of lymphoma, reflex screening of all "lymphocyte-rich" effusions is not of particular value and generally not recommended [29]. However, flow cytometry is helpful and indicated in serous fluid specimens suspicious for a low-grade NHL, particularly in cases of unexplained recurrent effusions or if there is a high index of clinical suspicion (e.g., persistent lymphadenopathy or peripheral blood lymphocytosis). A subsequent positive flow cytometry result can then help guide additional tissue sampling to fully characterize the lymphoma.

For serous effusions containing a predominant population of medium- to large-sized atypical lymphoid cells, the malignant nature of the lymphoid cells is almost always obvious on cytomorphology. In these cases, it is important to confirm the lymphoid nature of these cells and exclude other hematologic lines of differentiation (e.g., exclude involvement by acute myeloid leukemia or plasma cell neoplasm) as well as other diagnoses, such as poorly differentiated carcinoma, small cell carcinoma, melanoma, and sarcoma. In these cases, a cell block preparation and a general panel of IC stains can initially be performed. Once the lymphoid nature of the malignant cells is confirmed, then a more tailored panel of IC stains (as outlined above) can be performed and specialist hematopathological input sought for diagnosis and further supplementary ancillary studies. Flow cytometry in the setting of suspected large-cell lymphomas/high-grade NHL is not recommended because of the high risk for false-negative results. The neoplastic cells are particularly fragile and susceptible to destruction with artificial loss of surface antigens during cell sorting; equally, the presence of extensive necrosis can consequently lead to failure and noncontributory flow cytometry results [22, 24, 26, 31].

Although technically a *primary* cavity-based malignant effusion, one hematologic malignancy that deserves special mention in this subsection is the diagnosis of primary effusion lymphoma (PEL). According to the WHO classification, PEL is classified under the HHV8-associated lymphoproliferative disorders and is characterized by lymphomatous effusions of the pleural, pericardial, and peritoneal cavities but without a detectable solid extra-cavitary tumor mass in immunocompromised patients, mostly with HIV infection [32]. While the disease is localized to body cavities in the majority of cases, there may rarely be local extension of disease to adjacent organs (e.g., lung, soft tissue, or regional lymph nodes) or involvement of the bone marrow [32]. The cytological appearances are those of medium- to large-sized atypical lymphoid cells, ranging from immunoblastic (with prominent central nucleoli), anaplastic (with multinucleated and Reed-Sternberg-like cells), and plasmablastic (with eccentric nuclei and abundant cytoplasm) morphologies (Fig. 7.14) [32]. PEL has a distinctive immunophenotype with neoplastic cells expressing CD45 and activation-associated antigens (e.g., HLA-DR, CD30, CD38, and CD138) but lack expression of B-cell antigens (e.g., CD20 and C19) and surface immunoglobulins. Neoplastic cells are also positive for HHV8 and invariably positive for EBER [26, 32]. The IC panel suggested

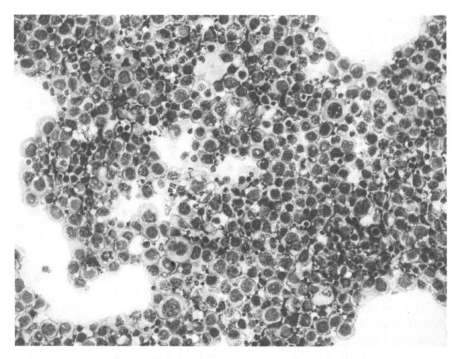

Fig. 7.14 Primary effusion lymphoma (PEL). Monomorphic population of discohesive, medium- to large-sized, atypical lymphoid cells (including occasional binucleate forms), interspersed by numerous apoptotic bodies, indicating involvement by a high-grade NHL. Ancillary studies are required for accurate subtyping. *(Pleural fluid, Papanicolaou stain, medium magnification)*

above for medium- and large-sized B-cell lymphomas can be used and slightly modified to include these extra markers. The prognosis is poor with low overall survival rates [33].

Classical Hodgkin Lymphoma

It is important to note that, not uncommonly, patients with classical HL will develop effusions during the clinical course of the disease [19, 34], but the actual finding of a positive serous effusion specimen with classical HL is rare with only case reports described in the literature [35–37].

Cytological Criteria
- Few singly scattered large atypical cells, either binucleated/multinucleated forms (Reed-Sternberg cells) or mononuclear variants (Hodgkin cells), with abundant cytoplasm and large nuclei with prominent nucleoli
- Background of mixed inflammatory cells comprising small mature lymphocytes, neutrophils, eosinophils, plasma cells, and histiocytes
- *Suggested IC panel on cell block preparation: CD45, PAX5, CD20, CD79a, CD3, CD30, CD15, MUM1, ALK1, EMA, MIB1, EBER*

Explanatory Notes

Although rare, if a diagnosis of classical HL is suspected in a serous effusion specimen, then a cell block preparation is recommended, and appropriate IC stains can be performed. The material should not be sent for flow cytometry because the neoplastic cells (i.e., Hodgkin/Reed-Sternberg [H/RS] cells) can be difficult to characterize due to their relative paucity and the accompanying rich reactive background, leading to false-negative results. The combination of cytomorphology and the characteristic immunophenotype of the neoplastic cells, in conjunction with clinical information, is required for a diagnosis of classical HL.

Based solely on cytomorphological features, H/RS cells in serous effusions may mimic large pleomorphic cells found in malignant effusion of non-hematolymphoid lineage, such as melanoma or poorly differentiated carcinoma [36]. H/RS cells may equally be confused with other atypical lymphoid cells seen in NHL, such as anaplastic large cell lymphoma (ALCL) [38, 39]. In both classical HL and ALCL, there are CD30 positive large pleomorphic cells as well as a mixed inflammatory background. However, the neoplastic cells in ALCL express T-cell markers, with 60–80% of cases expressing ALK1. Furthermore, reactive mesothelial cells exhibiting binucleation/multinucleation or megakaryocytes in serous effusions associated with extramedullary hematopoiesis may resemble H/RS cells [36, 40, 41]. In all instances, a select panel of IC stains will help resolve these diagnostic issues.

Plasma Cell Neoplasm

While lymphomas account for the great majority of serous effusion specimens involved by a hematolymphoid malignancy, plasma cell neoplasms may also involve the serous cavities. For instance, although affecting less than 1% of patients diagnosed with plasma cell myeloma, myelomatous involvement of serous fluids can occur, usually as a late complication of disseminated disease, and is associated with a poor prognosis [42, 43].

Cytological Criteria
- Predominant population of plasma cells (Fig. 7.15)
- Variable degree of atypia, ranging from those with recognizable mature plasma cell morphology (e.g., with eccentrically placed, round to oval nuclei) to those with plasmablastic morphology (e.g., high nuclear-to-cytoplasmic ratios, coarse chromatin, and prominent nucleoli) to anaplastic forms (e.g., marked nuclear pleomorphism, including binucleation/multinucleation)
- Hemorrhagic or necrotic background
- *Suggested IC panel on cell block preparation: CD20, CD79a, MUM1, CD138, CD38, CD56, Cyclin D1, CD117, EMA, kappa, lambda, IgG, IgA, IgM*

Explanatory Notes
Neoplastic plasma cells in serous effusion specimens may exhibit a wide spectrum of cytomorphological appearances; as a result, ancillary studies (e.g., flow cytometry or IC staining on a cell block preparation) are essential to confirm the clonal

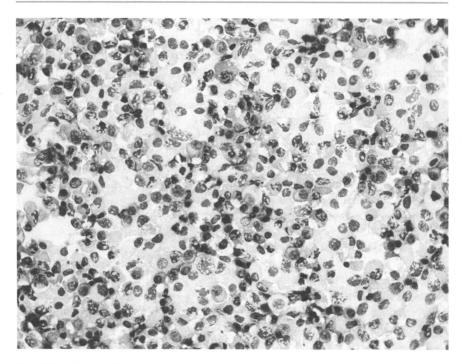

Fig. 7.15 Plasma cell myeloma. Numerous, mature-appearing plasma cells with eccentrically placed, round to oval nuclei. *(Pleural fluid, modified Giemsa stain, medium magnification)*

nature of the plasma cells. A specimen that contains mainly mature-appearing plasma cells can be sent for flow cytometric analysis [44]. However, if a specimen contains plasma cells that are poorly differentiated (e.g., those exhibiting plasmablastic or anaplastic morphological appearances), then IC staining on a cell block preparation is recommended. For such cases, the differential diagnosis includes non-hematolymphoid malignancies (such as melanoma or poorly differentiated carcinoma) as well as lymphoid neoplasms (such as plasmablastic lymphoma, ALCL, or PEL) [42]. The IC panel suggested above can be modified to include markers to help resolve these diagnostic issues. However, CD138 expression by a poorly differentiated neoplasm should be interpreted with caution, as it can be expressed by some B-cell lymphomas and is positive in a number of metastatic carcinomas [32].

Malignant Effusions of Melanocytic Origin

Melanoma

Involvement of the serous cavity by melanoma is exceedingly rare. The pleural cavity is the most commonly affected site and has been reported in less than 2% of metastatic melanoma cases [45]. The cytomorphological features of melanoma in serous fluids are similar to those of melanoma metastatic to other sites (Fig. 7.16).

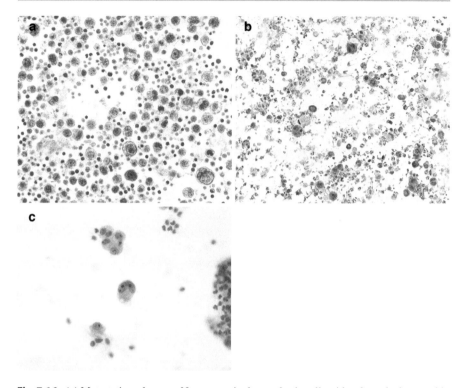

Fig. 7.16 (**a**) Metastatic melanoma. Numerous single neoplastic cells with enlarged, pleomorphic nuclei, prominent nucleoli, and intranuclear inclusions. *(Peritoneal fluid, Papanicolaou stain, high magnification).* (**b**) Metastatic melanoma. Many single malignant cells showing binucleation/multinucleation. *(Pleural fluid, Papanicolaou stain, medium magnification).* (**c**) Metastatic melanoma. A binucleated cell with eccentrically located nuclei, large "cherry-red" nucleoli, and dense to granular cytoplasm. *(Pleural fluid, Papanicolaou stain, high magnification)*

Cytological Criteria
- Predominantly single or loosely cohesive cells
- Epithelioid, plasmacytoid, or spindled cells
- Enlarged, oval, elongated, eccentrically placed, or pleomorphic nuclei
- Macronucleoli
- Intranuclear inclusions
- Binucleation/multinucleation
- Granular, eosinophilic cytoplasm that may contain brown melanin pigment

Explanatory Notes
Careful examination of the cytomorphological features, together with the clinical history and a panel of IC stains (e.g., SOX10, Melan-A, S100, HMB45), is usually sufficient to arrive at the correct diagnosis of metastatic melanoma.

Malignant Effusions of Mesenchymal Origin

Sarcomas

Sarcomas account for 3–6% of malignant effusions [46]. Although the vast majority of sarcomas involving the serous cavities are metastases, it is important to note that primary serosal sarcomas may also, very rarely, account for these cases. Only a few studies have examined the cytomorphological features of sarcomas in serous effusion specimens, and the most common observations are summarized below [46].

Cytological Criteria
- Often scant cellularity
- Tumor cells arranged singly or in loose clusters
- Variable cellular morphology (may be pleomorphic, epithelioid/polygonal, small and round, or spindled) (Fig. 7.17)
- Proteinaceous and/or hemorrhagic background

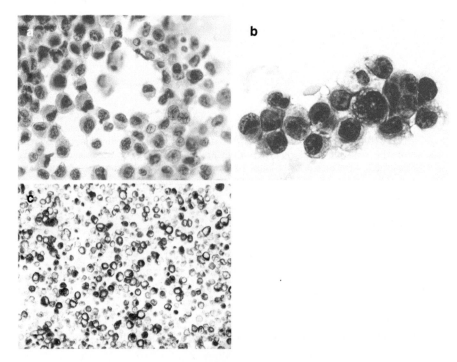

Fig. 7.17 (**a**) Metastatic alveolar rhabdomyosarcoma. Numerous discohesive single cells with epithelioid morphology and eccentrically placed, irregular nuclei, coarse chromatin, and prominent nucleoli. The mesenchymal origin of these malignant cells would be difficult to ascertain based on cytomorphology alone, and ancillary studies are required. *(Pleural fluid, Papanicolaou stain, high magnification).* (**b**) Metastatic alveolar rhabdomyosarcoma. Neoplastic cells with epithelioid morphology and enlarged, pleomorphic nuclei, coarse chromatin, and prominent nucleoli. *(Pleural fluid, modified Giemsa stain, high magnification).* (**c**) Metastatic alveolar rhabdomyosarcoma. Numerous discohesive single cells showing cytoplasmic expression of desmin. *(Pleural fluid, cell block, desmin stain, medium magnification)*

Explanatory Notes

Diagnostic subtyping of sarcomas in serous effusion specimens is particularly challenging. In comparison to fine-needle aspiration specimens of primary soft tissue tumors where subclassification can be guided by tumor cell morphology (e.g., spindled, pleomorphic, epithelioid/polygonal, small round cell) and the type of accompanying stromal elements [47, 48], the cytomorphology of the tumor cells in serous effusion specimens may differ from that of the original primary tumor since the tumor cells have a tendency to round up in fluid specimens [46]. Furthermore, the stromal patterns that may be observed in fine-needle aspiration specimens and provide clues to subtyping are not observed in serous fluid specimens. As a result, emphasis should be placed on recognizing the malignant nature of the tumor cells and confirming their mesenchymal origin while excluding the main differential diagnosis, including melanoma, poorly differentiated carcinoma, malignant mesothelioma, and small round blue cell tumors (in cases of sarcomas with small round cell morphology) [46].

Malignant Effusions of Germ Cell and Sex Cord-Stromal Origin

Germ Cell Tumors and Sex Cord-Stromal Tumors

As with sarcomas and melanomas, involvement of the serous cavity by metastatic germ cell tumors is exceedingly rare and usually presents in patients with advanced-stage disease. Studies examining the cytomorphological features of germ cell tumors in serous effusion specimens are lacking in the literature. The most common cytopathological features in the literature are summarized below [49].

Cytological Criteria

Seminoma/dysgerminoma

- Large discohesive cells
- Enlarged, round, vesicular nuclei
- Coarse chromatin
- Prominent nucleoli
- Small amounts of delicate to clear cytoplasm

Non-seminomatous germ cell tumors (embryonal carcinoma, yolk sac tumor, choriocarcinoma, malignant teratoma)

- Clusters and single large cells
- Pleomorphic, irregular nuclei
- Prominent nucleoli, often multiple
- Pale, finely granular chromatin
- Variable amounts of delicate to dense cytoplasm
- Syncytiotrophoblastic giant cells (primarily in choriocarcinoma but may occasionally be seen in embryonal carcinoma)

Sex cord-stromal tumor (adult granulosa cell tumor)

- Isolated cells or cohesive cell clusters
- Small- to medium-sized, uniform bland cells resembling mesothelial cells
- Round, monomorphic nuclei
- Pale chromatin
- Small, inconspicuous nucleoli
- Nuclear grooves
- Ill-defined cytoplasm

Explanatory Notes

Diagnosis of germ cell tumors in serous effusions based on cytomorphology alone can be challenging. Recognition of the tumor cells as malignant and confirming their origin based on the clinical history and IC stains will help arrive at the correct diagnosis. Both seminoma and embryonal carcinoma are positive for PLAP, OCT4, SALL4, and NANOG. Seminoma/dysgerminoma additionally stains positive for D2-40 and CD117, while embryonal carcinoma is characterized by positive staining for CD30 and SOX2. Yolk sac tumor is positive for AFP, glypican 3, SALL4, and HNF1β and negative for OCT4, NANOG, CD30 and SOX2. Choriocarcinoma is positive for pan-cytokeratin, CK7, and HCG; patients with choriocarcinoma typically have markedly elevated serum HCG levels. Although IC stains are usually not utilized in the diagnosis of teratoma, various elements in these tumors can stain positive for AFP, glypican 3, SOX2 and SALL4 (the latter two especially in primitive neuroectodermal components). OCT4 is typically negative in teratomas. Sex cord-stromal differentiation is supported by positive staining with calretinin, inhibin, SF1, and FOXL2 [50–52].

Rate and Risk of Malignancy/Clinical Management

As previously noted, the rate of malignancy varies widely in the literature, and reports may include both primary (mesothelioma) and secondary (metastatic) cases. Further targeted studies are necessary to highlight the prevalence of metastatic tumors overall in serous fluids and the propensity of tumors to target specific body cavities, since these values can change over time with changes in disease prevalence.

The risk of malignancy (ROM) in cases interpreted as malignant (MAL) is 99% in a recent meta-analysis [53], indicating the high accuracy of cytology for this diagnostic category.

Sample Reports

Example 7.1

Pleural fluid:
Satisfactory for evaluation

Malignant effusion, consistent with metastatic adenocarcinoma of primary breast origin
Category: Malignant-secondary

Note: The cytospin preparations are highly cellular and show many large, three-dimensional ("cannonball") groups of malignant cells with enlarged, pleomorphic nuclei, coarse chromatin, and prominent nucleoli. The cytomorphological features are those of metastatic adenocarcinoma, consistent with primary origin from the patient's known history of breast carcinoma.

Example 7.2

Ascitic fluid:
Satisfactory for evaluation
Malignant effusion, consistent with metastatic high-grade serous carcinoma
Category: Malignant-secondary

Note: The cytospin preparations are highly cellular and show numerous papillary fragments and clusters of malignant cells with enlarged, hyperchromatic nuclei, prominent nucleoli, and cytoplasmic vacuolation. Immunohistochemical staining performed on the cell block preparation shows the malignant cells to diffusely express Ber-EP4, PAX8, WT1, and ER, with complete absence of p53 expression (null phenotype). The cytomorphological and immunophenotypic features are those of metastatic high-grade serous carcinoma of ovarian, tubal, or peritoneal origin.

Example 7.3

Pleural fluid:
Satisfactory for evaluation
Malignant effusion, consistent with involvement by chronic lymphocytic leukemia/
    small lymphocytic lymphoma
Category: Malignant-secondary

Note: The cytospin preparations show a monotonous population of small lymphoid cells with uniform round to ovoid nuclei and coarse clumped chromatin. Flow cytometry confirms a predominant B-cell population expressing CD19, CD20(dim), CD43, CD5, CD23, and CD200 and showing kappa light chain restriction. They are negative for CD10 and FMC7. The cytomorphological and immunophenotypic features are those of chronic lymphocytic leukemia/small lymphocytic lymphoma.

Example 7.4

Pleural fluid:
Satisfactory for evaluation
Malignant effusion, consistent with metastatic melanoma
Category: Malignant-secondary

Note: The cytospin preparations show numerous discohesive malignant cells with moderate amounts of granular cytoplasm with focal intracytoplasmic pigment, pleomorphic nuclei, and macronucleoli. A few binucleate/multinucleate forms are also seen. Immunohistochemical staining performed on the cell block preparation shows the malignant cells to express S100, Melan-A, and HMB-45. They are negative for AE1/AE3 and CD45. The cytomorphological and immunophenotypic features are those of metastatic melanoma.

References

1. Lepus CM, Vivero M. Updates in effusion cytology. Surg Pathol Clin. 2018;11(3):523–44.
2. Starr RL, Sherman ME. The value of multiple preparations in the diagnosis of malignant pleural effusions. A cost-benefit analysis. Acta Cytol. 1991;35(5):533–7.
3. Motherby H, Nadjari B, Friegel P, Kohaus J, Ramp U, Böcking A. Diagnostic accuracy of effusion cytology. Diagn Cytopathol. 1999;20(6):350–7.
4. Johnston WW. The malignant pleural effusion. A review of cytopathologic diagnoses of 584 specimens from 472 consecutive patients. Cancer. 1985;56(4):905–9.
5. Monte SA, Ehya H, Lang WR. Positive effusion cytology as the initial presentation of malignancy. Acta Cytol. 1987;31(4):448–52.
6. Sears D, Hajdu SI. The cytologic diagnosis of malignant neoplasms in pleural and peritoneal effusions. Acta Cytol. 1987;31(2):85–97.
7. Pereira TC, Saad RS, Liu Y, Silverman JF. The diagnosis of malignancy in effusion cytology: a pattern recognition approach. Adv Anat Pathol. 2006;13(4):174–84.
8. Davidson B, Firat P, Michael CM. Serous effusions – etiology, diagnosis, prognosis and therapy. London: Springer; 2018.
9. LePhong C, Hubbard EW, Van Meter S, Nodit L. Squamous cell carcinoma in serous effusions: avoiding pitfalls in this rare encounter. Diagn Cytopathol. 2017;45(12):1095–9.
10. Huang CC, Michael CW. Cytomorphological features of metastatic squamous cell carcinoma in serous effusions. Cytopathology. 2014;25(2):112–9.
11. Chen L, Caldero SG, Gmitro S, Smith ML, Petris G, Zarka MA. Small orangiophilic squamous-like cells: an underrecognized and useful morphological feature for the diagnosis of malignant mesothelioma in pleural effusion cytology. Cancer Cytopathol. 2014;122(1):70–5.
12. DeMay RM. Fluids. In: The art and science of cytopathology, vol. Vol. 1. 2nd ed. Chicago: ASCP Press; 2012. p. 286–7.
13. Chhieng DC, Ko EC, Yee HT, Shultz JJ, Dorvault CC, Eltoum IA. Malignant pleural effusions due to small-cell lung carcinoma: a cytologic and immunocytochemical study. Diagn Cytopathol. 2001;25(6):356–60.
14. Das DK, Al-Juwaiser A, George SS, et al. Cytomorphological and immunocytochemical study of non-Hodgkin's lymphoma in pleural effusion and ascitic fluid. Cytopathology. 2007;18(3):157–67.
15. Das DK. Serous effusions in malignant lymphomas: a review. Diagn Cytopathol. 2006;34(5):335–47.
16. García-Riego A, Cuiñas C, Vilanova JJ. Malignant pericardial effusion. Acta Cytol. 2001;45(4):561–6.
17. Wong JW, Pitlik D, Abdul-Karim FW. Cytology of pleural, peritoneal and pericardial fluids in children. A 40-year summary. Acta Cytol. 1997;41(2):467–73.
18. Hallman JR, Geisinger KR. Cytology of fluids from pleural, peritoneal and pericardial cavities in children. A comprehensive survey. Acta Cytol. 1994;38(2):209–17.
19. Alexandrakis MG, Passam FH, Kyriakou DS, Bouros D. Pleural effusions in hematologic malignancies. Chest. 2004;125(4):1546–55.

20. Berkman N, Breuer R, Kramer MR, Polliack A. Pulmonary involvement in lymphoma. Leuk Lymphoma. 1996;20(3–4):229–37.
21. McGrath EE, Blades Z, Anderson PB. Chylothorax: aetiology, diagnosis and therapeutic options. Respir Med. 2010;104(1):1–8.
22. Tong LC, Ko HM, Saieg MA, Boerner S, Geddie WR, da Cunha Santos G. Subclassification of lymphoproliferative disorders in serous effusions: a 10-year experience. Cancer Cytopathol. 2013;121(5):261–70.
23. Bangerter M, Hildebrand A, Griesshammer M. Combined cytomorphologic and immunophenotypic analysis in the diagnostic workup of lymphomatous effusions. Acta Cytol. 2001;45(3):307–12.
24. Yu GH, Vergara N, Moore EM, King RL. Use of flow cytometry in the diagnosis of lymphoproliferative disorders in fluid specimens. Diagn Cytopathol. 2014;42(3):664–70.
25. Barroca H, Marques C. A basic approach to lymph node and flow cytometry fine-needle cytology. Acta Cytol. 2016;60(4):284–301.
26. Bode-Lesniewska B. Flow cytometry and effusions in lymphoproliferative processes and other hematologic neoplasias. Acta Cytol. 2016;60(4):354–64.
27. Czader M, Ali SZ. Flow cytometry as an adjunct to cytomorphologic analysis of serous effusions. Diagn Cytopathol. 2003;29(2):74–8.
28. Iqbal J, Liu T, Mapow B, Swami VK, Hou JS. Importance of flow cytometric analysis of serous effusions in the diagnosis of hematopoietic neoplasms in patients with prior hematopoietic malignancies. Anal Quant Cytol Histol. 2010;32(3):161–5.
29. Laucirica R, Schwartz MR. Clinical utility of flow cytometry in body fluid cytology: to flow or not to flow? That is the question. Diagn Cytopathol. 2001;24(5):305–6.
30. Simsir A, Fetsch P, Stetler-Stevenson M, Abati A. Immunophenotypic analysis of non-Hodgkin's lymphomas in cytologic specimens: a correlative study of immunocytochemical and flow cytometric techniques. Diagn Cytopathol. 1999;20(5):278–84.
31. Kesler MV, Paranjape GS, Asplund SL, McKenna RW, Jamal S, Kroft SH. Anaplastic large cell lymphoma: a flow cytometric analysis of 29 cases. Am J Clin Pathol. 2007;128(2):314–22.
32. Jaffe E, Arber DA, Campo E, Harris NL, Quintanilla-Fend L, editors. Hematopathology. 2nd ed. Philadelphia: Elsevier; 2017.
33. El-Fattah MA. Clinical characteristics and survival outcome of primary effusion lymphoma: a review of 105 patients. Hematol Oncol. 2017;35(4):878–83.
34. Bashir H, Hudson MM, Kaste SC, Howard SC, Krasin M, Metzger ML. Pericardial involvement at diagnosis in pediatric Hodgkin lymphoma patients. Pediatr Blood Cancer. 2007;49(5):666–71.
35. Peterson IM, Raible M. Malignant pleural effusion in Hodgkin's lymphoma. Report of a case with immunoperoxidase studies. Acta Cytol. 1991;35(3):300–5.
36. Olson PR, Silverman JF, Powers CN. Pleural fluid cytology of Hodgkin's disease: cytomorphologic features and the value of immunohistochemical studies. Diagn Cytopathol. 2000;22(1):21–4.
37. Kito M, Munakata W, Ono K, Maeshima AM, Matsushita H. The infiltration of classical Hodgkin lymphoma cells into pleural effusion. Int J Hematol. 2018;107(1):1–2.
38. Das DK, Chowdhury V, Kishore B, Chachra K, Bhatt NC, Kakar AK. CD-30 (Ki-1)-positive anaplastic large cell lymphoma in a pleural effusion. A case report with diagnosis by cytomorphologic and immunocytochemical studies. Acta Cytol. 1999;43(3):498–502.
39. Jiménez-Heffernan JA, Viguer JM, Vicandi B, et al. Posttransplant CD30 (Ki-1)-positive anaplastic large cell lymphoma. Report of a case with presentation as a pleural effusion. Acta Cytol. 1997;41(5):1519–24.
40. Irwin RS, Saunders RL, Isaac PC, Marcus JB, Corrao WM. Sternberg-Reed-like cells in a pleural effusion secondary to pulmonary emboli with infarction: a cytological observation. Arch Pathol Lab Med. 1978;102(2):76–8.
41. Silverman JF. Extramedullary hematopoietic ascitic fluid cytology in myelofibrosis. Am J Clin Pathol. 1985;84(1):125–8.

42. Harbhajanka A, Brickman A, Park JW, Reddy VB, Bitterman P, Gattuso P. Cytomorphology, clinicopathologic, and cytogenetics correlation of myelomatous effusion of serous cavities: a retrospective review. Diagn Cytopathol. 2016;44(9):742–7.
43. Chen H, Li P, Xie Y, Jin M. Cytology and clinical features of myelomatous pleural effusion: three case reports and a review of the literature. Diagn Cytopathol. 2018;46(7):604–9.
44. Palmer HE, Wilson CS, Bardales RH. Cytology and flow cytometry of malignant effusions of multiple myeloma. Diagn Cytopathol. 2000;22(3):147–51.
45. Chen JT, Dahmash NS, Ravin CE, et al. Metastatic melanoma to the thorax: report of 130 patients. Am J Roentgenol. 1981;137(2):293–8.
46. Abadi MA, Zakowski MF. Cytologic features of sarcomas in fluids. Cancer. 1998;84(2):71–6.
47. González-Cámpora R, Muñoz-Arias G, Otal-Salaverri C, et al. Fine needle aspiration cytology of primary soft tissue tumors. Morphologic analysis of the most frequent types. Acta Cytol. 1992;36(6):905–17.
48. Palmer HE, Mukunyadzi P, Culbreth W, Thomas JR. Subgrouping and grading of soft-tissue sarcomas by fine-needle aspiration cytology: a histopathologic correlation study. Diagn Cytopathol. 2001;24(5):307–16.
49. Cibas E, Ducatman B. Chapter 4 – pleural, pericardial, and peritoneal fluids. In: Cytology: diagnostic principles and clinical correlates. 4th ed. Philadelphia: Elsevier Saunders; 2014. p. 150–1.
50. Jones TD, Ulbright TM, Eble JN, Cheng L. OCT4 staining in testicular tumors. A sensitive and specific marker for testicular seminoma and embryonal carcinoma. Am J Surg Pathol. 2004;28(7):935–40.
51. Rabban JT, Zaloudek CJ. A practical approach to immunohistochemical diagnosis of ovarian germ cell tumours and sex cord-stromal tumours. Histopathology. 2013;62(1):71–88.
52. Kaspar HG, Crum CP. The utility of immunohistochemistry in the differential diagnosis of gynecologic disorders. Arch Pathol Lab Med. 2015;139(1):39–54.
53. Farahani SJ, Baloch Z. Are we ready to develop a tiered scheme for the effusion cytology? A comprehensive review and analysis of the literature. Diag Cytopathol. 2019;47(11):1145–59.

Ancillary Studies for Serous Fluids

Lukas Bubendorf, Pinar Firat, Ibrahim Kulac,
Pasquale Pisapia, Spasenija Savic-Prince, Gilda Santos,
and Giancarlo Troncone

Background

While IC is available and well-established in most pathology and cytology laboratories, the high variability of technical procedures for collection, handling, fixation, and types of preparations of cytological specimens remains a challenge. The use of IC markers and panels for refined diagnosis and classification of malignancies is well-established. An increasing number of molecular ancillary tests to detect numerical as well as structural chromosomal aberrations and gene mutations have also been added to diagnostic algorithms. As an example, homozygous 9p21 deletion shown by fluorescence in situ hybridization (FISH) in atypical mesothelial cells is diagnostic of mesothelioma, making this type of FISH analysis indispensable in many cases with suspicion of mesothelioma. In hematolymphoid proliferations found in effusions, analysis of multiple markers by flow cytometry can be instrumental to exclude or diagnose hematolymphoid neoplasms and may be supplemented by FISH analysis for specific gene rearrangements as needed in some

L. Bubendorf (✉) · S. Savic-Prince
Institute of Pathology, University Hospital Basel, Basel, Switzerland
e-mail: Lukas.Bubendorf@usb.ch

P. Firat
Department of Pathology, School of Medicine, Koç University, Istanbul, Turkey

I. Kulac
Koc University Schoold of Medicine, Istanbul, Turkey

P. Pisapia
University of Naples Federico II, Public Health, Naples, Italy

G. Santos
Department of Cellular Pathology, Royal Victoria Hospital, Belfast Health and Social Care Trust, Belfast, UK

G. Troncone
Department of Public Health, University of Naples "Federico II", Naples, Italy

© Springer Nature Switzerland AG 2020
A. Chandra et al. (eds.), *The International System for Serous Fluid Cytopathology*, https://doi.org/10.1007/978-3-030-53908-5_8

lymphoma subtypes. The importance of analysis of malignant effusions increases with the steadily growing number of new predictive markers and approval of related new drugs, particularly evident for lung cancer but also applied to many other tumor types. The alterations range from abnormal expression (e.g., estrogen receptor, mismatch repair deficiency proteins, and programmed death-ligand 1 [PD-L1]) to gene mutations, rearrangements, and copy number changes (e.g., amplifications). The main methods used for the detection of these alterations include IC, FISH, quantitative polymerase chain reaction (PCR) assays, and DNA- and/or RNA-based next-generation sequencing (NGS), which can all be performed using cytological material. However, the large variability in cytological specimen types, preanalytical conditions, and the dichotomy between cell block (CB) and non-CB cytology require tailored approaches and protocols. Besides serving as a valuable substrate for state-of-the-art molecular testing, effusions provide exciting opportunities for research and technology development. For example, the supernatant of malignant effusion may contain precious information waiting to be exploited. This includes protein signatures, cell-free DNA, and living tumor cells that can be used for ex vivo systems for studying tumor biology or individual drug sensitivity testing.

Predictive Immunocytochemistry (IC)

The discovery of molecular alterations in many cancer types has led to a major shift from classical chemotherapy toward targeted therapies for cancer patients. Over time, selective tyrosine kinase inhibitors have become first-line options. These developments in cancer treatment require specific testing for molecular alterations. Along with other methods for identifying molecular alterations such as FISH, sequencing, and PCR-based assays, IC is a fast and reliable method for prescreening or detection of some of these alterations (Table 8.1). In addition, IC has become even more important after the development of immune check point inhibitors, since PD-L1 expression is one of the main predictors of immunotherapy response.

Predictive IC assays validated for use on formalin-fixed and paraffin-embedded (FFPE) tissues are readily available, as are guidelines and recommendations for validation of comparable laboratory-developed tests [1–3]. Staining patterns and cutoffs for positivity are well-established, allowing for selection of eligible patients for related therapies. Cytology is an invaluable source for testing these biomarkers; however, cytologic samples need further laboratory validation, since their preanalytical factors are more variable and less standardized than tissue samples. Different preservatives, fixatives (e.g., ethanol and methanol), and staining techniques are used. Cytologic preparation techniques range from direct smears to cytospins and liquid-based preparations [4]. FFPE cytology cell blocks (CBs) are frequently preferred for immunostaining since the processing is similar to FFPE histology specimens. Because different cytology CB preparation methods exist, IC protocols used for FFPE histology specimens should be revalidated for cytology CBs [5]. If only formalin fixation is used for the CB preparation, without prefixation with ethanol- or methanol-based solutions, then the results will be highly concordant with the histologic samples. CBs may be less cellular than smears or cytospins, causing a problem with interpretation of predictive IC,

Table 8.1 Established predictive immunochemistry (IC) markers

IC[a] marker	Indication	Minimum # of cells required	IC[a] Staining pattern	FISH[b] verification	PCR[c]/NGS[d] verification
PDL1[e]	Immunotherapy	100	Membranous (cell block); more diffuse in non-cell block preparations	Not applicable	Not applicable
ALK[f]	Tyrosine kinase inhibitor therapy	Not applicable	Cytoplasmic and membranous	Not mandatory	Not mandatory
ROS1[g]	Tyrosine kinase inhibitor therapy	Not applicable	Cytoplasmic and membranous	Required	Required
Pan-TRK[h]	Tyrosine kinase inhibitor therapy	Not applicable	Nuclear, perinuclear, cytoplasmic, and membranous	Required	Required
HER2[i]	Anti-ERBB2 therapy	Not applicable	Membranous	Required if IC is equivocal (2+)	Not applicable
ER[j]/ PR[k]	Hormonal therapy	Not applicable	Nuclear	Not applicable	Not applicable
MMR[l]	Immunotherapy	Not applicable	Nuclear	Not applicable	Not mandatory

[a]*IC* Immunochemistry
[b]*FISH* Fluorescent in situ hybridization
[c]*PCR* Polymerase chain reaction
[d]*NGS* Next-generation sequencing
[e]*PDL1* Programmed death-ligand 1
[f]*ALK* Anaplastic lymphoma kinase
[g]*ROS1* c-Ros oncogene 1
[h]*Pan-TRK* Pan-tropomyosin receptor kinase
[i]*HER2* Human epidermal growth factor 2
[j]*ER* Estrogen receptor
[k]*PR* Progesterone receptor
[l]*MMR* Mismatch repair proteins

especially for heterogeneously expressed biomarkers such as PD-L1. In addition, CB material is not always available. Laboratories should therefore be prepared to reliably apply predictive biomarkers on non-CB cytologic specimens, such as smears, if possible. In a recent review, Jain et al. discussed the preanalytical, analytical, and postanalytical factors that influence the results of predictive IC in various cytology preparations in detail, which may help to guide the validation processes for cytology samples in laboratories [5].

PD-L1

PD-L1 is a transmembrane protein expressed by many cell types that interact with its receptor PD-1 on immune cells. This interaction suppresses immune response. In normal cells, PD-L1 prevents the erroneous destruction of host cells by the immune system. Many cancer types express PD-L1 as a strategy of the cancer cells to escape from immune response to tumor neoantigens. Blocking this interaction with mono-clonal antibodies against PD-1/PD-L1 results in substantial clinical improvement in some cancer types such as non-small cell lung cancer (NSCLC).

Response to therapy mostly depends on the level of PD-L1 expression in the tumor cells. Immunochemical PD-L1 testing does not give a black and white result but often provides continuous expression ranging from 1% to 100% of the tumor cells. Different scoring systems and cutoffs are used to select patients for therapy in different clinical trials for various tumor types [6]. Not only tumor cell but inflam-matory cell expression has been included in some scoring systems for particular indications. Several antibodies for PD-L1 testing have been developed, and some have been commercialized as validated assays: SP263 and SP142 Ventana assay and 22C3 and 22-8 PharmDx assay. Among these four assays, SP263, 22C3, and 22-8 show high concordance with each other, whereas SP142 is found to be less sensitive than the others [7–9].

For NSCLC, the efficacy of response is determined by the level of expression of PD-L1 on tumor cells. Tumor proportion score (TPS) is a measure of expression defined as the number of positive tumor cells divided by the number of total tumor cells. Any membranous staining, regardless of the intensity, complete or partial, is considered positive. At least 100 viable tumor cells are needed for evaluation. Criteria to evaluate PD-L1 expression on tumor cells are standardized throughout all indications and tumor types, but expression on inflammatory cells is more diffi-cult to interpret. In some tumors and/or indications, not only tumor cells but also inflammatory cells are evaluated for PD-L1 expression, and different scoring sys-tems are recommended for therapy plans. For NSCLC, TPS 50% is an important cutoff for treatment decisions regarding first-line single-agent treatment using pem-brolizumab. Staining of neighboring immune cells is irrelevant for this indication, which makes scoring possible and reliable on cytology. In contrast, accurate scoring of immune cells is virtually impossible in cytologic specimens due to the lack of architectural context.

There are several studies in the literature showing high concordance between CBs and histology samples for PD-L1 testing [10–12]. There is also emerging evidence suggesting that direct smears and liquid-based preparations might be equally suitable for PD-L1 testing, but more studies are needed [6, 13]. Criteria to define PD-L1-positive tumor cells in smears, cytospins, or liquid-based cytology (LBC) might differ from those in biopsy or CB sections, since membranous accentuation in uncut tumor cells is less distinct due to physical reasons [14]. Malignant effusions are a common substrate for PD-L1 testing, since they are often obtained from advanced disease patients and often highly cellular (Fig. 8.1). Positive cells should be interpreted with caution. Tumor cells in effusion speci-mens are usually admixed with macrophages, which are physiologically PD-L1-positive. Differentiation of PD-L1-positive macrophages from tumor cells can be challenging and cause false-positive results, especially if not analyzed by trained individuals for the interpretation of PD-L1 testing and with sufficient experience in cytology [12, 15, 16].

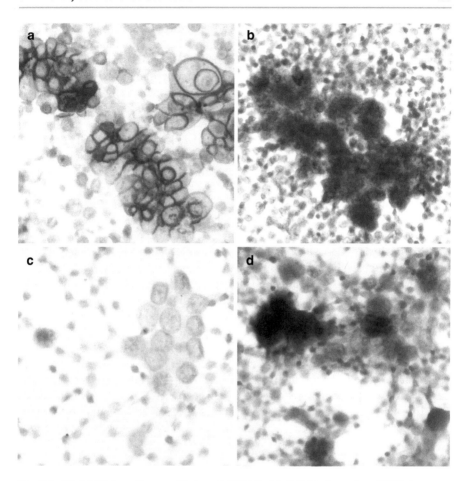

Fig. 8.1 PD-L1 IC in malignant effusion of NSCLC. (**a**) Cell block section. SP263 Assay on Ventana Benchmark. Distinct membranous PD-L1 staining in all tumor cells and weakly positive macrophages in the background. (**b–d**) Previously Papanicolaou-stained ethanol-fixed smears, laboratory developed test (LDT) with SP263 antibody on Leica Bond. (**b**) Diffuse staining of tumor cells without membranous accentuation. (**c**) PD-L1-negative tumor cells and an adjacent macrophage serving as a positive internal control. (**d**) Heterogenous PD-L1 staining with focal membranous accentuation

ALK

ALK (Anaplastic lymphoma kinase) is a receptor tyrosine kinase that functions as an important inducer of cellular development. Fusion of the *ALK* gene prevails as a driver alteration in approximately 5% of NSCLC, and it has also rarely been found in mesothelioma [17, 18]. ALK inhibitors have shown high response rates in treatment of tumors with *ALK* fusion [19]. Since detection of an *ALK* gene rearrangement is required for treatment with ALK inhibitors, guidelines mandate *ALK* testing for all NSCLC patients [1].

FISH has been the standard method for detecting *ALK* fusion. Based on the high concordance of IC with FISH, IC has now become the standard for ALK testing when using the commercial Ventana ALK (D5F3) assay [1, 20]. Two ALK clones are widely accepted as FISH equivalent; one has been approved as an assay (clone D5F3 by Ventana), and the other (clone 5A4) gives comparable results [5]. Even cases with positive ALK IC but negative FISH result respond well to ALK inhibitors, most probably due to false-negative FISH results [21]. On the other hand, ALK FISH-positive and ALK IC-negative NSCLC respond poorly, which has been explained by either false-positive FISH results or, less commonly, by rare complex rearrangements that do not lead to *ALK* overexpression. Given these pitfalls, it has been proposed to use IC and FISH concurrently for *ALK* testing, as it is the case for ROS proto-oncogene 1, receptor tyrosine kinase (*ROS1*), and neurotrophic receptor tyrosine kinase (*NTRK*) testing, as discussed below [22].

ALK-positive tumors show granular cytoplasmic staining without membranous blush. The cytoplasmic staining is particularly strong and granular when using the D5F3 assay but less so when using laboratory developed tests based on the 5A4 clone. Although Zhang et al. proposed a required minimum of 200 cells for ALK IC testing, there is currently no consensus recommendation for the minimum number of cells for ALK IC, since ALK is known to be diffusely positive throughout the tumor [5, 23].

CBs or other cytological samples can be accurately used for ALK IC (Fig. 8.2). Many studies showed very high concordance with low false-positive and false-negative results; the results tended to be even better when D5F3 clone was used [24, 25]. Effusion specimens have also been studied for ALK fusion either by FISH or IC, and these studies showed a high concordance of cytology with tissue samples [26–28].

ROS1

ROS1 is a receptor tyrosine kinase that is activated in various cancer types including NSCLC. *ROS1* fusion frequency is reported in 1–2% of all NSCLCs in various studies [29, 30]. Targeted inhibitors of ROS1 had high response rates. Current guidelines mandate ROS1 testing for all NSCLC [1]. FISH or real-time PCR (RT-PCR) is regarded as a gold standard for testing ROS1 fusions, and RNA-based next-generation sequencing (NGS) methods are increasingly being used to cover multiple rearrangements when there is limited specimen [31].

ROS1 IC is currently being used as a screening test, not as a definite indicator of fusion, due to lack of standardized reporting. The expression of ROS1 in tumor cells with *ROS1* gene rearrangement is dynamic, and the heterogeneous staining intensity of these tumors causes difficulties with interpretation. Any positivity should be further tested by FISH, RT-PCR, or NGS. Unlike ALK IC, the higher rates of false

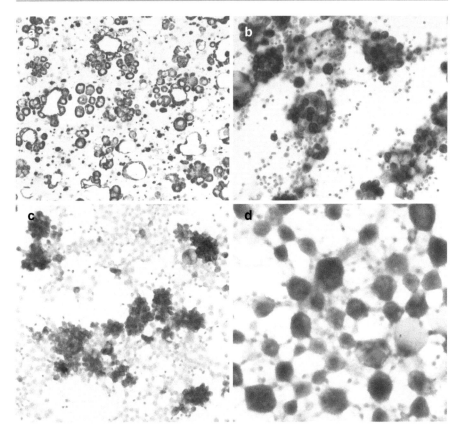

Fig. 8.2 ALK IC in malignant effusions from pulmonary adenocarcinomas with confirmed ALK rearrangements showing consistent cytoplasmic staining using DAB (**a**, **b**) or AEC (**c**, **d**) as a chromogen. (**a**) Cell block section. D5F3 Assay on Ventana Benchmark. (**b–d**) Previously Papanicolaou-stained ethanol-fixed smears using 5A4 LDT on Leica Bond. (**b**) Same case as (**a**)

positivity with ROS1 antibody require confirmation with a highly specific method [29, 32–34]. In general, an H-score of 100 or 150 has been proposed as a reliable threshold for detecting ROS1 rearrangement. However, there are also series claiming 100% correlation between immune staining and other molecular tests, and indeed these results have been obtained on cytological specimens [35]. Almost all cytological samples (including CBs and smears) can be used for ROS1 IC testing, as reported by several studies (Fig. 8.3) [32, 35]. There are two commercially available ROS1 antibodies: SP384 (Ventana, Tucson, Arizona) and D4D6 (Cell Signaling, Danvers, Massachusetts). A recent multicenter study reported recommendations for specific cutoffs and staining protocols for Ventana ROS1 (SP384) antibody [36]. Notably, there is physiological ROS1 expression of activated type 2 alveolar cells and macrophages, the latter of which requires attention in malignant effusion to avoid false-positive IC results.

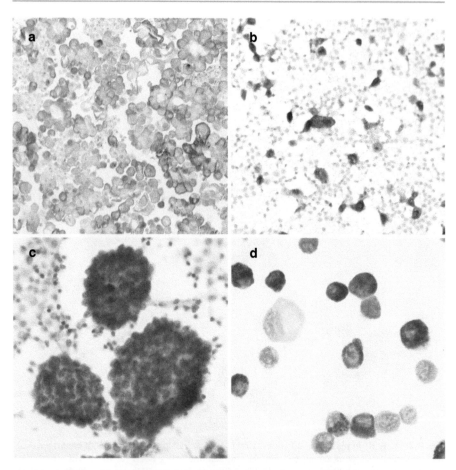

Fig. 8.3 ROS1 IC using cell signaling D4D6 antibody on Ventana Benchmark (**a**) and Leica Bond (**b–d**) in malignant effusions from pulmonary adenocarcinomas with confirmed ROS1 rearrangements. Note the variable staining intensity between tumor cells in (**a, b**) and (**d**). (**a**) Cell block section and (**b–d**) previously Papanicolaou-stained ethanol-fixed smears. (**d**) Cell line HCC-78 serving as positive external control

Pan-TRK

Fusions of *NTRK* isoforms *(NTRK1, NTRK2, NTRK3)* have gained much interest lately. Although rare (<0.5% of lung cancers), *NTRK* fusions are seen in a variety of tumors [37]. For example, rare *NTRK* as well as *ALK* and *ROS1* rearrangements is enriched in right-sided, Kirsten rat sarcoma viral oncogene homolog (*KRAS*) wild-type and microsatellite unstable colorectal adenocarcinomas [38]. Recently the Food and Drug Administration (FDA) has approved a tumor-agnostic anti-NTRK drug for any tumor type with NTRK fusion [39].

The standard method of detecting *NTRK* fusions is RNA-based NGS because it sequences all three isoforms. Fluorescence in situ hybridization may seem like a reasonable method, but it would be inefficient, laborious, and expensive to detect all three isoforms by FISH, given their very low prevalence. A recently developed pan-TRK antibody, which is capable of detecting all three fusions, has been recommended as a fast and reliable screening method for all tumor types [40]. Since it is a fairly reliable surrogate for the fusion of these three isoforms, pan-TRK IC seems to be promising and practical.

There is a FDA-approved assay for pan-TRK IC (Ventana-Clone EPR17341) and two additional commercial antibodies (Clone EPR17341 and Clone A7H6R). According to currently published data, these antibodies can be used for screening *NTRK* [41], although a proportion of *NTRK3* fusions might be missed by IC [42]. Staining can be seen in the nucleus, the nuclear membrane, or the cellular membrane [40]. Although not fully established yet, any staining above 1% of tumor cells should be interpreted as positive, and all positive results must be confirmed by molecular techniques. Although cytological samples seem like a suitable resource for pan-TRK immunostaining, currently there are not enough data on the concordance with tissue counterparts.

HER2

HER2 (Erb-B2 receptor tyrosine kinase 2 [ERBB2]) is a growth factor receptor and a member of the receptor tyrosine kinase family. Amplification of *HER2* gene is a relatively common event in breast cancer, gastric cancer, and tumors of the gastro-esophageal junction but is also rarely found in other tumors such as NSCLC, cholangiocarcinoma, or endometrial carcinoma. Amplified *HER2* gene qualifies patients for approved anti-HER2 treatment or clinical trials, depending on the tumor type. HER2 IC has a very high concordance with FISH; therefore, IC is recommended as a first-line method for *HER2* amplification [43]. Criteria for the evaluation of *HER2* amplification by IC have been defined for tumor types through specific guidelines [44, 45].

Studies have shown that HER2 IC can reliably be performed on CBs of cytological samples (Fig. 8.4) [46]. Analysis and scoring of HER2 IC are less well studied in other cytologic preparations and therefore not recommended [47]. Guidelines specific to the tumor type should be followed for accurate assessment of HER2 IC.

ER and PR

Estrogen receptor (ER) and/or progesterone receptor (PR)-positive breast cancer patients are candidates for hormonal therapy. Evaluation of ER and PR is based on the percentage of positive tumor cells. Biopsy specimens are routinely tested for ER

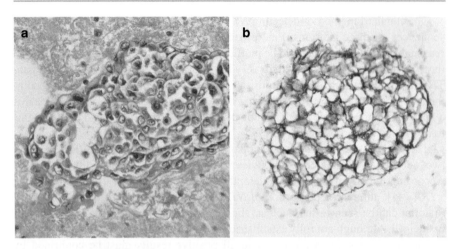

Fig. 8.4 Pleural metastasis of breast cancer (cell block). (**a**) H&E. (**b**) HER2 (3+) IC showing circumferential membranous staining in all tumor cells

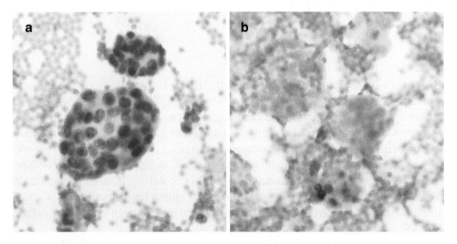

Fig. 8.5 Pleural metastasis of breast cancer. IC on Leica Bond using previously Papanicolaou-stained ethanol-fixed smears. (**a**) Estrogen receptor (ER) positive in >90% if tumor cells. (**b**) Only focal expression of progesterone receptor (PR)

and PR expression, and IC is the only method used. Cytologic specimens are effective for ER and PR testing on metastatic sites and commonly used to determine the receptor status of metastatic breast carcinoma (Fig. 8.5). Studies reported very high concordance between aspirations and subsequent surgical resections, so cytology can safely be used and is highly reliable for ER/PR testing [48, 49]. Cytospin slides, liquid-based preparations, or CBs prepared from effusions are good and reliable alternatives for testing the expression of steroid receptors, as shown by multiple studies [50, 51].

Mismatch Repair (MRR) Proteins

Microsatellite instability (MSI) is one of the useful predictive markers to select patients for immunotherapy, along with PD-L1 expression and tumor mutation burden, especially for colorectal cancer and other types of adenocarcinomas [52, 53]. Although direct sequencing of microsatellite regions is the gold standard in order to classify a tumor as microsatellite stable (MSS) or microsatellite instable (MSI), immunochemical detection of loss of the mismatch repair (MMR) proteins postmeiotic segregation increased 2 (PMS2), mutL homologue 1 (MLH1), mutS homologue 2 (MSH2), and mutS homologue 6 (MSH6) is a practical and less costly option [54]. The current recommendation is to perform all four antibodies, though some laboratories perform only two antibodies (PMS2 and MSH6). Certain combinations of the loss of these proteins (loss of PMS2 and MLH1 combined, loss of MSH2 and MSH6 combined, loss of MSH6, loss of PMS2) are indicators of a MSI tumor, as defined by guidelines [55, 56].

There are no recommendations for using cytologic specimens to test for the loss of MMR protein. One should be extremely careful while using CBs or other cytologic samples, since the level of MMR protein expression may vary in a tumor and this may result in false negativity due to the paucity of tumor cells.

ARID1A

The list of potentially predictive IC markers is continuously growing, along with increasing knowledge on disease mechanisms and new drug developments. The AT-rich interaction domain 1A (*ARID1A*) is one of these promising candidate biomarkers [57, 58]. *ARID1A* is a chromatin remodeling gene with tumor suppressor functions. Mutations or loss of the *ARID1A* gene mostly leads to its inactivation and ARID1A protein loss [57]. *ARID1A* is one of the most frequently mutated tumor suppressor genes across all solid tumor types, and mutations are particularly common in urothelial carcinoma (up to 20%) and in ovarian clear-cell carcinoma (50%). Importantly, ARID1A deficiency has been proposed as a potential predictive marker of response to immune checkpoint inhibitors, which is at least partly explained by increased mutability and PD-L1 overexpression [59]. In ovarian clear-cell carcinoma, ARID1A deficiency also appears to be associated with better response to chemotherapy with gemcitabine. Intriguingly, a recent study also suggested higher vulnerability of ARID1A-deficient cancer cells to inhibition of the antioxidant glutathione, which might provide a new therapeutic opportunity in the future [60]. Loss of ARID1A expression by IC has been shown to strongly correlate with inactivating *ARID1A* mutations both in cytologic and histologic specimens [61, 62]. Thus, ARID1A IC might serve as a convenient surrogate marker for pathogenic *ARID1A* mutations, which could be particularly useful in ovarian malignant effusions (Fig. 8.6).

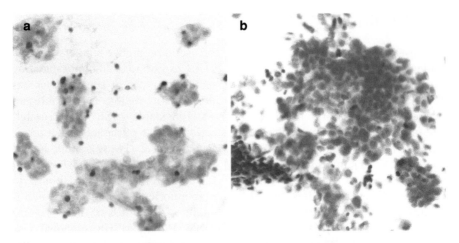

Fig. 8.6 ARID1A IC on previously Papanicolaou-stained ethanol-fixed smears using D2A8U antibody (cell signaling) on Leica Bond. (**a**) Ovarian clear-cell carcinoma from peritoneal effusion and (**b**) urothelial carcinoma from bladder washing showing complete loss of nuclear ARID1A expression. Admixed benign cells serve as positive internal staining control

Fluorescence In Situ Hybridization (FISH) Analysis

Genomic aberrations are a characteristic feature of malignant cells [63]. Normal cell nuclei are diploid and contain a set of paired autosomal chromosomes (2N) that provide two copies of each gene. Aneuploidy refers to numerical chromosomal abnormalities with gains (polysomy) or losses of single (monosomy) or multiple chromosomes. Polysomy commonly prevails in malignant neoplasms as a sign of general chromosomal instability. Structural chromosomal abnormalities like deletions, amplifications, or rearrangements point toward pathological gene function with inactivation of tumor suppressor genes and activation of oncogenes, respectively. These numerical and structural aberrations can readily be detected by FISH on interphase nuclei. Fluorescently labelled probes targeting DNA sequences near the centromere are used for enumeration of specific chromosomes, whereas locus-specific probes detect gains or losses of small chromosomal regions on which tumor suppressor genes or oncogenes are located. Finally, dual color break-apart or fusion probes allow for the detection of chromosomal rearrangements. FISH has become increasingly important for diagnostic and predictive biomarker testing in a wide range of malignant tumors.

Technical Aspects

Most laboratories, especially in the USA, rely on CB for molecular testing, IC, and FISH, which is partly explained by reimbursement restrictions and technical pipelines that are tailored to FFPE material. CB can be prepared from cell-rich cytology material after applying an aggregating agent to the centrifuged cell sediment followed by formalin fixation and paraffin embedding [64]. CB has the advantage of being processed in the histology laboratory with the same protocols established for histological specimens. CB is a valid option for FISH testing; however, ethanol-fixed smears, cytospins, or liquid-based preparations are superior for FISH analysis. Because these preparations lack nuclear truncation, the true number of FISH signals is revealed and the hybridization is not affected by the adverse impact of formalin fixation on the quality of the DNA [65].

FISH analysis provides an interesting opportunity for cytotechnologists, since a profound expertise in both morphology and FISH technique is essential. Some important prerequisites need to be considered for successful FISH on cytological specimen. In order to prevent cell loss during pretreatment and DNA denaturation, one should use adhesive slides with electrostatic positive charge. When tumor cells for FISH evaluation (e.g., malignant cells or atypical cells) are sparse and intermixed with benign cells, it is difficult to manually relocate these cells on the DAPI counterstain after hybridization. Automatic relocation of the target cells using a relocation software coupled with an automated stage and photo-documentation of the cells before uncovering and hybridization of the specimen can easily solve this problem if resources are available. This targeted FISH evaluation under visual control of the photo-documented cells improves the sensitivity and specificity of FISH analyses [66].

FISH is amenable to a wide range of cytological specimens, including conventional or liquid-based preparations, Papanicolaou or Giemsa-stained slides, and specimens already used for IC. For IC slides, red 3-amino-9-ethylcarbazole (AEC) should be used as a chromogen, since brown diaminobenzidine (DAB) causes nuclear autofluorescence. After selecting and marking an appropriate area on the slide and removing the coverslip in xylene, a standard FISH protocol for cytological specimens can be applied [67, 68]. FISH signals are visualized under a fluorescence microscope with appropriate filters. Z-stacked imaging throughout the cell nucleus facilitates signal evaluation on a computer screen and allows for systematic documentation of FISH findings.

Diagnostic FISH Testing in Mesothelioma

Diagnosis of mesothelioma is one of the most difficult areas in cytology due to the morphologic overlap between reactive mesothelial cells and mesothelioma, as outlined in Chap. 6, Malignant-Primary [69, 70]. Immunochemical markers can be very helpful but are not always specific or sensitive enough to reliably distinguish reactive from malignant mesothelial cells [71]. Lack of IC expression of BAP1 in mesothelial cells is diagnostic of mesothelioma but only present in 60–70% of pleural mesotheliomas [72].

Homozygous deletion of 9p21 is the most commonly reported genomic alteration in mesothelioma, prevailing in 56–79% of mesothelioma in pleural effusion cytology (Fig. 8.7) [71]. In peritoneal mesothelioma, 9p21 deletion is less common, with a prevalence of only 25% [73]. A smaller fraction of mesothelioma reveals

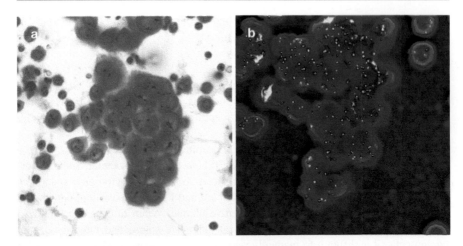

Fig. 8.7 FISH analysis of previously Papanicolaou-stained ethanol-fixed smears of malignant pleural mesothelioma using UroVysion® multi-probe FISH assay (Abbott Mol.). (**a**) Papanicolaou stain and (**b**) FISH showing increased copy numbers of chromosomes 3 (red), 7 (green), and 17 (aqua), and homozygous loss of 9p21 signals (gold). Note some benign cells with retained 9p21 signals

heterozygous 9p21 deletion with one preserved allele that is often inactivated by methylation [74]. 9p21 deletion can easily be detected by FISH on conventional cytologic specimens by a commercial multitarget FISH test used in urinary cytology (UroVysion®, Abbot Laboratories, Abbott Park, IL, USA) or by a dual FISH probe including a reference probe for centromere 9 and a locus-specific probe for 9p21 [75]. Whereas detection of a homozygous deletion is equally straightforward in histologic or CB sections and cytologic smears, identification of heterozygous deletion is less reliable in CB sections due to artificial loss of single signals following nuclear truncation, causing a false impression of heterozygous deletion. The presence of 9p21 deletion is specific for mesothelioma in cells of mesothelial origin but commonly occurs in many other cancer types such as NSCLC [74, 76]. Therefore, it is crucial to first ascertain the mesothelial origin of the atypical cells in question and exclude carcinoma by IC.

There is now a general consensus that a definitive diagnosis of mesothelioma can be made by cytology and small biopsies if supported by either loss of BRCA1-associated protein 1 (*BAP1*) expression or homozygous 9p21 deletion in the right clinical and radiological context [69, 71]. Analysis of *BAP1* and 9p21 status is often complementary, and the use of both of these approaches together increases the sensitivity to 80–90% for pleural mesothelioma [69, 76]. Pleural effusion can occur with mesothelioma in situ and other early stages of mesothelioma before the tumor becomes apparent by imaging studies [77]. In these situations, an atypical mesothelial proliferation with a positive 9p21 FISH result should prompt a video-assisted thoracoscopic biopsy. Immunochemical analysis of methylthioadenosine phosphorylase (*MTAP*), which is discussed in more detail in Chap. 6 Malignant-Primary, has been proposed as an alternative for 9p21 FISH testing [78]. The *MTAP* gene is located close to cyclin-dependent kinase inhibitor 2A (*CDKN2A*) p16 at the 9p21.3

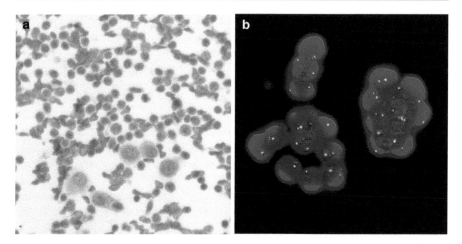

Fig. 8.8 Pleural manifestation of a known follicular B-cell lymphoma. (**a**) Atypical lymphoid cells (Papanicolaou stain). (**b**) Break-apart signals with separate red and green signals in several nuclei. Normal signals occur in admixed benign T-lymphocytes

locus and deleted in tandem with *CDKN2A* in the vast majority (91%–100%) of cases with 9p21 deletion determined by FISH [76]. Therefore, a complete loss of *MTAP* expression in mesothelial cells is an indicator of 9p21 deletion and malignancy, as also demonstrated in effusion cytology CB specimens [78]. These emerging data need further validation. FISH remains the gold standard for detection of 9p21 deletion.

Diagnostic FISH Testing in Other Tumor Types

Other than the diagnosis of mesothelioma, FISH in conjunction with IC profiling can also be used to diagnose or subtype hemolymphatic neoplasia with pleural manifestation [79]. Testing for *MYC*, *BCL2*, and *BCL6* translocations is standard practice for high-grade B-cell lymphomas in order to identify double-hit or triple-hit subtypes (Fig. 8.8). In T-cell lymphomas, testing for *ALK* rearrangements by IC and/or FISH identifies *ALK*-positive anaplastic large cell lymphoma, whereas *TCL1* rearrangements help in diagnosing T-prolymphocytic lymphoma.

Predictive FISH Testing

FISH serves as a standard and widely used method to detect predictive receptor tyrosine kinase gene rearrangements and oncogene amplifications. Highly cellular specimens are increasingly analyzed by RNA-based rearrangement panels covering a large number of different rearrangements with one analysis. This is more efficient and economic than testing for multiple different rearrangements by

FISH. Nevertheless, FISH remains indispensable for specimens not amenable to NGS testing as FISH is not limited by low cellularity and is applicable to paucicellular specimens with as few as 50–100 tumor cells.

Gene Rearrangements

The most commonly tested rearrangements in diagnostic practice include *ALK*, *ROS1*, rearranged during transfection (*RET*), and *NTRK1-3*, which are all linked to effective drugs that are already approved or regarded as emerging targets, with the option of trial inclusion or off-label use (*RET*) in NSCLC and other cancer types (Fig. 8.9) [80–82]. The role of IC for pretesting of these rare rearrangements has been discussed in the section on predictive IC. From a technical perspective, the scoring rules for assessment of microscopic or digitalized FISH signals are essentially identical for all rearrangements. Based on published evidence from *ALK* testing, at least 50–100 tumor cells must be evaluated. A case is regarded as positive for rearrangement when at least 15% of tumor cells show the typical signal patterns of rearrangement, i.e., a break-apart pattern, with the distance between the matched red and green signals being at least the size of two signal diameters or a deletion pattern with a single 3′ signal (linked to the tyrosine kinase domain) without the matched 5′ signal. Further discussion of the details and challenges related to rearrangement FISH testing is beyond the scope of this chapter and has been adequately addressed in the literature [14, 75, 83].

Gene Amplifications

Testing of *HER2* amplification is a diagnostic standard in breast cancer and gastro-esophageal adenocarcinoma to select patients for treatment with HER2-targeted drugs, with an approximate prevalence of 20% and 15%, respectively [45, 84, 85]. HER2-targeted therapies are also being explored in patients with other solid tumors harboring *HER2* amplification, including biliary tract, colorectal, NSCLC, and bladder cancers [85]. Guidelines for testing procedures and interpretation have been developed [44, 45]. In breast cancer, the recent guidelines require formalin fixation for HER2 testing by IC and in situ hybridization, and exceptions to this process should be included in the report [44]. Reflex testing by in situ hybridization should be performed for histologic or CB specimens with equivocal IC results. Since standardization of non-CB ethanol-fixed cytologic specimens for HER2 IC is challenging, we advise the initial use of FISH for *HER2* testing in these specimens. The definition of a positive FISH result varies based on tumor types and includes increased gene copy number and amplification. A true gene amplification is defined as a substantial *relative* increase of the number of gene copies as compared to the copy number of the respective chromosome. A gene/CEP ratio of ≥2 with a mean gene copy number of at least four or five is generally regarded as biologically meaningful and therefore used as a threshold to define gene amplification (Fig. 8.10). The *HER2* status remains highly conserved as breast cancers metastasize to the pleura and other distant sites. Nevertheless, discrepancies of FISH status between primary

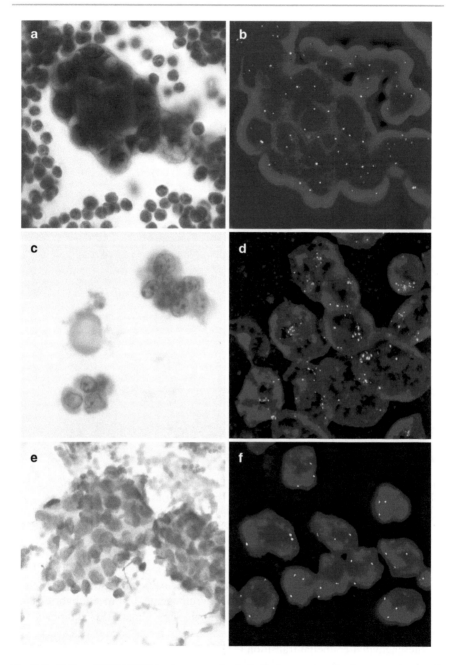

Fig. 8.9 ALK and ROS1 FISH testing on cytological effusion smears of pulmonary adenocarcinomas (compressed z-stacked images showing the projection of all FISH signals in the intact cell nuclei). (**a, b**) ALK-positive cancer with one or two single 3′ red signals with no corresponding 5′ green signal, in addition to one or two fused signals per tumor cell nucleus. Note a group of benign cells with normal disomic FISH pattern (right upper corner). (**b**) is an identical cell group as (**a**). (**c, d**) ALK-negative adenocarcinoma with a highly increased number *ALK* signals per tumor cell nucleus but no rearrangement. (**e, f**) ROS1-negative adenocarcinoma by IC using D4D6 antibody and (**f**) by FISH showing three normal ROS1 fusion signals per tumor cell nucleus

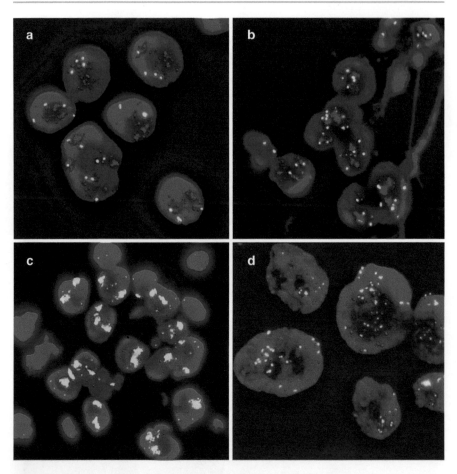

Fig. 8.10 Detection of gene amplification by FISH in malignant effusions. (**a, b**) High-level HER2-amplification with dense clusters of red HER2 gene and a low number of green CEP17 reference signals. (**a**) Breast cancer and (**b**) pulmonary adenocarcinoma. (**c, d**) MET amplification in pulmonary adenocarcinomas with a MET (green)/CEP7 (red) ratio of **a**) >5 (high-level, too many to count) and (**b**) 2.8 (intermediate)

tumors and distant metastases can occur and have been reported with a prevalence of 8%. These discrepant *HER2* FISH results can be caused by difficulties in result interpretation or tumor heterogeneity [86]. Chromogenic dual in situ hybridization (CISH) is a valid alternative to FISH for laboratories without FISH equipment and has been shown to be applicable to CB specimens of metastatic breast cancer [87].

Mesenchymal-epithelial transition (*MET*) amplification is currently regarded as an emerging biomarker in NSCLC, since it has been shown to predict response to MET inhibitors [88–90]. *MET* amplification is rare in untreated NSCLC (2–4%) but is found in up to 20% of patients with epidermal growth factor receptor (*EGFR*)-mutated tumors as a mechanism of acquired resistance to EGFR tyrosine kinase inhibitors (Fig. 8.10c, d) [88]. The highest response rates are observed in patients with high-level amplification defined by tight *MET* gene clusters too numerous to count or a MET/CEP7 ratio >5. Besides its potential as a predictive biomarker at the time of diagnosis, *MET* amplification is a good example of how molecular retesting of progressive tumor, such as subsequent malignant effusion, can help to adjust the treatment.

DNA Testing

Predictive DNA Mutation Analysis in Effusions

In this era of personalized medicine, malignant effusions (ME) have gained great importance as substrates for predictive biomarker testing, including mutations. In clinical practice, this is particularly helpful for advanced cancers that are initially diagnosed by effusion cytology or for subsequent tumor resistance to a targeted treatment. In absolute numbers, mutation testing of ME cytology is mostly accounted for by metastatic NSCLC followed by other different tumor types, as summarized in Table 8.2. Irrespective of tumor type and specific mutations, there are different techniques and challenges to be considered, as discussed below.

Table 8.2 Testing predictive mutations, alterations in malignant effusions (common examples), and principal molecular techniques with reference ranges

Gene	Tumor type	Targeted treatment	Status
Primary driver mutations			
EGFR[a]	Non-small cell lung carcinoma (NSCLC)	EGFR[a] TKIs[b]	FDA[c] approved
BRAF[d] (p.V600E)	NSCLC, melanoma	BRAF[d] inhibitors	FDA[c] approved
KRAS[e] (p.G12C)	NSCLC	AMG 510	Emerging
HER2[g]/ERBB2[h]	NSCLC	anti-HER2[g]	Emerging
METex14[i]	NSCLC	MET inhibitors	Emerging
BRCA1/2[k]	Ovarian, breast, and prostate cancer	PARP inhibitors	FDA[c] approved
STK11[m]/LKB1[n]	NSCLC	Immune checkpoint inhibitors	Emerging
MSI[o]	All tumor types	Immune checkpoint inhibitors	FDA[c] approved
TMB[p]	Different tumor types	Immune checkpoint inhibitors	Emerging
Gene	*Tumor type*	*Targeted treatment*	*Status*
Resistance mutations			
EGFR[a] (p.T790M, p.C797S)	NSCLC	Later-generation EGFR[a] TKIs[b]	FDA[c] approved
ALK[q]	NSCLC	Later-generation ALK TKIs[b]	Emerging

(continued)

Table 8.2 (continued)

ROS1[r]	NSCLC	Later-generation ROS1[r] TKIs[b]	Emerging
NTRK[s]	NSCLC	Later-generation NTRK TKIs[b]	Emerging
STK11[m]/LKB1[n]	NSCLC	Immune checkpoint inhibitors	Emerging
Molecular techniques		*Reference range*	*Logarithm of odds (LOD)*
Sanger sequencing		All the mutations in the analyzed gene regions	10–20%
RT-PCR[t]		Only hotspot mutations	1–5%
dPCR[u]		Only hotspot mutations	0.1–1%
Next-generation sequencing (NGS)		All the mutations in the analyzed gene regions	0.01–5%

[a]*EGFR* Epidermal growth factor receptor
[b]*TKIs* Tyrosine kinase inhibitors
[c]*FDA* Food and Drug Administration
[d]*BRAF* V-Raf Murine Sarcoma Viral Oncogene Homolog B1
[f]*AMG510* Amgen acrylamide-derived KRAS inhibitor
[h]*ERBB2* Erb-B2 receptor tyrosine kinase 2
[g]*HER2* Human epidermal growth factor receptor 2
[i]*METex14* MET exon 14 deletion mutation
[j]*MET* Mesenchymal-epithelial transition factor
[k]*BRCA 1,2* Breast cancer genes 1 and 2 susceptibility protein
[l]*PARP* Poly (ADP-ribose) polymerase
[n]*LKB1* Liver kinase B1 (also known as serine/threonine-protein kinase)
[o]*MSI* Microsatellite instability
[p]*TMB* Tumor mutational burden
[q]*ALK* Anaplastic lymphoma kinase
[r]*ROS1* ROS proto-oncogene 1
[s]*NTRK* Neurotrophic receptor tyrosine kinase
[t]*RT-PCR* Reverse transcription polymerase chain reaction
[u]*dPCR* Digital polymerase chain reaction
[e]*KRAS* Kirsten rat sarcoma
[m]*STK11* Serine threonine kinase 11

Tumor Cell Enrichment

Thoracentesis is a minimally invasive, safe, repeatable, and cost-effective procedure compared to tissue biopsy [91]. Pleural malignant effusion (ME) is a frequent complication of NSCLC, affecting approximately 40% of patients during the course of the disease [92]. Its occurrence defines advanced stage (IVa) lung disease [93]. From a biological perspective, the ME anchorage-independent and movable tumor cells feature a more complex genomic landscape than tumor cells obtained from the primary site [94]. According to the guideline issued by the College of American Pathologists (CAP), the International Association for the Study of Lung Cancer (IASLC), the Association for Molecular Pathology (AMP), and endorsed by the

National Comprehensive Cancer Network (NCCN) and the American Society of Clinical Oncology (ASCO), NSCLC patients presenting with ME must have molecular testing. *EGFR, ALK, ROS1*, and v-Raf murine sarcoma viral oncogene homolog B (*BRAF*) represent those "must test genes" to evaluate for targeted treatment with tyrosine kinase inhibitors (TKIs) [95–97]. Similarly, immunotherapy regimens require PD-L1 assessment [95–97]. Thus, ME is relevant in both diagnostic and therapeutic terms (Fig. 8.11). The feasibility to predict treatment response to first-generation TKI gefitinib by using a PCR approach on ME was demonstrated as early as in 2005 [98]. Similarly, Liu et al. showed that *EGFR* mutational status evaluated on ME is usually concordant with that derived on paired biopsy specimens [99]. However, ME is an unique biospecimen featuring specific technical requirements. While morphomolecular techniques, such as IC, make it possible to evaluate the protein expression of *ALK, ROS1*, and PD-L1 even in those samples featuring tumor cells as a minor cellular component, the rate of ME samples rejected for molecular testing due to insufficient tumor cellularity may be as high as 20% [100, 101]. Thus, genomic biomarkers may require enrichment for tumor cells using macro-/microdissection [102]. Laser capture microdissection (LCM) has been shown to be a robust and useful tool to visually and selectively dissect small groups of scattered cancer cells from routine Papanicolaou-stained effusion smears. This approach has a high (93.0%) success rate. Although *EGFR* point mutations in exon 21 (p.L858R) were identified in as few as 30 cells, the most reliable results were obtained in samples from which at least 100 cells were analyzed [103]. Instead of selecting neoplastic cells, subtracting contaminating cells (e.g., removing

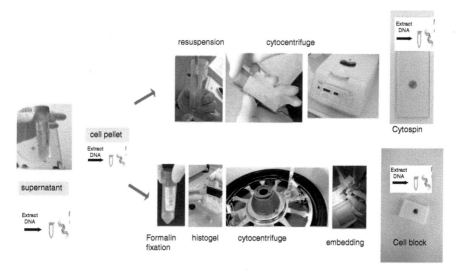

Fig. 8.11 DNA analysis from malignant pleural effusion. After centrifugation, cell pellet may be resuspended in either alcohol-based fixative, in order to obtain a cytospin, or formalin, in order to obtain a cell block. After morphological analysis DNA can be extracted from cyto-preparations or directly from either cell pellets or supernatant

leukocytes after immunostaining with anti-CD53 antibody) has been described as an alternative approach [104]. Similarly, others have selected malignant cells by their high metabolic activity and elevated glucose uptake by labeling nucleated cells with allophycocyanin (APC)-conjugated anti-CD45 antibody [105].

Sanger Sequencing

Genomic biomarkers can be assessed in ME by sequencing relevant hotspot regions by Sanger sequencing, pyrosequencing, or NGS. Sanger sequencing, also known as "sequencing by termination," is based on the use of fluorescent-labeled dideoxy-nucleotide [106]. Despite its lower sensitivity with respect to more advanced molecular technologies, Sanger sequencing can be useful to confirm novel or uncommon alterations detected by NGS [107]. Many studies carried out in prior decades showed that detecting *EGFR* mutations by Sanger sequencing correlates with a favorable response to TKI treatment [108]. As a general rule, Sanger sequencing should be applied to cellular specimens, because false-negative results occur with cell-free pleural fluids [109]. As expected, Sanger sequencing showed a lower *EGFR* mutant detection rate compared to mutant-enriched PCR (34.6% vs 50.0%) [109]. Similarly, PNA-mediated RT-PCR was more sensitive in detecting *KRAS* mutations in different malignancies involving the pleural cavity [110]. A fair concordance rate (83.3%) between Sanger sequencing and ADx amplification refractory mutation system (ADx-ARMS) was reported (10/24 vs 14/24, 41.7% vs 58.3%, respectively) [111].

Next-Generation Sequencing (NGS)

While Sanger sequencing is based on the "sequencing by termination" principle, NGS adopts a "sequencing by synthesis" approach enabling the evaluation of multiple genes simultaneously in different patients [112]. In addition to multiplexing power, NGS is more sensitive than Sanger sequencing [112]. The workflow is characterized by four steps: (1) library generation; (2) clonal amplification of single fragment; (3) massive parallel sequencing; and (4) data analysis [112]. NGS is evolving at a rapid pace. The Ion Torrent (Thermo Fisher Scientific, Waltham, MA) technology exploits the release of hydrogen ion (H+), and subsequently pH changes to evaluate base incorporation [113]. The Illumina (Illumina, San Diego, CA) platform uses nucleotide labeled with reversible dye terminators and adopts a "bridge amplification" system [114].

NGS can be useful to detect *EGFR* mutations in paucicellular (<10% tumor cells) ME samples [115]. Deep-sequencing workflow may reach a sensitivity comparable to that of ARMS RT-PCR [99]. However, ultrasensitive NGS may yield considerable background noise, making it difficult to distinguish between low levels of true mutant alleles and sequencing artifacts that may occur when processing paraffin-embedded samples such as CBs. ME CBs' false-positive results were minimized by using sequence tag-based analysis of microbial population dynamics

(STAMP), based on CAncer Personalized Profiling by deep Sequencing (CAPP-Seq) methodology [116]. NGS is also useful to detect drug-resistant molecular mechanisms, such as *MET* amplifications in subclones arising after treatment with icotinib [117]. Since effusion represents a natural medium, primary tumor cell cultures can be established from floating neoplastic cells, thereby enriching the malignant component to allow for selective evaluation of oncogenic molecular changes. By this approach, Sneddon et al. performed whole exome and transcriptome sequencing, and Roscilli et al. carried out targeted NGS analysis [118, 119].

Methylation

Epigenetic modifications are associated with human cancer progression [120–122]. In particular, hypermethylation occurring in CpG-rich regions may interfere with gene transcription and cause the dysfunction of tumor suppressor genes [120–122]. In addition, the DNA methylation profile may have a significant diagnostic and predictive role in cancer of unknown primary [123]. Using a microarray DNA methylation signature (EPICUP) assay has been shown to enhance the correct diagnosis in a majority of cases (87.0%) in which the primary origin was originally unknown [123]. ME may represent a suitable biospecimen for the assessment of epigenetic changes. In particular, methylation analysis can aid cytopathologists faced with challenging diagnoses, such as differentiating between benign reactive effusion cells and neoplasia. In particular, in hypermethylation of the promoters of the DNA repair gene O6-methylguanine-DNA methyltransferase (*MGMT*), *p16INK4a*, RAS association domain family 1A (*RASSF1A*), apoptosis-related genes, death-associated protein kinase (*DAPK*), and retinoic acid receptor β (*RARβ*) are relevant biomarkers [124]. Interestingly, the methylation status of the *DAPK* and *RASSF1A* genes is significantly associated with tobacco smoke ($p < 0.05$ and $p < 0.05$, respectively) [124]. Multiplex-nested methylation-specific PCR yields an upgrade in sensitivity in respect to conventional morphological cytological evaluation [125–128]. More standardized epigenetic assays are currently available, such as the Epi proLung® BL Reflex Assay (Epigenomics AG, Berlin, Germany) kit; this latter test is very specific (96.2%) but has a low sensitivity (39.5%) [129]. Thus, large panels of epigenetic biomarkers need to be developed and validated in clinical samples.

Digital PCR

Digital PCR (dPCR) is an evolution of the traditional PCR that allows an absolute quantitative evaluation by detecting and counting each single event [130–132]. Two different platforms are available: digital droplet PCR (ddPCR) in which the amplification is carried out by generating droplets of water in oil reverse emulsion and digital solid PCR (dsPCR) based on the use of chips in which each single amplification reaction is compartmentalized [130–132]. Similar to RT-PCR, fluorescent-labeled probes are adopted, and the absolute count of mutant copies is calculated by

Poisson distribution [130–132]. The dPCR high sensitivity has been exploited to process and detect mutations from the supernatant obtained from ME rather than on cell sediment [133]. By this approach, the *EGFR* mutation rate is much higher than that obtained by direct sequencing (75.4% vs 43.8%, $P < 0.0001$) [133]. In a setting where very high sensitivity is required, dPCR may be an alternative to deep sequencing [134]. Although the higher sensitivity of dPCR and ability to detect a low level of mutant alleles may raise questions regarding its clinical relevance, patients harboring *EGFR* mutations detected by ddPCR showed longer progression-free survival and higher objective response rates [133].

Other Ancillary Tests

RNA Quantity and Quality Evaluation

The RNA molecule has crucial relevance in conveying information encoded in the genomic DNA. However, RNA is rapidly degraded by RNase enzymes. Thus, following RNA extraction from ME cells, a quantitative and qualitative assessment should be performed. Traditionally, RNA integrity relied on identifying the presence of two bands (28S and 18S ribosomal RNA) using agarose gel electrophoresis stained with ethidium bromide. However, this approach is not entirely consistent and does not allow for quantitative assessment. Gene expression measurement techniques, such as reverse transcription polymerase chain reaction (RT-PCR), are more objective but time-consuming. RT-PCR is able to identify the presence of mRNA, pre-mRNA, or other types of RNA, such as noncoding RNA [135]. The key point of this technique is represented by the use of the enzyme reverse transcriptase (RT) that allows for generation of a complementary DNA strand (cDNA) from a RNA template [135]. A more cost-effect, rapid, and recent technique is RNA electrophoretic molecular weight separation using microfluidic techniques in channels of the microfabricated chips, with subsequent RNA detection using laser-induced fluorescence [136]. The results are visualized as a virtual electropherogram (Fig. 8.12).

RNA Testing of Predictive Biomarkers in Effusions

ME cell-derived RNA is suitable for detection of both gene point mutations and structural genomic alterations. *EGFR* direct sequencing using RT-PCR can be even more sensitive than DNA-based assays [137]. The RT-PCR methodology is most suitable to detect *ALK* gene rearrangements in ME specimens [138, 139] with high concordance rates (98.1%) demonstrated on matched histological and ME CB samples [25]. CBs are a valid source of RNA for *ALK* gene fusion testing by RT-PCR [24, 140]. Beyond *ALK* gene fusions, other targetable genomic structural alterations can be detected in ME samples by RT-PCR, such as *RET* gene fusions [141].

More recently, multiplex technologies are required for the simultaneous detection of *ALK*, *ROS1*, *RET*, and *NTRK1* using limited amounts of material. NGS

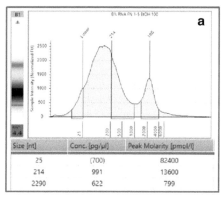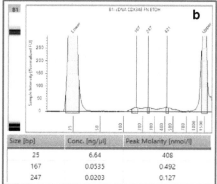

Size [nt]	Conc. [pg/µl]	Peak Molarity [pmol/l]
25	(700)	82400
214	991	13600
2290	622	799

Size [bp]	Conc. [ng/µl]	Peak Molarity [nmol/l]
25	6.64	408
167	0.0535	0.492
247	0.0203	0.127

Fig. 8.12 Virtual electropherograms display results in terms of quality and quantity in extracted RNA (panel (**a**)) and corresponding cDNA (panel (**b**)) from a malignant effusion sample, by using TapeStation 4200 (Agilent Technologies, Santa Clara, CA) platform

requires only 10 ng of RNA using semiconductor technology and commercially available panels, such as the Ion AmpliSeq™ RNA Fusion Lung Cancer Panel (Thermo Fisher Scientific, Waltham, Massachusetts) [142]. Another fascinating technology is represented by nCounter (NanoString Technologies, Seattle, Washington) [143]. nCounter analysis has been successfully performed on two CB samples where *ROS1* fusions have been detected [143].

Micro RNA

MicroRNAs (miRNAs) are critical regulators of gene expression. Since miRNA dysregulation has been identified in many human cancers, they have the potential to perform as ancillary markers but have not yet entered diagnostic practice [144, 145]. miRNAs can be extracted directly from the supernatant (cell-free miRNAs) of ME, and studies have demonstrated that cell-free miRNAs are regulated differently in malignant compared to benign effusions. A wide range of miRNAs have been investigated, and both upregulation and downregulation have been documented. For example, upregulation has been reported for cell-free miR-24, miR-26a, and miR-30d [146, 147] and downregulation for miR-198, miR-134, miR-185, and miR-22 [148, 149].

Besides lung cancer, miRNA may also be useful to diagnose mesothelioma in difficult cases. Mesothelioma cells significantly overexpress miR-19a, miR-19b, and miR-21, whereas miR-126 is upregulated in reactive cells [150]. miR-130a has been reported as useful for the differential diagnosis between mesothelioma and lung adenocarcinoma [151].

Analysis of miRNAs in exosomes from ME revealed that certain miRNAs were highly expressed in exosomes from lung cancer patients as compared to patients with pneumonia or tuberculosis [152]. Other studies showed that different miRNAs were detectable in exosomes from lung adenocarcinoma [153, 154]. The level of expression of miR-182 and miR-210 in exosomes was found to be higher in malignant than in benign pleural fluids [155].

Cell-Free DNA

Along with plasma samples, other fluids, such as effusion, can be considered "liquid biopsies" [156]. Effusions contain floating nucleic acids released by cellular components, including neoplastic cells. cfDNA can be precious for molecular analysis, especially when patients with advanced cancer are not biopsy candidates. Studies show that molecular testing in ME can be performed not only on cell pellets but directly on effusion cfDNA. Hummelink et al. were able to detect more driver mutations (*EGFR* or *KRAS*, 79.5%) in cfDNA than in cell pellets (70.5%) [157]. cfDNA is very suitable for NGS testing. Due to the sometimes limited amounts of nucleic acid in biopsy specimens, hybrid capture enrichment for library preparation is not always feasible, but cfDNA can be more readily tested on effusions. In a study that used matched metastatic pleural tumor tissue, supernatant, and cell block [158], ME supernatant was as informative as tissue with a sensitivity and specificity of 84% and 91%, respectively. In another study, cfDNA had a specificity of 100% (no false positives) and a sensitivity of 92% [159], although a lower sensitivity (44%) has been reported by others [160].

Cell-Based Research

Malignant effusions have vast potential in translational and experimental research. Clinicians should provide as much fluid volume as possible to not only guarantee an accurate diagnosis and predictive biomarker testing but to provide material for biobanking and research. It is rewarding to freeze and biobank surplus pellet material for future translational studies [4]. Archived CB specimens serve as an excellent resource for retrospective biomarkers studies [50, 161, 162]. The same is true for traditional ethanol-fixed and -stained non-CB cytology slides, as long as the nucleic acids and protein epitopes are protected from humidity and oxygen by an appropriate mounting medium [163]. Effusions are the prototypic cytology material to study metastatic disease in cancer, since body cavities are a common site of cancer spread and they often contain a high number of tumor cells. Comparing the molecular and genomic features of primary tumors and matched metastases in serous cavities can provide fundamental insights into the mechanisms of progression, resistance to treatment, and the patterns of genomic clonal evolution using state-of-the-art NGS and bioinformatic analysis [164, 165]. From a practical point of view, it is important to know to what degree a biomarker analyzed in a primary tumor is representative of the marker status in a distant metastasis. There is mounting evidence that most known genetic driver mutations, rearrangements, and amplifications are truncal and therefore ubiquitous across all tumor manifestations [86, 164, 166]. However, it has been shown that potentially targetable driver mutations can also appear in the metastases only [167]. This is a particular challenge in cases of adaptive-resistance mutations, which can be restricted to individual distant tumor manifestations [168].

In the field of immune oncology, biomarkers to better select patients for therapy with immune checkpoint inhibitors are a research area of continued interest. The interaction of tumor cells with immune cells in effusions is likely to differ from the situation in tissue. Thus, the analysis of the microenvironment and the immune profile in malignant effusions has emerged as an interesting area of investigations [161, 169, 170]. For example, tissue microarrays from malignant effusions have recently been used to establish prognostic immune cell profiles using computational immunochemical analysis [161]. New technical tools for multiplexing immunofluorescence biomarker analysis and imaging on tissue and cytology specimens promise to greatly enhance the granularity at which the interaction of the tumor microenvironment can be explored [171, 172].

Malignant effusions are mostly exudates, rich in proteins and cellular nutrients, and serve as a personalized growth medium facilitating preservation of live tumor cells during transport to the laboratory. Cells remain viable for 1–2 days if kept on ice or refrigerated. This provides an excellent opportunity for ex vivo cell culturing. Malignant effusions have been an important source of commercially available cell lines, mainly from lung and breast cancers, for use in research. In addition, protocols for 2D cultures from malignant effusions have been proposed as a promising tool to serve as avatars for personalized in vitro drug sensitivity testing based on the individual molecular tumor profile [119, 173–175]. Technically advanced impedance-based or live cell imaging systems for real-time measurement of cell proliferation or other properties greatly facilitate these experiments [176]. Ex vivo cell culturing can be accelerated by conditional reprogramming (CR), which involves co-culture of irradiated mouse fibroblast feeder cells with human cancer cells in the presence of Rho kinase inhibitor [174, 177]. Moreover, CR allows for the propagation of epithelial cells indefinitely in vitro, enabling unexhausted cell cultures for living cell banks for future basic and translational research demands. CR can also be used to enrich cancer cells from urine and pleural effusions [178, 179].

Organotypic spherical 3D ex vivo cancer models (i.e., organoids) are in vitro-cultured 3D structures that recapitulate the key aspects of in vivo organs, including genetic and phenotypic heterogeneity [180] (Fig. 8.13). In cancer research, they have become important tools to experimentally model cancer cells and facilitate personalized drug sensitivity screening [181, 182]. Other than 2D cell cultures, organoids grow in an extracellular hydrogel matrix and depend on different components of specified growth media. They have been generated mostly from tissue specimens, but they can also be grown from malignant effusions [183]. As in histologic specimens, the challenge lies in defining optimal protocols and growth conditions to select for cancer cells and avoid overgrowth by benign epithelial cells. The analysis of malignant effusion as a source of organoids remains underinvestigated, despite its high promise.

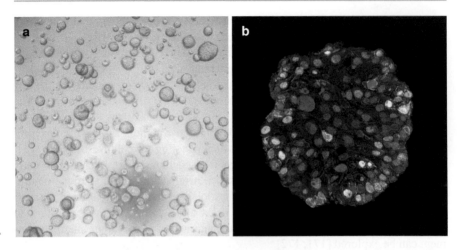

Fig. 8.13 Spherical organoids for three-dimensional ex vivo study of cancer cells. (**a**) Multiple organoids consisting of urothelial carcinoma cells growing in hydrogel matrix. (**b**) Organoid stained by nuclear DAPI and immunofluorescence (CK5 and CK8) for cell characterization

Conclusions

Ancillary biomarker testing has become a fascinating and challenging aspect of cytology in general and of effusion cytology in particular. It provides new opportunities for cytopathologists and cytotechnologists to broaden their expertise beyond traditional and morphology-based cytology and play an active part not only in optimal patient care but also in continuing medical progress.

References

1. Lindeman NI, Cagle PT, Aisner DL, et al. Updated molecular testing guideline for the selection of lung cancer patients for treatment with targeted tyrosine kinase inhibitors: guideline from the College of American Pathologists, the International Association for the Study of Lung Cancer, and the Association for Molecular Pathology. J Thorac Oncol. 2018;13(3):323–58.
2. Cheung CC, Barnes P, Bigras G, et al. Canadian Association of Pathologists-Association Canadienne Des Pathologistes' National Standards Committee for high complexity, fit-for-purpose PD-L1 biomarker testing for patient selection in immuno-oncology: guidelines for clinical laboratories from the Canadian Association of Pathologists-Association Canadienne Des Pathologistes (CAP-ACP). Appl Immunohistochem Mol Morphol. 2019;27(10):699–714.
3. Torlakovic EE, Nielsen S, Francis G, et al. Standardization of positive controls in diagnostic immunohistochemistry: recommendations from the International Ad Hoc Expert Committee. Appl Immunohistochem Mol Morphol. 2015;23(1):1–18.
4. Engels M, Michael C, Dobra K, Hjerpe A, Fassina A, Firat P. Management of cytological material, pre-analytical procedures and bio-banking in effusion cytopathology. Cytopathology. 2019;30(1):31–8.
5. Jain D, Nambirajan A, Borczuk A, et al. Immunocytochemistry for predictive biomarker testing in lung cancer cytology. Cancer Cytopathol. 2019;127(5):325–39.

6. Savic Prince S, Bubendorf L. Predictive potential and need for standardization of PD-L1 immunohistochemistry. Virchows Arch. 2019;474(4):475–84.
7. Hirsch FR, McElhinny A, Stanforth D, et al. PD-L1 immunohistochemistry assays for lung cancer: results from phase 1 of the blueprint PD-L1 IHC assay comparison project. J Thorac Oncol. 2017;12(2):208–22.
8. Savic S, Berezowska S, Eppenberger-Castori S, et al. PD-L1 testing of non-small cell lung cancer using different antibodies and platforms: a Swiss cross-validation study. Virchows Arch. 2019;475(1):67–76.
9. Tsao MS, Kerr KM, Kockx M, et al. PD-L1 immunohistochemistry comparability study in real-life clinical samples: results of blueprint phase 2 project. J Thorac Oncol. 2018;13(9):1302–11.
10. Wang G, Ionescu DN, Lee CH, et al. PD-L1 testing on the EBUS-FNA cytology specimens of non-small cell lung cancer. Lung Cancer. 2019;136:1–5.
11. Torous VF, Rangachari D, Gallant BP, Shea M, Costa DB, VanderLaan PA. PD-L1 testing using the clone 22C3 pharmDx kit for selection of patients with non-small cell lung cancer to receive immune checkpoint inhibitor therapy: are cytology cell blocks a viable option? J Am Soc Cytopathol. 2018;7(3):133–41.
12. Heymann JJ, Bulman WA, Swinarski D, et al. PD-L1 expression in non-small cell lung carcinoma: comparison among cytology, small biopsy, and surgical resection specimens. Cancer Cytopathol. 2017;125(12):896–907.
13. Munari E, Zamboni G, Sighele G, et al. Expression of programmed cell death ligand 1 in non-small cell lung cancer: comparison between cytologic smears, core biopsies, and whole sections using the SP263 assay. Cancer Cytopathol. 2019;127(1):52–61.
14. Bubendorf L, Lantuejoul S, de Langen AJ, Thunnissen E. Nonsmall cell lung carcinoma: diagnostic difficulties in small biopsies and cytological specimens: number 2 in the series "pathology for the clinician" edited by Peter Dorfmuller and Alberto Cavazza. Eur Respir Rev. 2017;26(144):170007.
15. Xu J, Han X, Liu C, et al. PD-L1 expression in pleural effusions of pulmonary adenocarcinoma and survival prediction: a controlled study by pleural biopsy. Sci Rep. 2018;8(1):11206.
16. Jain D, Sukumar S, Mohan A, Iyer VK. Programmed death-ligand 1 immunoexpression in matched biopsy and liquid-based cytology samples of advanced stage non-small cell lung carcinomas. Cytopathology. 2018;29(6):550–7.
17. Mian I, Abdullaev Z, Morrow B, et al. Anaplastic lymphoma kinase gene rearrangement in children and young adults with mesothelioma. J Thorac Oncol. 2020;15(3):457–61.
18. Hung YP, Dong F, Watkins JC, et al. Identification of ALK rearrangements in malignant peritoneal mesothelioma. JAMA Oncol. 2018;4(2):235–8.
19. Kwak EL, Bang YJ, Camidge DR, et al. Anaplastic lymphoma kinase inhibition in non-small-cell lung cancer. N Engl J Med. 2010;363(18):1693–703.
20. Peters S, Camidge DR, Shaw AT, et al. Alectinib versus crizotinib in untreated ALK-positive non-small-cell lung cancer. N Engl J Med. 2017;377(9):829–38.
21. Pekar-Zlotin M, Hirsch FR, Soussan-Gutman L, et al. Fluorescence in situ hybridization, immunohistochemistry, and next-generation sequencing for detection of EML4-ALK rearrangement in lung cancer. Oncologist. 2015;20(3):316–22.
22. Savic S, Diebold J, Zimmermann AK, et al. Screening for ALK in non-small cell lung carcinomas: 5A4 and D5F3 antibodies perform equally well, but combined use with FISH is recommended. Lung Cancer. 2015;89(2):104–9.
23. Zhang C, Randolph ML, Jones KJ, Cramer HM, Cheng L, Wu HH. Anaplastic lymphoma kinase immunocytochemistry on cell-transferred cytologic smears of lung adenocarcinoma. Acta Cytol. 2015;59(2):213–8.
24. Liu L, Zhan P, Zhou X, Song Y, Zhou X, Yu L, Wang J. Detection of EML4-ALK in lung adenocarcinoma using pleural effusion with FISH, IHC, and RT-PCR methods. PLoS One. 2015;10(3):e0117032.

25. Zhou J, Yao H, Zhao J, et al. Cell block samples from malignant pleural effusion might be valid alternative samples for anaplastic lymphoma kinase detection in patients with advanced non-small-cell lung cancer. Histopathology. 2015;66(7):949–54.
26. Fiset PO, Labbe C, Young K, et al. Anaplastic lymphoma kinase 5A4 immunohistochemistry as a diagnostic assay in lung cancer: a Canadian reference testing center's results in population-based reflex testing. Cancer. 2019;125(22):4043–51.
27. Wang Z, Wu X, Han H, et al. ALK gene expression status in pleural effusion predicts tumor responsiveness to crizotinib in Chinese patients with lung adenocarcinoma. Chin J Cancer Res. 2016;28(6):606–16.
28. Wang W, Tang Y, Li J, Jiang L, Jiang Y, Su X. Detection of ALK rearrangements in malignant pleural effusion cell blocks from patients with advanced non-small cell lung cancer: a comparison of Ventana immunohistochemistry and fluorescence in situ hybridization. Cancer Cytopathol. 2015;123(2):117–22.
29. Sholl LM, Sun H, Butaney M, et al. ROS1 immunohistochemistry for detection of ROS1-rearranged lung adenocarcinomas. Am J Surg Pathol. 2013;37(9):1441–9.
30. Davies KD, Le AT, Theodoro MF, et al. Identifying and targeting ROS1 gene fusions in non-small cell lung cancer. Clin Cancer Res. 2012;18(17):4570–9.
31. Lozano MD, Echeveste JI, Abengozar M, et al. Cytology smears in the era of molecular biomarkers in non-small cell lung cancer: doing more with less. Arch Pathol Lab Med. 2018;142(3):291–8.
32. Bubendorf L, Buttner R, Al-Dayel F, et al. Testing for ROS1 in non-small cell lung cancer: a review with recommendations. Virchows Arch. 2016;469(5):489–503.
33. Shan L, Lian F, Guo L, et al. Detection of ROS1 gene rearrangement in lung adenocarcinoma: comparison of IHC, FISH and real-time RT-PCR. PLoS One. 2015;10(3):e0120422.
34. Yoshida A, Tsuta K, Wakai S, et al. Immunohistochemical detection of ROS1 is useful for identifying ROS1 rearrangements in lung cancers. Mod Pathol. 2014;27(5):711–20.
35. Vlajnic T, Savic S, Barascud A, et al. Detection of ROS1-positive non-small cell lung cancer on cytological specimens using immunocytochemistry. Cancer Cytopathol. 2018;126(6):421–9.
36. Huang RSP, Smith D, Le CH, et al. Correlation of ROS1 immunohistochemistry with ROS1 fusion status determined by fluorescence in situ hybridization. Arch Pathol Lab Med. 2019; https://doi.org/10.5858/arpa.2019-0085-OA.
37. Cocco E, Scaltriti M, Drilon A. NTRK fusion-positive cancers and TRK inhibitor therapy. Nat Rev Clin Oncol. 2018;15(12):731–47.
38. Pietrantonio F, Di Nicolantonio F, Schrock AB, et al. ALK, ROS1, and NTRK rearrangements in metastatic colorectal cancer. J Nat Cancer Instit. 2017;109(12) https://doi.org/10.1093/jnci/djx089.
39. Drilon A, Laetsch TW, Kummar S, et al. Efficacy of larotrectinib in TRK fusion-positive cancers in adults and children. N Engl J Med. 2018;378(8):731–9.
40. Hechtman JF, Benayed R, Hyman DM, et al. Pan-Trk immunohistochemistry is an efficient and reliable screen for the detection of NTRK fusions. Am J Surg Pathol. 2017;41(11):1547–51.
41. Bourhis A, Redoulez G, Quintin-Roue I, Marcorelles P, Uguen A. Screening for NTRK-rearranged tumors using immunohistochemistry: comparison of 2 different pan-TRK clones in melanoma samples. Appl Immunohistochem Mol Morphol. 2020;28(3):194–6.
42. Gatalica Z, Xiu J, Swensen J, Vranic S. Molecular characterization of cancers with NTRK gene fusions. Mod Pathol. 2019;32(1):147–53.
43. Bahreini F, Soltanian AR, Mehdipour P. A meta-analysis on concordance between immunohistochemistry (IHC) and fluorescence in situ hybridization (FISH) to detect HER2 gene overexpression in breast cancer. Breast Cancer. 2015;22(6):615–25.
44. Wolff AC, Hammond MEH, Allison KH, et al. Human epidermal growth factor receptor 2 testing in breast cancer: American Society of Clinical Oncology/College of American Pathologists clinical practice guideline focused update. J Clin Oncol. 2018;36(20):2105–22.
45. Bartley AN, Washington MK, Colasacco C, et al. HER2 testing and clinical decision making in gastroesophageal adenocarcinoma: guideline from the College of American Pathologists,

American Society for Clinical Pathology, and the American Society of Clinical Oncology. J Clin Oncol. 2017;35(4):446–64.

46. Shabaik A, Lin G, Peterson M, et al. Reliability of Her2/neu, estrogen receptor, and progesterone receptor testing by immunohistochemistry on cell block of FNA and serous effusions from patients with primary and metastatic breast carcinoma. Diagn Cytopathol. 2011;39(5):328–32.

47. Wolff AC, Hammond MEH, Allison A, et al. Human epidermal growth factor receptor 2 testing in breast cancer: American Society of Clinical Oncology/College of American Pathologists Clinical practice guideline focused update. Arch Pathol Lab Med. 2018;142(11):1364–82.

48. Pareja F, Murray MP, Jean RD, et al. Cytologic assessment of estrogen receptor, progesterone receptor, and HER2 status in metastatic breast carcinoma. J Am Soc Cytopathol. 2017;6(1):33–40.

49. Srebotnik Kirbis I, Us Krasovec M, Pogacnik A, Strojan FM. Optimization and validation of immunocytochemical detection of oestrogen receptors on cytospins prepared from fine needle aspiration (FNA) samples of breast cancer. Cytopathology. 2015;26(2):88–98.

50. Pu RT, Giordano TJ, Michael CW. Utility of cytology microarray constructed from effusion cell blocks for immunomarker validation. Cancer. 2008;114(5):300–6.

51. Mossler JA, McCarty KS Jr, Johnston WW. The correlation of cytologic grade and steroid receptor content in effusions of metastatic breast carcinoma. Acta Cytol. 1981;25(6):653–8.

52. Zhao P, Li L, Jiang X, Li Q. Mismatch repair deficiency/microsatellite instability-high as a predictor for anti-PD-1/PD-L1 immunotherapy efficacy. J Hematol Oncol. 2019;12(1):54.

53. Chang L, Chang M, Chang HM, Chang F. Microsatellite instability: a predictive biomarker for cancer immunotherapy. Appl Immunohistochem Mol Morphol. 2018;26(2):e15–21.

54. Luchini C, Bibeau F, Ligtenberg MJL, et al. ESMO recommendations on microsatellite instability testing for immunotherapy in cancer, and its relationship with PD-1/PD-L1 expression and tumour mutational burden: a systematic review-based approach. Ann Oncol. 2019;30(8):1232–43.

55. Longacre TA, Broaddus R, Chuang LT, et al. for the C.o.A.P. members of the Cancer Biomarker Reporting Committee. Template for reporting results of biomarker testing of specimens from patients with carcinoma of the endometrium. Arch Pathol Lab Med. 2017;141(11):1508–12.

56. Bartley AN, Hamilton SR, Alsabeh R, et al. for the C.o.A.P. members of the Cancer Biomarker Reporting Workgroup. Template for reporting results of biomarker testing of specimens from patients with carcinoma of the colon and rectum. Arch Pathol Lab Med. 2014;138(2):166–70.

57. Okamura R, Kato S, Lee S, Jimenez RE, Sicklick JK, Kurzrock R. ARID1A alterations function as a biomarker for longer progression-free survival after anti-PD-1/PD-L1 immunotherapy. J Immunother Cancer. 2020;8(1) https://doi.org/10.1136/jitc-2019-000438.

58. Hu G, Tu W, Yang L, Peng G, Yang L. ARID1A deficiency and immune checkpoint blockade therapy: from mechanisms to clinical application. Cancer Lett. 2020;473:148–55.

59. Shen J, Ju Z, Zhao W, et al. ARID1A deficiency promotes mutability and potentiates therapeutic antitumor immunity unleashed by immune checkpoint blockade. Nat Med. 2018;24(5):556–62.

60. Sasaki M, Chiwaki F, Kuroda T, et al. Efficacy of glutathione inhibitors for the treatment of ARID1A-deficient diffuse-type gastric cancers. Biochem Biophys Res Commun. 2020;522(2):342–7.

61. Khalique S, Naidoo K, Attygalle AD, et al. Optimised ARID1A immunohistochemistry is an accurate predictor of ARID1A mutational status in gynaecological cancers. J Pathol Clin Res. 2018;4(3):154–66.

62. Dugas SG, Muller DC, Le Magnen C, et al. Immunocytochemistry for ARID1A as a potential biomarker in urine cytology of bladder cancer. Cancer Cytopathol. 2019;127(9):578–85.

63. Yu XM, Wang XF. The in vitro proliferation and cytokine production of Valpha24+Vbeta11+ natural killer T cells in patients with systemic lupus erythematosus. Chin Med J. 2011;124(1):61–5.

64. Nambirajan A, Jain D. Cell blocks in cytopathology: an update. Cytopathology. 2018;29(6):505–24.
65. Srinivasan M, Sedmak D, Jewell S. Effect of fixatives and tissue processing on the content and integrity of nucleic acids. Am J Pathol. 2002;161(6):1961–71.
66. Vlajnic T, Somaini G, Savic S, et al. Targeted multiprobe fluorescence in situ hybridization analysis for elucidation of inconclusive pancreatobiliary cytology. Cancer Cytopathol. 2014;122(8):627–34.
67. Wilkens L, Gerr H, Gadzicki D, Kreipe H, Schlegelberger B. Standardised fluorescence in situ hybridisation in cytological and histological specimens. Virchows Arch. 2005;447(3):586–92.
68. Bubendorf L, Grilli B. UroVysion multiprobe FISH in urinary cytology. Methods Mol Med. 2004;97:117–31.
69. Siddiqui MT, Schmitt F, Churg A. Proceedings of the American Society of Cytopathology companion session at the 2019 United States and Canadian Academy of Pathology Annual meeting, part 2: effusion cytology with focus on theranostics and diagnosis of malignant mesothelioma. J Am Soc Cytopathol. 2019;8(6):352–61.
70. Whitaker D. The cytology of malignant mesothelioma. Cytopathology. 2000;11(3):139–51.
71. Husain AN, Colby TV, Ordonez NG, et al. Guidelines for pathologic diagnosis of malignant mesothelioma 2017 update of the consensus statement from the International Mesothelioma Interest Group. Arch Pathol Lab Med. 2018;142(1):89–108.
72. Cigognetti M, Lonardi S, Fisogni S, et al. BAP1 (BRCA1-associated protein 1) is a highly specific marker for differentiating mesothelioma from reactive mesothelial proliferations. Mod Pathol. 2015;28(8):1043–57.
73. Chiosea S, Krasinskas A, Cagle PT, Mitchell KA, Zander DS, Dacic S. Diagnostic importance of 9p21 homozygous deletion in malignant mesotheliomas. Mod Pathol. 2008;21(6):742–7.
74. Savic S, Franco N, Grilli B, et al. Fluorescence in situ hybridization in the definitive diagnosis of malignant mesothelioma in effusion cytology. Chest. 2010;138(1):137–44.
75. Savic S, Bubendorf L. Common fluorescence in situ hybridization applications in cytology. Arch Pathol Lab Med. 2016;140(12):1323–30.
76. Berg KB, Dacic S, Miller C, Cheung S, Churg A. Utility of methylthioadenosine phosphorylase compared with BAP1 immunohistochemistry, and CDKN2A and NF2 fluorescence in situ hybridization in separating reactive mesothelial proliferations from epithelioid malignant mesotheliomas. Arch Pathol Lab Med. 2018;142(12):1549–53.
77. Churg A, Galateau-Salle F, Roden AC, et al. Malignant mesothelioma in situ: morphologic features and clinical outcome. Mod Pathol. 2020;33(2):297–302.
78. Berg KB, Churg AM, Cheung S, Dacic S. Usefulness of methylthioadenosine phosphorylase and BRCA-associated protein 1 immunohistochemistry in the diagnosis of malignant mesothelioma in effusion cytology specimens. Cancer Cytopathol. 2020;128(2):126–32.
79. Patel T, Patel P, Mehta S, Shah M, Jetly D, Khanna N. The value of cytology in diagnosis of serous effusions in malignant lymphomas: an experience of a tertiary care center. Diagn Cytopathol. 2019;47(8):776–82.
80. Rolfo C. NTRK gene fusions: a rough diamond ready to sparkle. Lancet Oncol. 2020;21(4):472–4.
81. Li AY, McCusker MG, Russo A, et al. RET fusions in solid tumors. Cancer Treat Rev. 2019;81:101911.
82. Schram AM, Chang MT, Jonsson P, Drilon A. Fusions in solid tumours: diagnostic strategies, targeted therapy, and acquired resistance. Nat Rev Clin Oncol. 2017;14(12):735–48.
83. Savic S, Bubendorf L. Role of fluorescence in situ hybridization in lung cancer cytology. Acta Cytol. 2012;56(6):611–21.
84. Meric-Bernstam F, Johnson AM, Dumbrava EEI, et al. Advances in HER2-targeted therapy: novel agents and opportunities beyond breast and gastric cancer. Clin Cancer Res. 2019;25(7):2033–41.
85. Oh DY, Bang YJ. HER2-targeted therapies - a role beyond breast cancer. Nat Rev Clin Oncol. 2020;17(1):33–48.

86. Tapia C, Savic S, Wagner U, et al. HER2 gene status in primary breast cancers and matched distant metastases. Breast Cancer Res. 2007;9(3):R31.
87. Edelweiss M, Sebastiao APM, Oen H, Kracun M, Serrette R, Ross DS. HER2 assessment by bright-field dual in situ hybridization in cell blocks of recurrent and metastatic breast carcinoma. Cancer Cytopathol. 2019;127(11):684–90.
88. Camidge DR, Davies KD. MET copy number as a secondary driver of epidermal growth factor receptor tyrosine kinase inhibitor resistance in EGFR-mutant non-small-cell lung cancer. J Clin Oncol. 2019;37(11):855–7.
89. Song Z, Wang H, Yu Z, et al. De novo MET amplification in Chinese patients with non-small-cell lung cancer and treatment efficacy with crizotinib: a multicenter retrospective study. Clin Lung Cancer. 2019;20(2):e171–6.
90. Mignard X, Ruppert AM, Antoine M, et al. c-MET overexpression as a poor predictor of MET amplifications or exon 14 mutations in lung sarcomatoid carcinomas. J Thorac Oncol. 2018;13(12):1962–7.
91. Corcoran JP, Psallidas I, Wrightson JM, Hallifax RJ, Rahman NM. Pleural procedural complications: prevention and management. J Thorac Dis. 2015;7(6):1058–67.
92. Antony VB, Loddenkemper R, Astoul P, et al. Management of malignant pleural effusions. Eur Respir J. 2001;18(2):402–19.
93. Detterbeck FC. The eighth edition TNM stage classification for lung cancer: what does it mean on main street? J Thorac Cardiovasc Surg. 2018;155(1):356–9.
94. Han HS, Eom DW, Kim JH, et al. EGFR mutation status in primary lung adenocarcinomas and corresponding metastatic lesions: discordance in pleural metastases. Clin Lung Cancer. 2011;12(6):380–6.
95. Ettinger DS, Aisner DL, Wood DE, et al. NCCN guidelines insights: non-small cell lung cancer, version 5.2018. J Natl Compr Cancer Netw. 2018;16(7):807–21.
96. Kalemkerian GP, Narula N, Kennedy EB, et al. Molecular testing guideline for the selection of patients with lung cancer for treatment with targeted tyrosine kinase inhibitors: American Society of Clinical Oncology endorsement of the College of American Pathologists/International Association for the Study of Lung Cancer/Association for Molecular Pathology clinical practice guideline update. J Clin Oncol. 2018;36(9):911–9.
97. Lindeman NI, Cagle PT, Aisner DL, et al. Updated molecular testing guideline for the selection of lung cancer patients for treatment with targeted tyrosine kinase inhibitors: guideline from the College of American Pathologists, the International Association for the Study of Lung Cancer, and the Association for Molecular Pathology. Arch Pathol Lab Med. 2018;142(3):321–46.
98. Huang MJ, Lim KH, Tzen CY, Hsu HS, Yen Y, Huang BS. EGFR mutations in malignant pleural effusion of non-small cell lung cancer: a case report. Lung Cancer. 2005;49(3):413–5.
99. Liu L, Shao D, Deng Q, et al. Next generation sequencing-based molecular profiling of lung adenocarcinoma using pleural effusion specimens. J Thorac Dis. 2018;10(5):2631–7.
100. Gupta V, Shukla S, Husain N, Kant S, Garg R. A comparative study of cell block versus biopsy for detection of epidermal growth factor receptor mutations and anaplastic lymphoma kinase rearrangement in adenocarcinoma lung. J Cytol. 2019;36(1):13–7.
101. Malapelle U, Bellevicine C, De Luca C, et al. EGFR mutations detected on cytology samples by a centralized laboratory reliably predict response to gefitinib in non-small cell lung carcinoma patients. Cancer Cytopathol. 2013;121:552–60.
102. Jiang SX, Yamashita K, Yamamoto M, et al. EGFR genetic heterogeneity of nonsmall cell lung cancers contributing to acquired gefitinib resistance. Int J Cancer. 2008;123(11):2480–6.
103. Savic S, Tapia C, Grilli B, et al. Comprehensive epidermal growth factor receptor gene analysis from cytological specimens of non-small-cell lung cancers. Br J Cancer. 2008;98(1):154–60.
104. Ellison G, Zhu G, Moulis A, Dearden S, Speake G, McCormack R. EGFR mutation testing in lung cancer: a review of available methods and their use for analysis of tumour tissue and cytology samples. J Clin Pathol. 2013;66(2):79–89.

105. Tang Y, Wang Z, Li Z, et al. High-throughput screening of rare metabolically active tumor cells in pleural effusion and peripheral blood of lung cancer patients. Proc Natl Acad Sci U S A. 2017;114(10):2544–9.
106. Sanger F, Nicklen S, Coulson AR. DNA sequencing with chain-terminating inhibitors. Proc Natl Acad Sci U S A. 1977;74(12):5463–7.
107. Beck TF, Mullikin JC, NISC Comparative Sequencing Program, Biesecker LG. Systematic evaluation of Sanger validation of next-generation sequencing variants. Clin Chem. 2016;62(4):647–54.
108. Kimura H, Fujiwara Y, Sone T, et al. EGFR mutation status in tumour-derived DNA from pleural effusion fluid is a practical basis for predicting the response to gefitinib. Br J Cancer. 2006;95(10):1390–5.
109. Zhang X, Zhao Y, Wang M, Yap WS, Chang AY. Detection and comparison of epidermal growth factor receptor mutations in cells and fluid of malignant pleural effusion in non-small cell lung cancer. Lung Cancer. 2008;60(2):175–82.
110. Kang JY, Park CK, Yeo CD, et al. Comparison of PNA clamping and direct sequencing for detecting KRAS mutations in matched tumour tissue, cell block, pleural effusion and serum from patients with malignant pleural effusion. Respirology. 2015;20(1):138–46.
111. Chu H, Zhong C, Xue G, et al. Direct sequencing and amplification refractory mutation system for epidermal growth factor receptor mutations in patients with non-small cell lung cancer. Oncol Rep. 2013;30(5):2311–5.
112. Vigliar E, Malapelle U, de Luca C, Bellevicine C, Troncone G. Challenges and opportunities of next-generation sequencing: a cytopathologist's perspective. Cytopathology. 2015;26(5):271–83.
113. Rothberg JM, Hinz W, Rearick TM, et al. An integrated semiconductor device enabling non-optical genome sequencing. Nature. 2011;475(7356):348–52.
114. Bentley DR, Balasubramanian S, Swerdlow HP, et al. Accurate whole human genome sequencing using reversible terminator chemistry. Nature. 2008;456(7218):53–9.
115. Buttitta F, Felicioni L, Del Grammastro M, et al. Effective assessment of EGFR mutation status in bronchoalveolar lavage and pleural fluids by next-generation sequencing. Clin Cancer Res. 2013;19(3):691–8.
116. Yang SR, Lin CY, Stehr H, et al. Comprehensive genomic profiling of malignant effusions in patients with metastatic lung adenocarcinoma. J Mol Diagn. 2018;20(2):184–94.
117. Wang CG, Zeng DX, Huang JA, Jiang JH. Effective assessment of low times MET amplification in pleural effusion after epidermal growth factor receptor-tyrosine kinase inhibitors (EGFR-TKIs) acquired resistance: cases report. Medicine (Baltimore). 2018;97(1):e9021.
118. Sneddon S, Dick I, Lee YCG, et al. Malignant cells from pleural fluids in malignant mesothelioma patients reveal novel mutations. Lung Cancer. 2018;119(5):64–70.
119. Roscilli G, De Vitis C, Ferrara FF, et al. Human lung adenocarcinoma cell cultures derived from malignant pleural effusions as model system to predict patients chemosensitivity. J Transl Med. 2016;14:61.
120. Baylin SB, Esteller M, Rountree MR, Bachman KE, Schuebel K, Herman JG. Aberrant patterns of DNA methylation, chromatin formation and gene expression in cancer. Hum Mol Genet. 2001;10(7):687–92.
121. Baylin SB, Herman JG, Graff JR, Vertino PM, Issa JP. Alterations in DNA methylation: a fundamental aspect of neoplasia. Adv Cancer Res. 1998;72:141–96.
122. Merlo A, Herman JG, Mao L, et al. 5' CpG island methylation is associated with transcriptional silencing of the tumour suppressor p16/CDKN2/MTS1 in human cancers. Nat Med. 1995;1(7):686–92.
123. Moran S, Martinez-Cardus A, Sayols S, et al. Epigenetic profiling to classify cancer of unknown primary: a multicentre, retrospective analysis. Lancet Oncol. 2016;17(10):1386–95.
124. Katayama H, Hiraki A, Aoe K, et al. Aberrant promoter methylation in pleural fluid DNA for diagnosis of malignant pleural effusion. Int J Cancer. 2007;120(10):2191–5.
125. Botana-Rial M, De Chiara L, Valverde D, et al. Prognostic value of aberrant hypermethylation in pleural effusion of lung adenocarcinoma. Cancer Bio Ther. 2012;13(14):1436–42.

126. Yang TM, Leu SW, Li JM, et al. WIF-1 promoter region hypermethylation as an adjuvant diagnostic marker for non-small cell lung cancer-related malignant pleural effusions. J Cancer Res Clin Oncol. 2009;135(7):919–24.

127. Benlloch S, Galbis-Caravajal JM, Martin C, et al. Potential diagnostic value of methylation profile in pleural fluid and serum from cancer patients with pleural effusion. Cancer. 2006;107(8):1859–65.

128. Brock MV, Hooker CM, Yung R, et al. Can we improve the cytologic examination of malignant pleural effusions using molecular analysis? Ann Thorac Surg. 2005;80(4):1241–7.

129. Ilse P, Biesterfeld S, Pomjanski N, Fink C, Schramm M. SHOX2 DNA methylation is a tumour marker in pleural effusions. Cancer Genomics Proteomics. 2013;10(5):217–23.

130. Malapelle U, de Luca C, Vigliar E, et al. EGFR mutation detection on routine cytological smears of non-small cell lung cancer by digital PCR: a validation study. J Clin Pathol. 2016;69(5):454–7.

131. Zhang BO, Xu CW, Shao Y, et al. Comparison of droplet digital PCR and conventional quantitative PCR for measuring EGFR gene mutation. Exp Ther Med. 2015;9(4):1383–8.

132. Vogelstein B, Kinzler KW. Digital PCR. Proc Natl Acad Sci U S A. 1999;96(16):9236–41.

133. Li X, Liu Y, Shi W, et al. Droplet digital PCR improved the EGFR mutation diagnosis with pleural fluid samples in non-small-cell lung cancer patients. Clin Chim Acta. 2017;471:177–84.

134. Gu J, Zang W, Liu B, et al. Evaluation of digital PCR for detecting low-level EGFR mutations in advanced lung adenocarcinoma patients: a cross-platform comparison study. Oncotarget. 2017;8(40):67810–20.

135. Rio DC. Reverse transcription-polymerase chain reaction, Cold Spring. Harb Protoc. 2014;2014(11):1207–16.

136. Schroeder A, Mueller O, Stocker S, et al. The RIN: an RNA integrity number for assigning integrity values to RNA measurements. BMC Mol Biol. 2006;7(1):3.

137. Tsai TH, Su KY, Wu SG, et al. RNA is favourable for analysing EGFR mutations in malignant pleural effusion of lung cancer. Eur Respir J. 2012;39(3):677–84.

138. Soda M, Isobe K, Inoue A, et al. North-East Japan Study, ALKLCS Group. A prospective PCR-based screening for the EML4-ALK oncogene in non-small cell lung cancer. Clin Cancer Res. 2012;18(20):5682–9.

139. Wu SG, Kuo YW, Chang YL, et al. EML4-ALK translocation predicts better outcome in lung adenocarcinoma patients with wild-type EGFR. J Thorac Oncol. 2012;7(1):98–104.

140. Chen YL, Lee CT, Lu CC, et al. Epidermal growth factor receptor mutation and anaplastic lymphoma kinase gene fusion: detection in malignant pleural effusion by RNA or PNA analysis. PLoS One. 2016;11(6):e0158125.

141. Tsai TH, Wu SG, Hsieh MS, Yu CJ, Yang JC, Shih JY. Clinical and prognostic implications of RET rearrangements in metastatic lung adenocarcinoma patients with malignant pleural effusion. Lung Cancer. 2015;88(2):208–14.

142. Vaughn CP, Costa JL, Feilotter HE, et al. Simultaneous detection of lung fusions using a multiplex RT-PCR next generation sequencing-based approach: a multi-institutional research study. BMC Cancer. 2018;18(1):828.

143. Ali G, Bruno R, Savino M, et al. Analysis of fusion genes by nanostring system: a role in lung cytology? Arch Pathol Lab Med. 2018;142(4):480–9.

144. Nicole L, Cappello F, Cappellesso R, VandenBussche CJ, Fassina A. MicroRNA profiling in serous cavity specimens: diagnostic challenges and new opportunities. Cancer Cytopathol. 2019;127(8):493–500.

145. Lin S, Gregory RI. MicroRNA biogenesis pathways in cancer. Nat Rev Cancer. 2015;15(6):321–33.

146. Xie L, Wang T, Yu S, et al. Cell-free miR-24 and miR-30d, potential diagnostic biomarkers in malignant effusions. Clin Biochem. 2011;44(2–3):216–20.

147. Xie L, Chen X, Wang L, et al. Cell-free miRNAs may indicate diagnosis and docetaxel sensitivity of tumor cells in malignant effusions. BMC Cancer. 2010;10:591.

148. Shin YM, Yun J, Lee OJ, et al. Diagnostic value of circulating extracellular miR-134, miR-185, and miR-22 levels in lung adenocarcinoma-associated malignant pleural effusion. Cancer Res Treat. 2014;46(2):178–85.

149. Han HS, Yun J, Lim SN, et al. Downregulation of cell-free miR-198 as a diagnostic biomarker for lung adenocarcinoma-associated malignant pleural effusion. Int J Cancer. 2013;133(3):645–52.

150. Cappellesso R, Nicole L, Caroccia B, et al. MicroRNA-21/microRNA-126 profiling as a novel tool for the diagnosis of malignant mesothelioma in pleural effusion cytology. Cancer Cytopathol. 2016;124(1):28–37.

151. Cappellesso R, Galasso M, Nicole L, Dabrilli P, Volinia S, Fassina A. miR-130A as a diagnostic marker to differentiate malignant mesothelioma from lung adenocarcinoma in pleural effusion cytology. Cancer Cytopathol. 2017;125(8):635–43.

152. Lin J, Wang Y, Zou YQ, et al. Differential miRNA expression in pleural effusions derived from extracellular vesicles of patients with lung cancer, pulmonary tuberculosis, or pneumonia. Tumour Biol. 2016; https://doi.org/10.1007/s13277-016-5410-6.

153. Hydbring P, De Petris L, Zhang Y, et al. Exosomal RNA-profiling of pleural effusions identifies adenocarcinoma patients through elevated miR-200 and LCN2 expression. Lung Cancer. 2018;124:45–52.

154. Wang Y, Xu YM, Zou YQ, et al. Identification of differential expressed PE exosomal miRNA in lung adenocarcinoma, tuberculosis, and other benign lesions. Medicine (Baltimore). 2017;96(44):e8361.

155. Tamiya H, Mitani A, Saito A, et al. Exosomal microRNA expression profiling in patients with lung adenocarcinoma-associated malignant pleural effusion. Anticancer Res. 2018;38(12):6707–14.

156. Siravegna G, Marsoni S, Siena S, Bardelli A. Integrating liquid biopsies into the management of cancer. Nat Rev Clin Oncol. 2017;14(9):531–48.

157. Hummelink K, Muller M, Linders TM, et al. ERJ Open Res. 2019;5(1) https://doi.org/10.1183/23120541.00016-2019.

158. Liu D, Lu Y, Hu Z, et al. Malignant pleural effusion supernatants are substitutes for metastatic pleural tumor tissues in EGFR mutation test in patients with advanced lung adenocarcinoma. PLoS One. 2014;9(2):e89946.

159. Lin J, Gu Y, Du R, Deng M, Lu Y, Ding Y. Detection of EGFR mutation in supernatant, cell pellets of pleural effusion and tumor tissues from non-small cell lung cancer patients by high resolution melting analysis and sequencing. Int J Clin Exp Pathol. 2014;7(12):8813–22.

160. Kawahara A, Fukumitsu C, Azuma K, et al. A combined test using both cell sediment and supernatant cell-free DNA in pleural effusion shows increased sensitivity in detecting activating EGFR mutation in lung cancer patients. Cytopathology. 2018;29(2):150–5.

161. Wu C, Mairinger F, Casanova R, Batavia AA, Leblond AL, Soltermann A. Prognostic immune cell profiling of malignant pleural effusion patients by computerized immunohistochemical and transcriptional analysis. Cancers (Basel). 2019;11(12) https://doi.org/10.3390/cancers11121953.

162. Bubendorf L. Tissue microarrays meet cytopathology. Acta Cytol. 2006;50(2):121–2.

163. Scott SN, Ostrovnaya I, Lin CM, et al. Next-generation sequencing of urine specimens: a novel platform for genomic analysis in patients with non-muscle-invasive urothelial carcinoma treated with bacille Calmette-Guerin. Cancer Cytopathol. 2017;125(6):416–26.

164. Lorber T, Andor N, Dietsche T, et al. Exploring the spatiotemporal genetic heterogeneity in metastatic lung adenocarcinoma using a nuclei flow-sorting approach. J Pathol. 2019;247(2):199–213.

165. Leichsenring J, Volckmar AL, Kirchner M, et al. Targeted deep sequencing of effusion cytology samples is feasible, informs spatiotemporal tumor evolution, and has clinical and diagnostic utility. Genes Chromosomes Cancer. 2018;57(2):70–9.

166. Birkeland E, Zhang S, Poduval D, et al. Patterns of genomic evolution in advanced melanoma. Nat Commun. 2018;9(1):2665.

167. Yates LR, Knappskog S, Wedge D, et al. Genomic evolution of breast cancer metastasis and relapse. Cancer Cell. 2017;32(2):169–184 e7.
168. Lim ZF, Ma PC. Emerging insights of tumor heterogeneity and drug resistance mechanisms in lung cancer targeted therapy. J Hematol Oncol. 2019;12(1):134.
169. Simonsohn U, Nelson LD, Simmons JP. P-curve won't do your laundry, but it will distinguish replicable from non-replicable findings in observational research: comment on Bruns & Ioannidis (2016). PLoS One. 2019;14(3):e0213454.
170. Tseng YH, Ho HL, Lai CR, et al. PD-L1 expression of tumor cells, macrophages, and immune cells in non-small cell lung cancer patients with malignant pleural effusion. J Thorac Oncol. 2018;13(3):447–53.
171. Francisco-Cruz A, Parra ER, Tetzlaff MT, Wistuba II. Multiplex immunofluorescence assays. Methods Mol Biol. 2020;2055:467–95.
172. Goltsev Y, Samusik N, Kennedy-Darling J, et al. Deep profiling of mouse splenic architecture with CODEX multiplexed imaging. Cell. 2018;174(4):968–981 e15.
173. Vinayanuwattikun C, Prakhongcheep O, Tungsukruthai S, et al. Feasibility technique of low-passage in vitro drug sensitivity testing of malignant pleural effusion from advanced-stage non-small cell lung cancer for prediction of clinical outcome. Anticancer Res. 2019;39(12):6981–8.
174. Ruiz C, Kustermann S, Pietilae E, et al. Culture and drug profiling of patient derived malignant pleural effusions for personalized cancer medicine. PLoS One. 2016;11(8):e0160807.
175. Cailleau R, Mackay B, Young RK, Reeves WJ Jr. Tissue culture studies on pleural effusions from breast carcinoma patients. Cancer Res. 1974;34(4):801–9.
176. Artymovich K, Appledorn DM. A multiplexed method for kinetic measurements of apoptosis and proliferation using live-content imaging. Methods Mol Biol. 2015;1219:35–42.
177. Liu X, Krawczyk E, Suprynowicz FA, et al. Conditional reprogramming and long-term expansion of normal and tumor cells from human biospecimens. Nat Protoc. 2017;12(2):439–51.
178. Palechor-Ceron N, Krawczyk E, Dakic A, et al. Conditional reprogramming for patient-derived cancer models and next-generation living biobanks. Cell. 2019;8(11) https://doi.org/10.3390/cells8111327.
179. Jiang S, Wang J, Yang C, et al. Continuous culture of urine-derived bladder cancer cells for precision medicine. Protein Cell. 2019;10(12):902–7.
180. Schutgens F, Clevers H. Human organoids: tools for understanding biology and treating diseases. Ann Rev Pathol. 2020;15:211–34.
181. Bleijs M, van de Wetering M, Clevers H, Drost J. Xenograft and organoid model systems in cancer research. EMBO J. 2019;38(15):e101654.
182. Tuveson D, Clevers H. Cancer modeling meets human organoid technology. Science. 2019;364(6444):952–5.
183. Mazzocchi A, Devarasetty M, Herberg S, et al. Pleural effusion aspirate for use in 3D lung cancer modeling and chemotherapy screening. ACS Biomater Sci Eng. 2019;5(4):1937–43.

Special Considerations for Peritoneal Washings

9

Christopher VandenBussche, Barbara Crothers,
Amanda Fader, Amanda Jackson, Zaibo Li,
and Chengquan Zhao

The Washing Procedure

The washing procedure utilizes a physiologic balanced saline solution to forcibly exfoliate cells within the cavity and to collect cells that have naturally exfoliated into the cavity prior to the procedure. The washing procedure occurs prior to the removal of pelvic neoplasms and before any significant manipulation of abdominopelvic organs. Ascitic fluid, if present, is first aspirated. 50–100 mLs of saline solution is then projected onto the mesothelial wall lining and subsequently aspirated. The results of cytologic examination are frequently reported on a diagnostic checklist if the neoplasm is found to be malignant or of uncertain malignant potential. Washings may be taken from the entire peritoneal or pelvic cavity or may be directed at designated anatomic areas, such as the left or right paracolic gutters and hemidiaphragms.

C. VandenBussche (✉)
Departments of Pathology and Oncology, The John Hopkins University of School of Medicine, Baltimore, MD, USA
e-mail: cjvand@jhmi.edu

B. Crothers
Gynecology, Breast and Cytopathology, Joint Pathology Center, Silver Spring, MD, USA

A. Fader
Department of Obstetrics and Gynecology, The Johns Hopkins Hospital, The Johns Hopkins University, Baltimore, MD, USA

A. Jackson
Department of Obstetrics and Gynecology, Walter Reed National Military Medical Center, Bethesda, MD, USA

Z. Li
Department of Pathology, The Ohio State University, Columbus, OH, USA

C. Zhao
Magee Women's Hospital, University of Pittsburgh Medical Center, Pittsburgh, PA, USA

© Springer Nature Switzerland AG 2020
A. Chandra et al. (eds.), *The International System for Serous Fluid Cytopathology*, https://doi.org/10.1007/978-3-030-53908-5_9

167

Staging and Clinical Relevance

The examination of pelvic washing specimens for neoplastic cells is used for the staging of gynecologic and non-gynecologic malignancies and to exclude occult malignancy in patients with apparent benign disease [1]. A list of entities in which peritoneal washings is reported and whether involvement impacts stage is summarized in Table 9.1. Even if the presence of neoplastic cells in a peritoneal washing does not impact tumor staging, a positive specimen may potentially impact clinical management on an individualized basis.

Positive peritoneal cytology was incorporated into the International Federation of Gynecologists and Obstetricians (FIGO) staging of ovarian and fallopian tube cancer in 1975 and continues to be part of staging today. Currently, positive cytology upgrades a FIGO Stage IA or IB ovarian tumor to Stage IC3 [2]. There is no role for cytology in the staging of ovarian cancer if the cancer has spread beyond Stage IC3. A retrospective study published in 2016 found that in Stage I ovarian tumors, 13% of the 102 Stage I cases in the study were upstaged by cytology alone [3]. A previous study demonstrated that regardless of stage, positive peritoneal cytology is an indicator of poor prognosis for epithelial ovarian cancers [4]. Intraoperative capsule rupture, even in Stage I disease, may portend a higher risk of recurrence and death from disease, depending upon tumor type

Table 9.1 Peritoneal washing and staging of carcinoma by tumor origin

Neoplasm	Staging impact of positive washing
Ovary/fallopian tube	Upstages to at least AJCC[a] Stage T1cC3 (FIGO[b] Stage IC3)
Uterus	Does not upstage (AJCC[a]); collected as a registry value; considered an independent risk factor for poor survival
Cervix	Does not upstage (AJCC[a]); studies have shown an association with a poor prognosis
Stomach	AJCC M1; Stage IV disease
Esophagus	Does not upstage (AJCC[a])
Pancreas	AJCC M1; Stage IV disease
Large and small intestine	Does not upstage (AJCC[a])
Gallbladder	Does not upstage (AJCC[a])
Appendix	Does not upstage (AJCC[a])
Liver (hepatocellular carcinoma)	Does not upstage (AJCC[a])
Cholangiocarcinoma	Does not upstage (AJCC[a])
Rectum	Does not upstage (AJCC[a])

[a]*AJCC* American Joint Committee on Cancer
Reference: Amin et al. [1]
[b]*FIGO* Federation of International Gynecology and Obstetrics
Reference: Prat J, FIGO Committee on Gynecologic Oncology [147]

[5]. Positive cytology and upstaging to Stage IC3 may be the difference between receiving adjuvant chemotherapy or not in Grade 1–2 endometrioid, mucinous, clear cell, and low-grade serous histology [2]. In 2013, Stage IC was divided into three groups based upon surgical spillage (IC1), capsule rupture or ovarian surface involvement (IC2), and positive peritoneal cytology (IC3). A study published in 2018 found no difference in progression-free survival or disease-specific survival between the three groups [6]. However, in our survey of gynecologic oncologists, 20% reported an observed difference in outcome between Stage IC1 and IC3, specifically a higher risk of recurrence in Stage IC3 patients [publication in progress]. This highlights the importance of careful collection and pathologic evaluation of peritoneal cytology in ovarian cancer patients.

The use of peritoneal washings in some gynecologic malignancies is controversial. In endometrial cancer, positive peritoneal cytology is no longer included as part of staging, but FIGO and the American Joint Committee on Cancer (AJCC) continue to recommend that pelvic washings be included as part of an initial staging procedure [7]. In the Gynecologic Oncology Group study #33, 12% of patients with disease suspected to be confined to the uterus had positive cytology, and of those patients, 25% had lymph node metastasis as compared to 7% with negative cytology [8]. Prior to 2009, FIGO staging classified patients with positive cytology alone as Stage IIIA. This classification changed in 2009 following the publication of studies that did not show a difference in survival outcome for patients with positive cytology alone in the absence of other high-risk factors [9–11]. There have been some conflicting studies published that have found positive peritoneal cytology to be an independent predictor of recurrence and poorer survival [12–14]. Optimal therapy for patients with Stage I endometrial cancer and positive peritoneal cytology is therefore undetermined. Sixty-four percent of gynecologic oncologists surveyed reported that they continue to collect peritoneal washings for their endometrial cancer patients, but there was a wide range of response when asked how they managed patients with positive cytology and no evidence of extrauterine disease. While the majority agreed they would manage according to the pathology results and ignore the cytology, a minority indicated they would follow these patients with closer surveillance or treat with progestins or even chemotherapy [publication in progress].

Cytology is not currently considered in cervical cancer staging. There is a higher incidence of positive peritoneal cytology in cervical adenocarcinoma and adenosquamous carcinoma, the prognostic relevance of which is unknown [15]. A study published in 2015 found a significant correlation between parametrial involvement and positive peritoneal cytology [16]. Peritoneal cytology is not considered a prognostic factor in cervical cancer, and its routine collection in surgery is unnecessary [15–17].

Pelvic washings are included as part of risk-reducing surgery for BRCA1- and BRCA2-positive patients for detection of occult malignancy [2]. In a retrospective

10-year study of 117 patients undergoing risk-reducing bilateral salpingo-oophorectomy for BRCA1 or BRCA2, one patient was found to have occult malignancy which was presumed to be primary peritoneal cancer, since no other evidence of disease was found in the surgical specimens [18]. She underwent four cycles of platinum-based chemotherapy and had no evidence of disease at 10-year follow-up. Three additional patients had cytology that was either atypical or suspicious for malignancy that was reclassified as benign after further review [18]. A large retrospective study did not find clinical utility in collecting pelvic washing specimens in patients undergoing gynecologic risk-reducing surgery [19]. The utility of collecting washings in these cases has therefore been questioned, as discordance between cytology and pathology results may lead to potentially unnecessary treatment and stress. Despite these studies, 82% of gynecologic oncologists surveyed found clinical utility in collecting washings at the start of risk-reducing surgeries [publication in progress].

Although positive peritoneal cytology is highly predictive of a poor prognosis for women with epithelial carcinoma of the gynecologic tract [4], it also has a high false-negative rate, presumably due to the encapsulation of persistent tumor by tissue repair mechanisms, resulting in cells that do not readily exfoliate with washings [20]. For other tumors, such as gastric and pancreatic adenocarcinoma, peritoneal lavage may detect tumor cells before they become visible macroscopically and help predict the presence or absence of disease in high-stage patients following neoadjuvant chemotherapy [21].

A Cytopathologic Approach to Peritoneal Washing Interpretation

The cytopathologic approach to peritoneal washing specimens relies on a combination of cytomorphologic examination, performance of ancillary studies, comparison with concurrent surgical specimens, and correlation with the clinician's observations during the procedure. Figure 9.1 shows the origin of cells in peritoneal washings. If performed, results from an intraoperative frozen section may be available for correlation with the initial cytomorphologic findings. Cytomorphologically, the cells seen in peritoneal washings can be broadly categorized into the following:
- Benign background elements
- Mesothelial proliferations
- Benign-appearing or low-grade epithelial cells (of uncertain origin)
- Malignant cells with high-grade morphology

Practical approaches to classifying these findings are outlined in Table 9.2. This table stresses the importance of correlating the cytology findings with a corresponding surgical specimen whenever possible, ideally by comparing the microscopic appearance to one another, and reporting that comparison. When the cellular features are

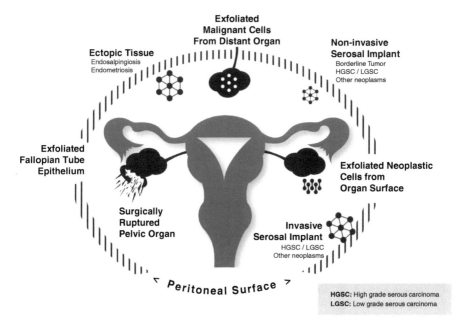

Fig. 9.1 Origin of gynecologic lesions in peritoneal fluids

compatible, the likelihood of them being of the same origin is high. For low-grade neoplasia such as borderline tumors, reporting these findings as atypia of undetermined significance (AUS), "consistent with borderline tumor," is preferred. If the cells are dissimilar, the surgical specimen may provide clues to their origin (e.g., endometriosis). For high-grade neoplasia, a definitive malignant diagnosis is preferred when all conditions are concordant. The terminology should be concise and match the tumor (e.g., metastatic high-grade serous carcinoma), rather than relying on descriptive text. If doubt remains regarding the lesion and surgical correlation is not possible, either an atypical/AUS (likely benign process) or a suspicious/SFM (likely malignant process) category is the option, with further clarification in a comment or an explanatory note that describes the problem and suggests steps toward resolution. Twenty-two percent of gynecologic oncologists surveyed indicated that they find the reporting of atypical cells that appear to be benign to be useful. Out of 119 free-text responses to a question on how they manage these patients, the majority indicated they would treat as benign in the absence of positive pathology. However, 13% indicated that they would either counsel the patient on the results, follow these patients more closely, or treat as malignant with either hormonal treatment or even chemotherapy [publication in progress]. Given the diversity of management styles, it may be useful to continue to report atypical results. Most of the malignant tumors detected will be metastatic from a primary

Table 9.2 Approach to reporting findings in peritoneal washings

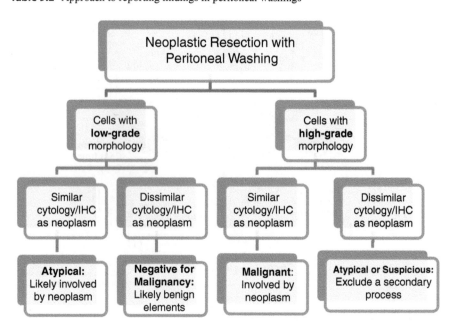

site other than the peritoneum. The most common primary peritoneal neoplasia is serous carcinoma, but it is not possible to distinguish this from metastatic serous carcinoma. The origin of Müllerian primary peritoneal tumors is still under investigation, but none can be cytologically distinguished from their ovarian counterpart. Additionally, primary uterine carcinoma (endometrioid, serous, clear cell carcinomas) cannot be cytologically distinguished from their ovarian counterparts, and the descriptions below cover the uterus as a possible primary site. Mentioning benign background elements, such as suture or hemostatic material, is optional, with notable exceptions. Background mucin, even in the absence of neoplastic cells, is important due to its association with pseudomyxoma peritonei. The presence of bile may indicate biliary tract leakage. Both should be reported in an explanatory note.

Benign Background Elements

Background

Benign background elements are usually increased in number in washing specimens. Additional benign findings may be seen only in washing specimens, such as collagen balls, sheets of mesothelial cells, and endosalpingiosis. Other epithelioid cells that may be rarely collected by procedures include decidual or trophoblastic cells from pregnant patients, histiocytes and giant cells in granulomatous processes, smooth muscle cells from leiomyomatosis, Walthard's rest or adrenal rest cells, and endocervical cells from endocervicosis. Familiarity with these findings is important, because it allows possible distractors to be dismissed. These findings should be reported as negative for malignancy (NFM) with a descriptive diagnosis as to their likely origin. In the current practices survey of international cytologists preceding this text, 76% of participants agreed that benign cells other than mesothelial cells should be reported along with the potential significance of the finding [publication in progress].

Mesothelial Cells

The most common finding in peritoneal washings is the presence of sheets of mesothelial cells. Normal mesothelial cell features are described in detail in Chap. 3, "Negative for Malignancy (NFM)." The peritoneal washing procedure exfoliates normal mesothelial cells primarily as monolayer sheets rather than individual mesothelial cells (Fig. 9.2).

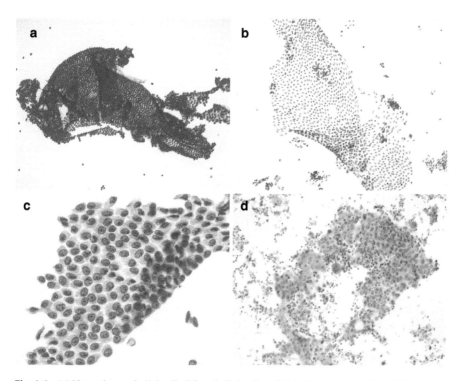

Fig. 9.2 (**a**) Normal mesothelial cells. Mesothelial cells exfoliated by pelvic washing fluid present as two-dimensional, large, flat monolayer sheets with pavement stone architecture. Cytospin; modified Giemsa stain. (**b**) Normal mesothelial cells in folded sheets. ThinPrep; Papanicolaou stain. (**c**) Normal mesothelial cells. Benign mesothelial cells with distinct cellular borders; uniform, evenly spaced nuclei; and finely granular, powdery chromatin. ThinPrep; Papanicolaou stain. (**d**) Mesothelial cells, isolated and forming loose sheets. Papanicolaou stain

Cytologic Criteria

- Two-dimensional, large, flat monolayer sheets with pavement stone architecture
- Crisp cytoplasmic sheet edges and distinct cellular borders or spaces between cells
- Uniform, evenly spaced nuclei with finely granular, powdery chromatin
- Nuclear longitudinal grooves possible
- Well-defined, smooth nuclear membrane, sometimes with slight indentations
- Absent to inconspicuous nucleoli
- Mesothelial sheet folding
- Single, polygonal mesothelial cells with uniform, round-to-oval central nuclei and moderate cytoplasm
- Reactive features include:
  - Large clusters, balls, or non-branching papillae
  - Plump cells with denser cytoplasm and cytoplasmic vacuoles
  - Enlarged nuclei with multinucleation and small- to medium-sized nucleoli
  - Normal mitotic figures

Explanatory Notes

Reactive mesothelial cells may be caused by a variety of conditions such as abdominal or pelvic masses, inflammatory conditions, endometriosis, and surgical procedures. Reactive mesothelial cells may show a broad spectrum of cellular changes in the same specimen. They are difficult to distinguish from reactive mesothelial hyperplasia and multilocular peritoneal inclusion cysts, which will shed identical cells, but may also have associated isolated or sheets of metaplastic squamous cells [22]. Reactive mesothelial cells should be differentiated from malignant mesothelioma (Chap. 6, "Malignant-Primary") and adenocarcinoma (Chap. 7, "Malignant-Secondary"). Reactive mesothelial cells do not require a diagnostic statement and should be reported as NFM rather than as AUS.

Collagen Balls

Collagen balls are tissue fragments composed of collagen covered by mesothelial cells. It has been speculated that they primarily derive from ovarian surfaces. They may appear in pelvic washing specimens and have no clinical importance (Fig. 9.3). As opposed to psammoma bodies, they have no calcification [23].

Cytologic Criteria

- Three-dimensional, large spherical to oval structures
- Central dense, hyalinized matrix (aqua on Papanicolaou; magenta on modified Giemsa)

- Surrounded by a single layer of attenuated, well-spaced benign mesothelial cells, visible on different planes of focus as single nuclei without cytoplasm

Endosalpingiosis

Endosalpingiosis is the ectopic presence of benign, often cystic, glands, lined by fallopian tube-type epithelium, on the peritoneal surface or other pelvic structures and within lymph nodes (Fig. 9.4).

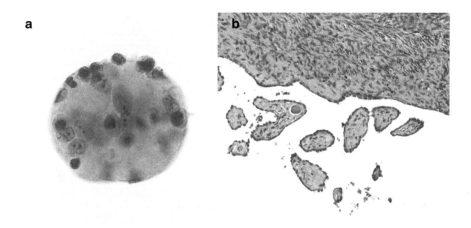

Fig. 9.3 (**a**) Collagen balls, peritoneal fluid. Three-dimensional, large spherical to oval structure with central dense, hyalinized matrix. ThinPrep; Papanicolaou stain. (**b**) Collagen balls, ovarian origin. The collagen balls are surrounded by a single layer of attenuated, well-spaced benign ovarian surface cells. H&E stain

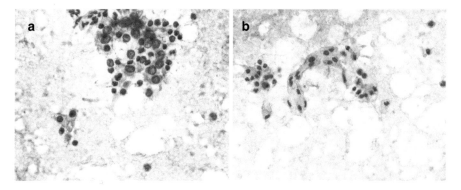

Fig. 9.4 (**a**) Endosalpingiosis. Clusters of small, uniform, evenly spaced tubal epithelial cells with small, round, uniform nuclei with fine chromatin and inconspicuous nucleoli. Cilia and terminal bar can be seen. Cytospin; modified Giemsa stain. (**b**) Endosalpingiosis. Clusters of small, uniform, evenly spaced tubal epithelial cells with small, round, uniform nuclei with fine chromatin and inconspicuous nucleoli. Eosinophilic cilia are prominent. Cytospin; modified Giemsa stain

Cytologic Criteria

- Cohesive aggregates of non-branching papillae
- Clusters of small, uniform, evenly spaced tubal epithelial cells
- Small, round, uniform nuclei with fine chromatin and inconspicuous nucleoli
- Ciliated or non-ciliated; terminal bar
- Psammoma bodies possible (but infrequent)

Explanatory Notes

The origin of endosalpingiosis is controversial. As an isolated finding, it is more frequent in postmenopausal women. It is also associated with other pelvic diseases such as leiomyomas, endometriosis, hydrosalpinx, and pelvic adhesions [24, 25]. It may present as a cystic or multicystic mass. The presence of cilia and/or a terminal bar supports a benign process, but ciliated carcinoma cells have been described [26, 27]. Psammoma bodies may be observed with these glands [28]. Rarely, the disruption of the ciliated terminal end of the tubal cells, usually due to cellular degeneration, can result in the phenomenon known as *ciliocytophthoria*, where the ciliated end of the now-enucleated "cell" can mimic a mobile parasite in unfixed, fresh specimens (Fig. 9.5) [29].

Inflammatory Cells, Including Macrophages

An abundance of inflammatory cells in peritoneal fluids always indicates disease, infection, or tissue repair and should be reported as acute inflammation (predominately neutrophils), chronic inflammation (predominately lymphocytes), granulomatous inflammation (macrophages, granulomas, and/or giant cells), or mixed

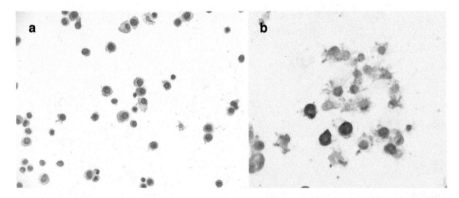

Fig. 9.5 (**a**) Ciliocytophthoria with ciliated terminal end of tubal cells detached in the background. Papanicolaou stain. (**b**) Ciliocytophthoria. Multiple cytoplasmic fragments with cilia. High magnification, Papanicolaou stain

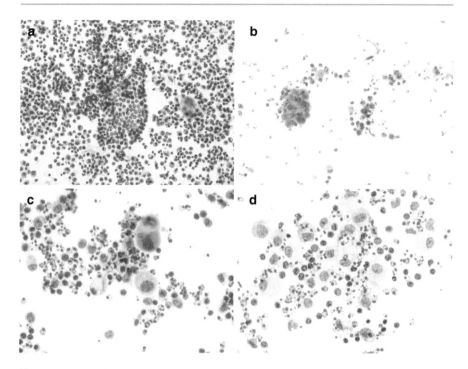

Fig. 9.6 (**a**) Mixed acute and chronic inflammation with sheets and single mesothelial cells. The debris may represent vegetable matter from a ruptured bowel. Cytospin, Papanicolaou stain. (**b**) Small cluster of mesothelial cells in a background of chronic (lymphocytic) inflammation. Lymphocytes cling to the cells and vacuoles are present in some mesothelial cells. Cytospin, Papanicolaou stain. (**c**) "Windows" (spaces) occur between mesothelial cells. Cytospin, Papanicolaou stain. (**d**) Histiocytes and lymphocytes. Histiocytes have oval- to kidney bean-shaped, uniform nuclei, reticular chromatin, and abundant, frothy, pale cytoplasm. Lymphocytes have scant cytoplasm and round nuclei with coarse, regular chromatin. Papanicolaou stain

(Fig. 9.6). Most benign inflammatory conditions show a polymorphous population of inflammatory cells with one cell type predominant.

Macrophages deserve special mention for their role in orchestrating tissue response. It is not uncommon to observe macrophages in peritoneal washing specimens, especially in inflammatory conditions. It is not always possible to distinguish macrophages from degenerating mesothelial cells in serous fluids. These cells can be single or clustered together with abundant cytoplasm and uniform nuclei. Use of CD68 or CD163 can confirm their identity. Occasionally, hemosiderin pigmentation (Fig. 9.7) can be observed in these cells.

Cytologic Criteria (Macrophages)

- Single (typically) or in loose clusters with distinct edges
- Oval- to kidney bean-shaped, uniform nuclei with reticular chromatin; multinucleation possible

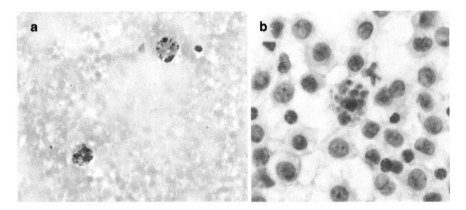

Fig. 9.7 (a) Hemosiderin-laden macrophages with dark purple hemosiderin pigment. Modified Giemsa stain. (b) Hemosiderin-laden macrophages with mesothelial cells from a patient with endometriosis. Hemosiderin pigment appears as dark greenish cytoplasmic material. Cytospin, Papanicolaou stain

- Indistinct nucleoli
- Abundant, frothy, pale cytoplasm (without "two-tone" staining)
- Cytoplasmic vacuoles of variable sizes with "fuzzy" borders
- Cytoplasmic inclusions such as other cells, cellular debris, bacteria, fungus, crystals, and pigment (bile, hemosiderin, melanin)

Explanatory Notes

The peritoneum plays a key role in regulating inflammatory processes in the abdomen and pelvis [30]. Causes of peritoneal inflammation include infectious salpingitis, ectopic pregnancy, endometriosis, appendicitis, bacterial infection (e.g., from ruptured colonic diverticula), bile leakage peritonitis, trauma, surgical procedures, and carcinomatosis. The usual offending organisms in acute peritonitis are Gram-positive *Staphylococcus epidermidis*, *Staphylococcus aureus*, or Gram-negative enteric bacteria, which induce large numbers of neutrophils. Chronic inflammation, as evidenced by primarily mature lymphocytes, may mimic low-grade lymphoma, and flow cytometry may be useful to differentiate between them. Granulomatous inflammation usually indicates a foreign body or fungal infection, such as histoplasmosis, but can also be caused by mycobacteria. Clusters of macrophages and giant cells may be present. Dialysis patients are particularly susceptible to the development of chronic peritonitis and infection [31]. The presence of specific elements within a macrophage can help in identification of disease. Hemosiderin (confirmed with an iron stain) and/or engulfed red blood cells indicate active or remote bleeding, as is common with endometriosis. Macrophages and giant cells with golden-green bile pigment and cholesterol crystals indicate bile leakage; extracellular stringy green mucus and microspheroliths are other findings [32]. Bile peritonitis is a serious condition with a high mortality and, when suspected, should be reported immediately.

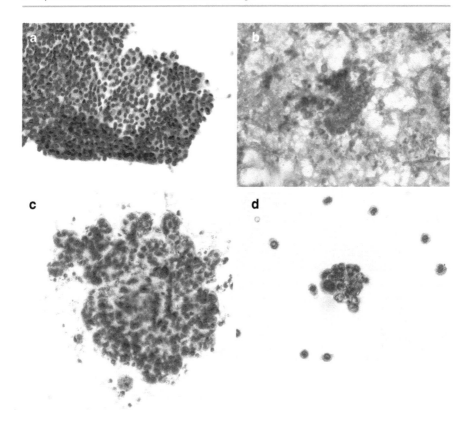

Fig. 9.8 (**a**) Endometriosis. Endometrial glandular cell sheets with honeycomb pattern and closely approximated, uniform, oval nuclei. ThinPrep; Papanicolaou stain. (**b**) Endometriosis. Tightly cohesive, three-dimensional balls of small endometrial cells with small round-to-oval nuclei and hyperchromatic chromatin. Papanicolaou stain. (**c**) Endometriosis. Tightly cohesive endometrial cells with round-to-oval nuclei, mild hyperchromasia, and cellular crowding. Degenerated red blood cells are present. Papanicolaou stain. (**d**) Endometriosis. A cluster of small endometrial cells in a three-dimensional configuration with background endometrial stromal cells. ThinPrep; Papanicolaou stain

Endometriosis

Endometriosis is characterized by the ectopic presence of endometrial glands and stroma outside of the endometrium (Fig. 9.8).

Cytologic Criteria

- Endometrial cell sheets with honeycomb pattern and closely approximated, uniform, oval nuclei
- Tightly cohesive, three-dimensional balls of small endometrial cells with round-to-oval nuclei and hyperchromatic chromatin
- Branching tubules of columnar endometrial cells with small to medium uniform nuclei

- Endometrial glandular cells may show mild nuclear enlargement, hyperchromasia, crowding, and disorganization
- Glandular cell atypia and mitoses uncommon
- Endometrial stromal cells in loose sheets with plump, oval to spindled nuclei and indistinct, syncytial cytoplasm
- Single endometrial stromal cells more frequently show oval nuclei, nuclear grooves, irregular membranes, and scant cytoplasm
- Endometrial stromal cells with decidual change related to pregnancy appear loosely cohesive and epithelioid with abundant eosinophilic cytoplasm
- Hemosiderin-laden macrophages (often prominent) and degenerating blood

Explanatory Notes

The origin of endometriosis is unclear, but may be related to ectopic growth of endometrium seeded through fallopian tubes, by surgical procedures or vascular channels, or evolve from Müllerian differentiation of the pelvic peritoneum. The histologic diagnosis of endometriosis requires the presence of at least two of the following findings: endometrial glands, endometrial stroma, and/or hemosiderin-laden macrophages. The cytopathologic diagnosis can usually be made with confidence with intraoperative findings of brown to maroon "chocolate cysts" along with benign-appearing endometrial cells and hemosiderin-laden macrophages. In peritoneal washings, benign endometrial cells appear identical to exfoliated benign endometrial cells on Pap tests, but may be better preserved, resulting in cytologic features that are more clearly visualized [33, 34]. Endometrial stromal cells are rarely identified in pelvic washing but may become more apparent in cell blocks (CB). CD10 can be useful to identify stromal cells in CB [35]. Hemosiderin-laden macrophages often predominate and, in the proper setting, are highly suggestive of endometriosis [33, 36]. The presence of hemosiderin-laden macrophages alone is not diagnostic because they may be seen in other conditions associated with bleeding. Endometriosis may be a cause of false-positive results [37].

Sample Reports

Example 1
Peritoneal fluid, washings:
- Satisfactory for evaluation.
- Negative for malignancy. Benign mesothelial cells and collagen balls.
- Category: Negative for malignancy.
  Note: Collagen balls and reactive mesothelial cells are present, but these are benign findings without clinical significance.

Example 2
Peritoneal fluid, washings:
- Evaluation limited by obscuring inflammation.
- Negative for malignancy. Acute inflammation.
- Category: Negative for malignancy.

Example 3

Peritoneal fluid, lavage:

- Satisfactory for evaluation.
- Negative for malignancy. Benign endometrial cells and hemosiderin-laden macrophages, consistent with endometriosis.
- Category: Negative for malignancy.

Nonepithelial Elements

Background

Nonepithelial elements are rare in peritoneal fluid. The most important of these are psammoma bodies, acellular mucin, and bile. Other nonepithelial elements that may appear unexpectedly include surgical products such as hemostatic microcrystalline collagen; talcum powder granules; mesh graft fibers; lubricant; oils; cellulose and cotton fibers or suture material; organisms such as bacteria, fungi, and parasites; debris from bowel rupture or trauma (including plant cell walls and vegetable matter) (Fig. 9.9); and spillage of amniotic fluid containing vernix

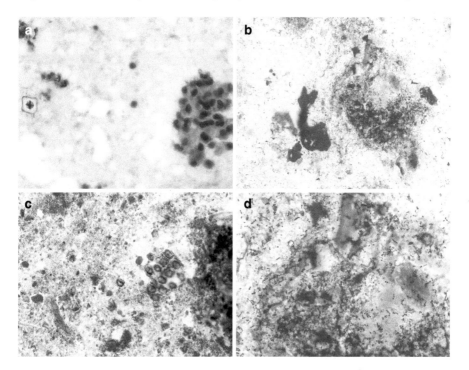

Fig. 9.9 (**a**) Talcum powder crystal in pelvic washing fluid with an irregular, refractile outline and a small "x" in the center. Modified Giemsa stain. (**b**) Intestinal contents due to bowel rupture. Noncellular debris and abundant bacteria are present. Modified Giemsa stain. (**c**) Intestinal contents due to bowel rupture. Plant material, acellular debris, bacteria, and crystals are present. Papanicolaou stain. (**d**) Intestinal contents due to bowel rupture. Abundant noncellular debris with coccobacilli and rodlike bacteria are present. Modified Giemsa stain

caseosa (keratin and benign squamous cells, sebum, and lanugo hair) or meconium from cesarean section.

Psammoma Bodies

Psammoma bodies can be seen in up to 20% of pelvic washing specimens (Fig. 9.10) [38].

Cytologic Criteria

- Spherical, dense, darkly stained calcifications with concentric lamination
- Variable sizes; sometimes fragmented or cracked
- No attached epithelial or mesothelial cells
- Low cellularity background

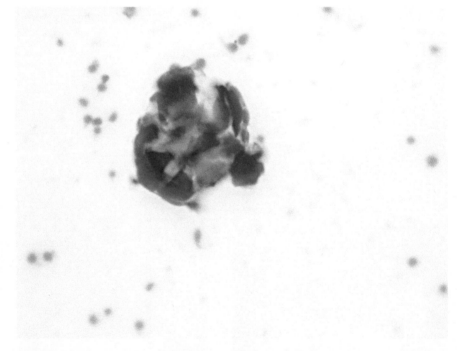

Fig. 9.10 Psammoma body. Spherical, dense, darkly stained calcifications with concentric lamination and attached mesothelial cells. Papanicolaou stain

Explanatory Notes

Psammoma bodies can be associated with benign or neoplastic processes. Benign conditions include endosalpingiosis, endometriosis, mesothelial hyperplasia, and benign ovarian tumors (primarily serous tumors) [38]. Free psammoma bodies without attached cells and without atypical cellular components are more likely to represent a benign process. Those associated with attached cells and a highly cellular background are more likely malignant. About half of peritoneal washing cases with psammoma bodies are associated with malignant tumors or borderline ovarian tumors, including serous carcinoma or serous borderline tumor (most common), endometrioid carcinoma (EC) (uncommon), and mesothelioma (rare) [39–41]. An abundance of psammoma bodies may be indicative of the so-called psammocarcinoma, a serous tumor comprised of greater than 75% psammoma bodies [42, 43], but this lesion is falling out of favor as a distinct entity and the diagnosis cannot be made cytologically.

Acellular Mucin

Acellular mucin is an abnormal finding that must be correlated with the clinical and operative findings to determine its significance and should be reported (Fig. 9.11).

Cytologic Criteria

- Sheets of thick to thin, finely granular, or smooth matrix
- Folds, rivulets, and undulations within the matrix
- Indistinct edges appear to merge with background; fuzzy edges
- No epithelial cells

Explanatory Notes

Pseudomyxoma peritonei (PMP) is a clinical condition in which mucin is present within the peritoneal cavity and is not a term used in diagnosis. Mucin is usually produced by a low-grade appendiceal mucinous neoplasm. Rupture of this lesion causes intraabdominal mucin with or without bland epithelial cells in peritoneal fluid, a phenomenon referred to as disseminated peritoneal adenomucinosis (DPAM) [44]. High-grade malignant cells from the gallbladder or other areas within the gastrointestinal tract may also produce mucin; these cells often have formed implants within the peritoneal cavity. Care must be taken to avoid over-calling artifact that can mimic mucin by confirming its presence with special stains such as PAS with and without diastase, Alcian blue, or mucicarmine. True mucin is mucicarmine positive and remains positive when PAS is subject to diastase digestion. Surgical collection suction devices may be lined with a material that can mimic mucin cytologically, but may show striations and blunt, thick edges that are not present in true mucin [45].

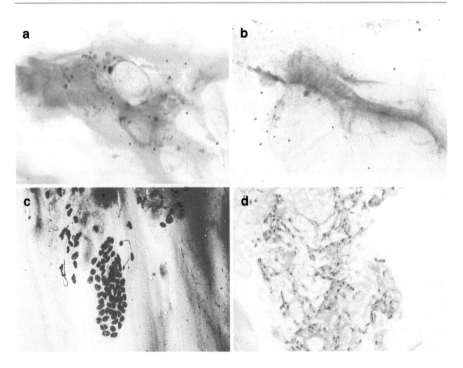

Fig. 9.11 (**a**) Acellular mucin. Sheets of thick to thin, finely granular, or smooth matrix. Papanicolaou stain. (**b**) Acellular mucin. Matrix folds and undulations help distinguish mucin from mimics. Papanicolaou stain. (**c**) Well-differentiated mucinous carcinoma. Atypical epithelial cells with mild nuclear irregularities and crowding are present in flat sheets and clusters or singly in a background of thick mucin. Modified Giemsa stain. (**d**) Thick mucin with atypical cells present in a cell block section. H&E stain

Bile

The presence of bile in peritoneal fluid is associated with bile leakage syndrome that occurs when bile escapes from the gallbladder and involves peritoneal surfaces (Fig. 9.12).

Cytologic Criteria

- Gold to green sheets of fibrillar material in clumps and pools (may appear stringy grossly)
- Variable numbers of inflammatory cells, mostly neutrophils with some lymphocytes
- Bile-laden macrophages
- Cholesterol crystals/clefts of various sizes, sometimes in giant cells
- Granulomatous inflammation, including giant cells
- Mesothelial cells

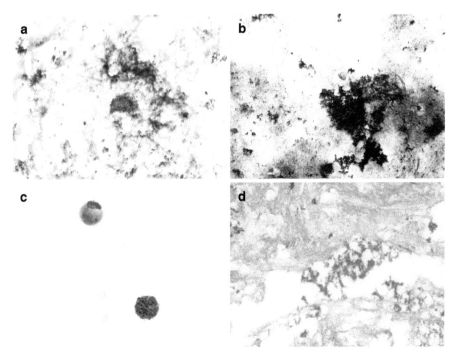

Fig. 9.12 (**a**) Bile spillage. Gold-green sheets of fibrillary material in clumps. Cytospin, Papanicolaou stain. (**b**) Bile spillage. Dark golden-brown clumps of fibrillary material. Cytospin, modified Giemsa stain. (**c**) Pigmented macrophages in pelvic washing fluid with bile spillage. Cytospin, modified Giemsa stain. (**d**) Bile spillage. Golden fibrillary material in pelvic washing fluid. Cell block, H&E stain

Explanatory Notes

Bile peritonitis is a severe, aseptic inflammatory response to bile that is debilitating and requires urgent surgical intervention. Histologically, it may not cause severe acute inflammation, but in more chronic conditions, is associated with granulomatous inflammation and giant cells engulfing cholesterol. Common causes are migrating gallstones, biliary obstruction, biliary tract inflammation, cholecystectomy, and perforated gallbladder or biliary tree [32]. The material is often positive for mucosubstances but negative for bilirubin [46].

Sample Reports

Example 1
Peritoneal washing:
- Evaluation limited by scant cellularity.
- Negative for malignancy. Psammoma bodies present (see note).
- Category: Negative for malignancy.

Note: Psammoma bodies without attached epithelial cells are present. In most cases, this finding is associated with benign processes such as endosalpingiosis, endometriosis, mesothelial hyperplasia, or benign ovarian tumors, but may also be associated with neoplastic processes such as borderline and malignant serous tumors. Clinical correlation is required.

Example 2

Peritoneal lavage:
- Satisfactory for evaluation.
- Atypical epithelial cells with psammoma bodies.
- Category: Atypia of undetermined significance.

Note: Psammoma bodies with attached epithelial cells showing features of Müllerian origin are present. The benign-appearing cells are reactive for PAX8, ER, and CK7 and may represent endosalpingiosis, endometriosis, or a benign/low-grade serous ovarian tumor, but a corresponding surgical specimen is unavailable for correlation. Clinical correlation is required.

Example 3

Abdominal cavity, peritoneal lavage:
- Evaluation limited by scant to absent cellularity.
- Negative for malignancy. Acellular mucin present (see note).
- Category: Negative for malignancy.

Note: The presence of acellular mucin has been confirmed by a positive PASD stain with appropriately reactive control specimens. This finding has been associated with pseudomyxoma peritonei. The presence or absence of cells is an important prognostic feature; in this case, cells are lacking, which often portends a better prognosis. Acellular mucin may also be associated with other gastrointestinal, pancreatic, or ovarian mucinous neoplasms. Clinical correlation is required.

Mesothelial Proliferations

Mesothelial proliferations that raise concern for mesothelioma should be assessed as described in Chap. 5, "Suspicious for Malignancy," and Chap. 6, "Malignant-Primary (Mesothelioma)." The most common mesothelial proliferation in women is benign peritoneal inclusion cysts (PIC), which may be unilocular or multilocular. Unilocular PIC are usually an incidental finding. Multilocular PIC can produce a large mass, can be painful, and are more frequently associated with a history of prior surgical intervention, endometriosis, or pelvic inflammatory disease [47]. In most cases, these cells are undistinguishable from other benign mesothelial cells in the peritoneum, but on occasion they may undergo squamous or mucinous metaplasia or develop reactive mild mesothelial atypia.

Well-Differentiated Papillary Mesothelioma

Well-differentiated papillary mesothelioma (WDPM) occurs primarily in female peritoneum as an incidental finding, either as single or multiple lesions, and is unassociated with asbestosis. It may be associated with endometriosis or abdominal surgical procedures. It is a low-grade neoplasm that behaves as a benign tumor, with rare recurrence or persistence in the peritoneum [48]. It does occur in the pleura both in women and men.

Cytologic Criteria

- Blunt, broad papillae with central, smoothly hyalinized or fibrous core, lined with a single layer of cuboidal mesothelial cells, often present as spheres
- Mesothelial cells flattened or hobnailed around papillae
- Monolayered, flat mesothelial sheets
- Nuclei round, uniform with fine chromatin and inconspicuous nucleoli
- Stromal histiocytes and multinucleated giant cells possible in cores
- Scattered, scant inflammatory cells
- Mild to absent cellular atypia
- No mitoses
- Psammoma bodies possible

Explanatory Notes

The cytologic features of WDPM in fluids [49] mirror those found in fine needle aspiration of this lesion [50], but fluid specimens may be less cellular and show more background mesothelial cells. The differential includes collagen balls, but WDPM papillae are more cellular. Cells lining the papillae are reactive for calretinin, D2-40, and HBME1. The cells are negative for epithelial markers such as BerEP4 and MOC-31. One diagnostic pitfall is that WDPM may be positive for PAX8, which may cause concern for a neoplasm of Müllerian origin. Malignant mesothelioma should be excluded (Fig 9.13). These lesions are best categorized as AUS. When comparison with a confirming surgical specimen is possible, interpretation can include "consistent with WDPM."

Sample Report

Example 1
Right pelvis, peritoneal washings:
- Satisfactory for evaluation.
- Atypical mesothelial cells consistent with well-differentiated papillary mesothelioma.

- Category: Atypical cells of undetermined significance.

   Note: The cytology was compared with the surgical excision of the peritoneal tumor and the findings are compatible. Tumor cell reactivity for calretinin, WT1, and D2-40 on the cell block confirms mesothelial origin.

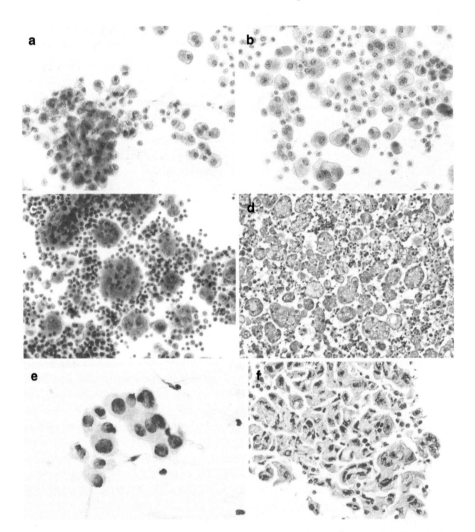

Fig. 9.13 (**a**) Mesothelioma. Blunt, broad papillae lined with cuboidal or hobnailed atypical mesothelial cells, which show round nuclei, fine chromatin, and inconspicuous or small nucleoli. Papanicolaou stain. (**b**) Mesothelioma. Single cells with pleomorphic, variable-sized nuclei and abundant cytoplasm. Binucleation and multinucleation are common. Papanicolaou stain. (**c**) Mesothelioma. Small clusters and hypercellular balls of cells in a background of lymphocytes. Papanicolaou stain. (**d**) Mesothelioma. Clusters of and single malignant cells with pleomorphic, variable-sized nuclei and abundant cytoplasm. Hobnailed cells are present at the periphery of cell clusters. Cell block, H&E stain. (**e**) Mesothelioma. A small cluster of cells with pleomorphic, variable-sized nuclei, abundant cytoplasm, and prominent nucleoli. Modified Giemsa stain. (**f**) Mesothelioma. Malignant cells with pleomorphic, variable-sized nuclei and abundant cytoplasm. Cell block, H&E stain

Low-Grade Neoplastic Cells

Bland-appearing epithelial cells are often found in peritoneal washing specimens and may represent benign processes (such as endosalpingiosis) or low-grade neoplastic processes (such as borderline ovarian tumors) (Table 9.3). Cells may or may not be associated with psammoma bodies; psammoma bodies from tumors are more likely associated with cellular specimens, including cell clusters without psammoma bodies. The presence of rare glandular fragments in serous fluids may cause diagnostic difficulty in patients with concurrent serous borderline tumors. Since many of the entities within the differential diagnosis are of Müllerian origin, immunohistochemical studies are not usually helpful in narrowing the diagnosis. Generally, the presence of a neoplasm results in a proliferative population of cells in a washing specimen when the lesion involves the ovarian or peritoneal surfaces. Comparison of the cytology with the surgical specimen is critical in confirming the origin; when compatible, they are likely from the same process.

Benign Ovarian Epithelial Tumors

Background
Benign ovarian epithelial tumors are not usually seen in peritoneal washing specimens unless there is intraprocedural rupture of the tumor (iatrogenic cause) or in rare cases where the tumor involves the ovarian surface, such as serous surface papillomas. Ovarian epithelial tumors fall into general categories defined by their epithelium: serous, mucinous, endometrioid, clear cell, seromucinous, or transitional (Brenner tumors). Benign tumors include papillomas, adenofibromas, and cystadenomas. The tendency of epithelial cells to form tight balls in serous fluids can make it difficult to identify distinguishing cell features such as cilia, mucin

Table 9.3 Differential diagnosis of bland epithelial or low-grade neoplastic cells

Process	Clues to diagnosis
Borderline serous tumor	Concordant with morphology of patient's established neoplasm
Low-grade serous carcinoma	Concordant with morphology of patient's established neoplasm
Endosalpingiosis/ fallopian tube epithelium	Columnar cells with terminal bars and/or cilia; often subclinical on pelvic washing specimens
Endometriosis	Cytomorphologically similar to endometrial cells seen on Pap test specimens; background contains degenerated blood and hemosiderin-laden macrophages; clinical impression of endometriosis before or during surgery
Cystadenofibroma/ adenofibroma	Columnar cells with terminal bars and/or cilia; often subclinical on pelvic washing specimens; concordant with morphology of patient's resected tumor (if available)
Benign mesothelial fragments	Positive for mesothelial markers (such as calretinin) and negative for MOC 31, MOC-31, and BerEP4

vacuoles, or characteristic nuclei. Degeneration of any cell in fluid can create cytoplasmic vacuoles that should not be interpreted as evidence of mucin production.

Serous Cystadenoma

Iatrogenic rupture of serous cystadenoma may cause a cellular peritoneal washing specimen with variable amounts of benign serous-type glands cytologically identical to endosalpingiosis, but much more cellular (Fig. 9.14). Cilia, although a distinctive feature, are often not apparent.

Mucinous Cystadenoma/Adenofibroma

Iatrogenic rupture of mucinous cystadenoma may result in a cellular peritoneal washing specimen with benign mucinous-type glands, in sheets or papillary clusters, with or without extracellular mucin (Fig. 9.15). The mucinous epithelial cells resemble endocervical cells or intestinal cells with intracellular mucin. Goblet cells may be present. Typically, it is not possible to differentiate between a benign and borderline mucinous tumor on cytology alone, although benign tumors shed fewer cells and specimens are less cellular [51]. Moreover, benign and borderline mucinous tumors are significantly less likely to cause a positive peritoneal fluid than serous low-grade tumors [52]. Ovarian mucinous cystadenomas have been associated with *pseudomyxoma peritonei*.

Seromucinous Cystadenoma/Adenofibroma

Seromucinous tumors (previously "endocervical-type" mucinous tumor) are a specific subtype of ovarian tumors comprised of two or more Müllerian type cells (serous, endocervical, endometrial, or clear cell), most often serous and endocervical mucinous cells, that occur in middle-aged women and are associated with endometriosis. Iatrogenic rupture of these tumors may cause spillage of benign seromucinous-type glands in seromucinous cystadenoma [53]. The cytologic features overlap with benign serous tumors but endocervical cells are also present.

Endometrioid Cystadenoma/Adenofibroma

Endometrioid tumors of the ovary are rare and often associated with endometriosis. Endometrioid cystadenomas and borderline tumors tend to be solid tumors with small cyst-like spaces or mural nodules in an endometriotic cyst. Cells shed from these tumors will be identical to those found in endometriosis, and it may not be possible to differentiate between them. There are usually fewer, if any, background hemosiderin-laden macrophages with tumors as opposed to endometriosis.

Brenner Tumor and Borderline Brenner Tumor

Brenner/borderline Brenner tumors are transitional (urothelial) cell neoplasms, sometimes associated with ovarian mucinous tumors, that rarely exfoliate cells into the peritoneal cavity due to their densely fibrous stroma. Infrequent sheets or clusters of evenly spaced urothelial epithelial cells from a benign Brenner tumor might occur in fluids; these closely mimic sheets of mesothelial cells and both show oval nuclei with longitudinal grooves and micronucleoli. Similar sheets of cells can be

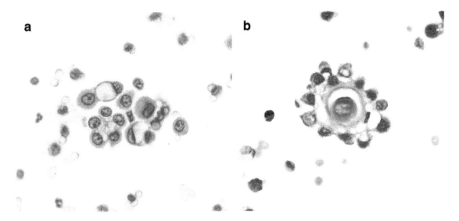

Fig. 9.14 (**a**) Serous cystadenoma. Small clusters of benign serous-type glandular cells. Small vacuoles may be present. Papanicolaou stain. (**b**) Serous cystadenoma. Small clusters of benign serous-type glandular cells with psammoma body in the center. Note the small nuclear sizes. Cell block, H&E stain

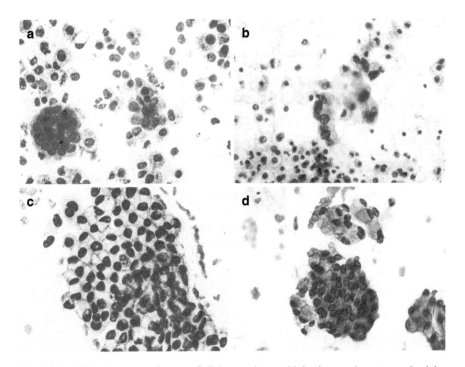

Fig. 9.15 (**a**) Mucinous cystadenoma. Cellular specimen with benign mucinous-type glandular cells in small papilla or single cells, some with mucin vacuoles. Cytospin, modified Giemsa stain. (**b**) Mucinous cystadenoma. Small cluster of mucinous glandular cells and single cells with background mucin. Cytospin, Papanicolaou stain. (**c**) Mucinous cystadenoma. Sheet of benign, honeycomb mucinous glandular cells. Cytospin, modified Giemsa stain. (**d**) Mucinous cystadenoma. Benign mucinous glandular cells in sheets and small clusters. Cell block, H&E stain

produced from Walthard's rests. It is less important to identify their origin than to recognize that they are benign. Borderline Brenner tumors have papillae with fibro-vascular cores lined with transitional epithelium, are more highly cellular, and might mimic fragments of urothelial carcinoma in fluids. Nuclei are uniformly enlarged, are more hyperchromatic, and have greater overlapping and crowding [54]. These tumors are rare and unlikely to be present in peritoneal washings.

Ovarian Borderline Tumors: Serous, Mucinous, and Endometrioid Types

Ovarian borderline tumors have uncertain malignant potential and tend to recur. These tumors have morphologic and architectural features between their benign and malignant counterparts that may be subtle in cytology specimens. Generally, bor-derline tumors are less cellular and more uniform cytologically than their malignant counterparts [35]. Peritoneal washing in this setting has the advantage of detecting subclinical intraperitoneal extension of borderline tumor due to wider sampling of the peritoneal surface [55]. Cell blocks and ancillary studies may be required to confirm tumor type and distinguish tumor from mesothelium and mesothelioma. The most important (and common) of these is serous borderline tumor.

Serous Borderline Tumor

Ovarian serous borderline tumors (SBT) are common, frequently bilateral ovarian tumors, most common in reproductive women. Long survival is the norm, but they are notorious for forming noninvasive and invasive implants on the peritoneal sur-faces. Positive peritoneal washings can be found in up to 30–40% of serous border-line tumors and usually correlate with the presence of implants within the peritoneal cavity (Fig. 9.16) [55, 56].

Cytologic Criteria
- Variable cellularity with medium to large, tightly cohesive papillary clusters
- Smooth, discrete, uniform papillary edges with uniformly situated cells
- Scant to no single cells
- Small cells with high nuclear-to-cytoplasmic ratio and well-defined cell borders
- Nuclei with hyperchromasia, coarse chromatin, and minimal to absent atypia
- Infrequent mitoses
- Cytoplasmic vacuoles (less frequent than in serous carcinoma)
- Frequent psammoma bodies
- Cell block shows papillae with a stromal core lined by tumor cells.

Explanatory Notes
The major differential is with serous carcinoma. It is not usually possible to cyto-logically distinguish between SBT and low-grade serous carcinoma, but one can usually exclude high-grade serous carcinoma (HGSC) [41]. The presence of tumor cells in peritoneal washings should be categorized as AUS if associated with a bor-derline tumor, and suspicious for malignancy or malignancy if associated with car-cinoma, based upon correlation with the surgical specimen. The best practice is to correlate with the histologic diagnosis before reporting the washing specimen.

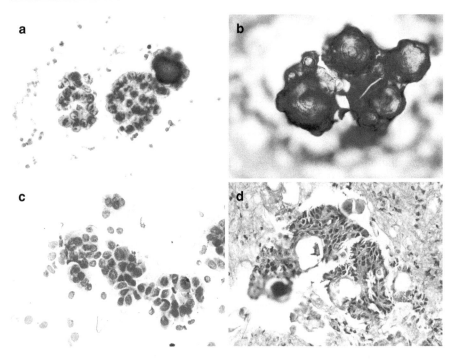

Fig. 9.16 (**a**) Serous borderline tumor. Tight papillary clusters of small cells with uniform nuclei, high nuclear-to-cytoplasmic ratio, and well-defined cell borders. Papillary edges are smooth, discrete, and uniform with uniformly situated cells. A psammoma body is present. Cytospin, Papanicolaou stain. (**b**) Serous borderline tumor. Laminated concretions of psammoma bodies. Cytospin, modified Giemsa stain. (**c**) Serous borderline tumor. Papillary clusters of small cells with high nuclear-to-cytoplasmic ratio and well-defined cell borders. Note the variation in nuclear sizes. Cytospin, modified Giemsa stain. (**d**) Serous borderline tumor. Sheets of small cells with high nuclear-to-cytoplasmic ratio and well-defined cell borders with psammoma bodies. Cell block, H&E stain

Mucinous Borderline Tumor

Mucinous tumors are mostly benign (80%), frequently bilateral, and very large. Ovarian mucinous borderline tumors (MBT) have been associated with *pseudomyxoma peritonei* and should be considered whenever abundant background mucin is present. Mucin-producing metastatic tumors (especially the colon, appendix, pancreas, gallbladder, and cervix) should be excluded. Ovarian MBT are more common than primary ovarian mucinous adenocarcinoma but rarely occur in peritoneal washings [52].

Cytologic Criteria

- Cell clusters with intracellular mucin (confirm with mucicarmine)
- Extracellular mucin possible
- Columnar cells may be inapparent and best appreciated at cluster edges
- Small- to medium-sized, uniform, eccentric nuclei with coarse chromatin

- Moderate vacuolated cytoplasm; goblet cells possible
- Minimal to no nuclear atypia
- Mitoses rare

Explanatory Notes

There is significant cytologic overlap between benign, borderline, and malignant mucinous tumors and metastases. Surgical excision with clinical correlation is required to distinguish between them. Even malignant mucinous tumors may have benign-appearing epithelium and are a source of false-negative interpretations [57]. Differentiation may be intestinal- or endocervical-like. Primary ovarian intestinal-type mucinous tumors tend to be strongly reactive for CK7 and usually negative or only focally positive for CK20, whereas gastrointestinal tumors are strongly reactive for CK20. CDX2 can be positive in about a third of primary ovarian mucinous tumors, but SATB2 reactivity can help to distinguish metastatic colonic and appendiceal tumors (positive) from primary ovarian mucinous carcinoma (MC) (negative) [58]. Endocervical-type ovarian mucinous tumors have a different IHC profile and are ER, PR, CA125, and mesothelin positive [59].

Endometrioid Borderline Tumor

Endometrioid borderline tumors (EBT) occur much less frequently than serous and mucinous borderline tumors [60]. Therefore, positive pelvic washings from EBT with implants are very rare [61]. In one study with 33 endometrioid borderline tumors, only one case had a positive pelvic washing [60]. EBT are often associated with endometriosis. There are no citations describing the cytologic features in peritoneal fluids. These tumors may be cytologically indistinguishable from endometriosis, benign endometrioid tumors, and low-grade endometrioid adenocarcinoma of the ovary or uterus. Morphologically, neoplastic cells in washings will resemble their counterpart in histologic sections and Pap tests with small endometrioid-type cells, minimal atypia, and infrequent mitosis (Fig. 9.17). Nuclei are round with distinct but small nucleoli and coarse, evenly distributed chromatin. Columnar cells are not typically seen. The cytoplasm may include vacuoles without intracytoplasmic neutrophils.

Sample Reports

Example 1

Pelvic cavity, peritoneal washings:
- Satisfactory for evaluation.
- Benign-appearing glandular cells in a background of mesothelial cells, histiocytes, and lymphocytes (see note).
- Category: Negative for malignancy.

Note: The specimen contains rare small fragments of bland-appearing glandular cells that are positive for BerEP4 and PAX8 and negative for calretinin. This profile is consistent with epithelial cells from a Müllerian origin. The patient's concurrent

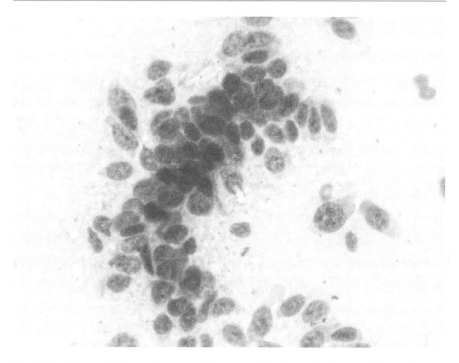

Fig. 9.17 Endometrioid borderline tumor. Clusters and single small endometrioid-type columnar cells with minimal atypia. Nuclei are oval with evenly distributed chromatin. Cytospin, modified Giemsa stain

surgical specimen was reviewed and demonstrates a borderline serous tumor associated with numerous psammomatous calcifications. Given the absence of associated psammoma bodies and paucity of glandular cells in the current pelvic washing specimen, we favor that it is not involved by the patient's borderline serous tumor. These glandular cells likely represent a benign process such as endosalpingiosis.

Example 2
Pelvic cavity, peritoneal lavage:
- Satisfactory for evaluation.
- Consistent with serous borderline tumor (see note).
- Category: Atypia of undetermined significance.
    Note: The specimen is hypercellular and contains numerous uniform neoplastic epithelial cells arranged in small papillary fragments and associated with psammomatous calcification. The patient's concurrent surgical specimen was reviewed; the neoplastic cells in both specimens have similar morphology. Studies have demonstrated that pelvic washings containing borderline serous tumor cells are strongly correlated with the presence of peritoneal implants.

Malignant Low-Grade Epithelial Tumors

Micropapillary Serous Carcinoma

The term micropapillary serous carcinoma (MPSC) refers to a subtype of ovarian serous tumor with a distinctive pattern of filigree cellular proliferation, with delicate elongated fibrovascular cores arising from blunt papillae, and lacking stromal invasion, thereby mimicking a serous borderline tumor [39]. This term is not universally accepted, as many pathologists regard this finding as a variation of borderline tumor. Its behavior is similar to low-grade serous carcinoma and it is likely to be associated with invasive peritoneal implants and recurrence.

Cytologic Criteria

- High cellularity
- Simple, small, tightly packed micropapillary fragments (<30 cells)
- Delicate fibrovascular core with minimal to absent branching
- Monotonous epithelial cells with scant cytoplasm
- Small, hyperchromatic nuclei with multiple small nucleoli
- Uniform hobnail or peripheral palisading of cells
- Rarely single or enlarged, atypical cells
- Infrequent mitoses
- Psammoma bodies common

Explanatory Notes

MPSC has features between benign and borderline ovarian tumors (low-grade nuclei and small, non-branching papillary groups) and serous carcinoma (focal blunt papillary branching, papillary tufts, focal atypia, and higher cellularity). MPSC shows only moderately intense p53 nuclear reactivity in over 50% of cells [62]. Nuclei of MPSC are closer to borderline tumors than serous carcinoma, and the cell group contours are more uniformly scalloped. Practically speaking, MPSC cannot be reliably distinguished from borderline tumor or LGSC in serous fluid specimens.

Low-Grade Serous Carcinoma (LGSC)

Low-grade serous carcinoma (LGSC) of the ovary is a less aggressive, less common serous carcinoma than its high-grade counterpart and is thought to arise from ovarian serous borderline tumors. Its origin from the peritoneum is debated, but the cytologic features of a primary peritoneal LGSC would be identical. It typically

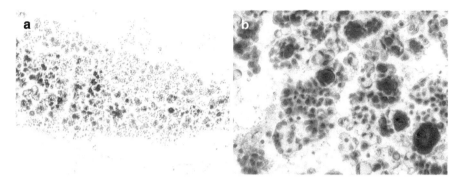

Fig. 9.18 (**a**) Low-grade serous carcinoma. Cellular specimen shows abundant small papillary clusters with uniform hobnailed or scalloped borders, often with embedded psammoma bodies. Cytospin, Papanicolaou stain. (**b**) Low-grade serous carcinoma. High magnification demonstrates small cells with round/oval nuclei, scant cytoplasm, occasional cytoplasmic vacuoles, and small, discrete nucleoli. Cytospin, Papanicolaou stain

presents in young women and is considered resistant to chemotherapy. It frequently presents with peritoneal implants (Fig. 9.18). Their prognosis is good due to an indolent growth pattern and survival is about 75% [63]. The amount of residual disease following surgery has been shown to be an important prognostic factor.

Cytologic Criteria

- Large, cohesive, branching papillary fragments of epithelioid cells
- Hobnailed, scalloped, uniform cluster borders
- Less nuclear pleomorphism than high-grade serous carcinoma (HGSC)
- Smaller cells than in HGSC
- Round-to-oval nuclei (2X increased nuclear size) with low nuclear-to-cytoplasmic ratio
- Moderate cytoplasm with rare cytoplasmic vacuoles
- Small, discrete nucleoli
- Psammoma bodies frequent

Explanatory Notes

There is cytologic overlap of low-grade serous carcinoma with borderline tumors [64], but it is usually not difficult to distinguish from high-grade serous tumors. LGSC frequently demonstrate wild-type expression (patchy, variable nuclear staining) of p53 and are less likely than high-grade serous carcinoma to demonstrate strong, diffuse p16 expression.

Endometrioid Carcinoma (EC)

Low-grade endometrial carcinoma cells may be derived from the uterus or from the ovary; these will appear cytologically identical. Low-grade endometrioid carcinomas are the most common epithelial malignancy of the uterus, usually occurring in postmenopausal women with vaginal bleeding. It is associated with unopposed endogenous and exogenous estrogen. Extrauterine disease (Stage III or IV) is uncommon, as is positive cytology. Peritoneal cytology has a reduced role in staging uterine endometrioid carcinoma as a result of contradictory studies on the significance of tumor cells in the fluid, and currently their presence does not contribute to staging, but they should be reported for prognostic purposes [65]. Ovarian endometrioid carcinomas comprise up to 25% of ovarian carcinomas, are usually low stage, and confer a better prognosis than HGSC. Because of this, a positive peritoneal washing is usually unexpected. Ovarian endometrioid tumors are closely associated with endometriosis (30–40%; from which they may arise), adenofibromas, and synchronous uterine endometrioid carcinoma (15%) [47].

Cytologic Criteria

- Cohesive clusters, some with microacinar formation
- High nuclear-to-cytoplasmic ratio
- Uniform oval, enlarged nuclei with mild variation
- Small, inconspicuous nuclei and coarse chromatin
- Scant granular to finely vacuolated cytoplasm
- Polygonal squamoid cells with distinct cell borders, variable nuclear sizes, and glassy or waxy cytoplasm
- Squamous metaplasia in sheets or morulas possible; may produce peritoneal keratin granulomas
- Focal mucinous differentiation possible

Explanatory Notes

Endometrioid adenocarcinoma in peritoneal fluid is more likely to be derived from the endometrium than the ovary or peritoneum. Features are similar to exfoliated endometrial cells found in Pap tests and may be difficult to distinguish from endometriosis. They are strongly reactive for ER, PR, BER-Ep4, and vimentin, but not for WT1 or p53 [66]. Cells may represent iatrogenic spread from surgical procedures, primarily from vaginal or laparoscopic procedures. For example, hysteroscopy procedures that introduce saline into the endometrial canal may result in transport of endometrial cells through the fallopian tubes to the peritoneal cavity [67, 68]. Insertion of a uterine manipulator (a Foley catheter-like device with an inflatable balloon) into the uterine canal to enable movement of the uterus during vaginal or laparoscopic hysterectomy has also been reported to result in transtubal migration of low-grade endometrial adenocarcinoma into the peritoneum in Stage I uterine tumors [69, 70]. Preventive measures have been subsequently implemented by many surgeons to prevent this phenomenon.

Endometrioid carcinoma, primarily of low and intermediate grades, may also produce peritoneal keratin granulomas due to squamous metaplasia produced by the neoplasm. This may result in multinucleated giant cells containing elongated, "ghost" squamous cells, numerous histiocytes, anucleate squamous cells, and keratinous eosinophilic material in the fluid or cell block [71]. The ghost cells are positive for AE1/AE3 and p63.

Low-Grade Mucinous Neoplasm (with Pseudomyxoma Peritonei)

Most low-grade mucinous neoplasia associated with *pseudomyxoma peritonei* (PMP) will be of appendiceal or gastrointestinal origin, and by consensus opinion, these have been termed "low-grade (appendiceal) mucinous neoplasm" to reflect their low-grade behavior. Most PMP is caused by low-grade mucinous neoplasia. Patients present with unremitting abdominal pain, bloating, increased girth, weight loss, and fatigue. Ten-year survival is approximately 45% due to complications [44].

Cytologic Criteria

- Abundant thick, mucinous background matrix with rivulets, creases, folds, and fuzzy edges
- Variable cellularity, from low to high (low-grade lesions have fewer epithelial cells)
- Epithelial clusters, sheets, and single cells
- Honeycomb sheets of uniform columnar cells with moderate mucinous cytoplasm
- Uniform, bland, round-to-oval nuclei
- Mild nuclear atypia possible
- Focal cytoplasmic vacuoles
- Fibroblast-like spindle cells entrapped in mucin
- Background mesothelial cells and histiocytes
- Rare mitoses

Explanatory Notes

The gross appearance of the fluid will be thick, gelatinous, and tenacious, creating difficulty with processing. By definition, these low-grade neoplasms lack infiltrative peritoneal invasion and are represented by islands of bland cells in a sea of mucin. The amount of mucin should be greater than 50%. These lesions can be diagnosed with confidence when extensive mucin and the corresponding cytologic features above are present [72]. PMP is a clinical term. The synonymous term "disseminated peritoneal adenomucinosis" can be used when invasion is not present. Because invasion cannot be determined without a biopsy, cytologic evaluation should focus on determining low-grade or high-grade features and the presence of excessive mucin noted. The presence of signet ring cells excludes a low-grade neoplasm. An immunochemical (IC) panel for mucin-producing tumors can help to identify the primary site.

Sample Reports

Example 1
Abdominal cavity, peritoneal lavage:
- Satisfactory for evaluation.
- Consistent with low-grade serous neoplasm (see note).
- Category: Suspicious for malignancy.

Note: The clinical appearance of multiple peritoneal nodules is noted. The cytologic findings are concordant with the peritoneal biopsies. In the absence of a primary site, a definitive interpretation cannot be rendered; the differential diagnosis includes an ovarian, fallopian tube, primary peritoneal, or endometrial origin.

Example 2
Abdominal cavity, peritoneal lavage:
- Satisfactory for evaluation.
- Features suspicious for low-grade mucinous neoplasm (see note).
- Category: Suspicious for malignancy.

Note: There is abundant extracellular mucin along with nests of bland mucin-producing cells with low-grade cytologic features. These findings suggest *pseudomyxoma peritonei* (disseminated peritoneal adenomucinosis) that is most often associated with primary appendiceal mucinous neoplasia, although other origins (gastrointestinal, ovarian, or pancreatic) are possible.

High-Grade Neoplastic Cells

Background

The presence of neoplastic cells with high-grade cytomorphology indicates that a peritoneal fluid is involved by malignancy. While this finding greatly increases the odds that a malignancy has formed implants within the peritoneum, only tissue biopsy can confirm implantation because malignant cells may have entered the cavity through iatrogenic or other means. In a large quality-controlled study over 12 years, Özkara [52] noted that positive peritoneal washing cytology rates for serous, clear cell, and undifferentiated carcinoma were higher than overall positive rates. Endometrioid and mucinous carcinomas had lower positive rates. Overall, malignant cases were more likely to yield positive results, significantly so when of higher grade, higher stage, and bilateral or with lymph node involvement.

In women, ovarian neoplasms are the most common cause of malignant ascites or positive peritoneal cytology [73]. In men, high-grade neoplastic cells are usually from a pancreaticobiliary or gastrointestinal primary and manifest as ascites [74]. Intraoperative collection of peritoneal washings is less common for non-gynecologic neoplasms; abdominal paracentesis or laparoscopic biopsies are often preferred. Intraoperative peritoneal washings are still used to detect gastric carcinoma since peritoneal metastasis is a common reason for treatment failure [75]. Molecular testing, such as for messenger RNA (mRNA) of carcinoembryonic antigen (CEA), is used as a complementary test and has superior sensitivity but less specificity than cytology [76]. Ascites associated with pancreatic carcinoma confers a poor prognosis [77] and may impact resection decisions [78, 79].

The frequency of neoplastic cells in peritoneal fluid varies over the decades with the incidence of high-stage disease and an increased ability to detect and treat tumors at a lower stage. The sensitivity of cytology for detecting malignancy in ascites is around 58–75% [74]. Nearly all patients with carcinomatosis have positive peritoneal fluid cytology, but carcinomatosis occurs in only about 2/3 of patients with ascites [80]. Of uncommon tumors in peritoneal fluid, hematopoietic are the most common, followed by squamous cell carcinoma (SCC) [73]. Urothelial carcinoma overlaps cytologically with squamous cell carcinoma and malignant Brenner tumor [81]. Testicular germ cell tumors, which may also involve the peritoneum in men, have identical cytologic features to their ovarian counterparts when present in peritoneal fluids.

High-Grade Serous Carcinoma (HGSC)

The most frequent intraperitoneal malignancy in women is high-grade serous carcinoma (HGSC), regardless of ovarian, fallopian tube, peritoneal, or endometrial origin. High-grade serous ovarian carcinoma (HGSOC) represents approximately 75% of all epithelial ovarian carcinomas and 80–90% of serous ovarian carcinomas [82–84]. It is usually associated with nonsynonymous p53 mutations and has marked genomic instability. Recent scientific evidence suggests that most "ovarian" HGSC arise from the fallopian tube, from which they disseminate [85]. Serous tubal intraepithelial carcinomas (STIC lesions) are thought to be the precursor lesion in these cases [84]. Ovarian HGSC are aggressive, are usually diagnosed at an advanced stage, and follow a relapse-response pattern until eventually becoming resistant to chemotherapy [84]. Serous endometrial carcinoma (SEC) is considered a high-risk histologic subtype of endometrial cancer. It is more likely to be diagnosed in older women and is not related to unopposed estrogen exposure or other risk factors that predispose women to develop endometrioid carcinoma. SEC follows a more aggressive course and is responsible for a disproportionate number of deaths from endometrial cancer [86].

Cytologic Criteria

- Pleomorphic epithelioid cells in small, loose clusters with acinar or papillary configurations
- Frequent single cells
- Hierarchical branching clusters with nonuniform, knobby outlines
- Large cells with enlarged, eccentric, hyperchromatic nuclei (>4X increase)
- Coarse chromatin with nuclear membrane irregularities
- Prominent macronucleoli; frequent multiple nucleoli
- Variable amount of cytoplasm; frequent large, discrete ("soap-bubble") vacuoles
- Occasional high nuclear-to-cytoplasmic ratio with scant, ill-defined cytoplasm
- Psammoma bodies less frequent than low-grade serous tumors
- Mitoses frequent

Explanatory Notes

HGSC is easily recognized as malignant (Fig. 9.19) [66]. Since the origin of ovarian high-grade serous tumors continues to be debated, it is best to cytologically identify high-grade serous features [87] and defer site of origin to the surgical excision or imaging studies. There is morphologic overlap between ovarian serous tumors in the borderline, low-grade, and high-grade categories. Attention to nuclear size and specimen cellularity is helpful. Endometrial serous carcinoma is also notorious for seeding the peritoneum and cannot be distinguished from tubo-ovarian serous tumors. HGSC typically shows strong, diffuse nuclear reactivity for p53 in greater than 75% of tumor cells or complete absence of staining (null phenotype), which helps to distinguish it from LGSC. It is positive for PAX8, WT1, ER, BerEP4, and MOC-31 [88].

Mucinous Carcinoma (MC)

Mucinous carcinoma of the ovary is rare. It is less common than metastatic mucin-producing adenocarcinoma of the gastrointestinal or pancreaticobiliary tract and endometrioid tumors with focal mucinous metaplasia. It may show a variety of patterns from benign-appearing to overtly malignant mucinous epithelium. Most primary ovarian mucinous carcinomas are low-grade, with significant cytologic overlap with mucinous borderline tumors (Fig. 9.20). Their behavior is similar to endometrioid ovarian carcinoma [47]. Malignant features overlap with a variety of other primary and metastatic tumors that should be excluded (Fig. 9.21).

Cytologic Criteria

- Moderate to high cellularity
- Variable cytologic features; three-dimensional clusters, sheets, single cells

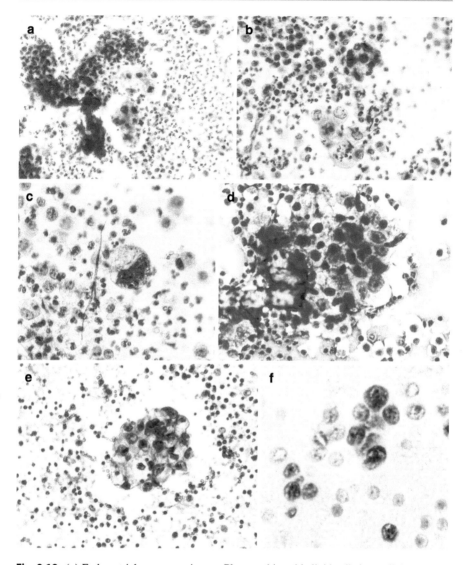

Fig. 9.19 (**a**) Endometrial serous carcinoma. Pleomorphic epithelioid cells in small, loose clusters with acinar or tight papillary configurations. Cytospin, Papanicolaou stain. (**b**) Endometrial serous carcinoma. Large cells with enlarged, eccentric, hyperchromatic nuclei, coarse chromatin, and marked nuclear membrane irregularities. Cytospin, Papanicolaou stain. (**c**) Endometrial serous carcinoma. One large epithelioid cell with a giant nucleus and coarse chromatin. Cytospin, Papanicolaou stain. (**d**) Endometrial serous carcinoma. Pleomorphic epithelioid cells in a loose cluster with variable finely vacuolated cytoplasm and variable nuclear sizes. Cytospin, modified Giemsa stain. (**e**) Endometrial serous carcinoma. Cluster of large cells with enlarged, eccentric, hyperchromatic nuclei and prominent macronucleoli. Large discrete ("soap-bubble") vacuoles are present. Cytospin, Papanicolaou stain. (**f**) Endometrial serous carcinoma. Carcinoma cells show p53 nuclear reactivity. Immunostain of p53

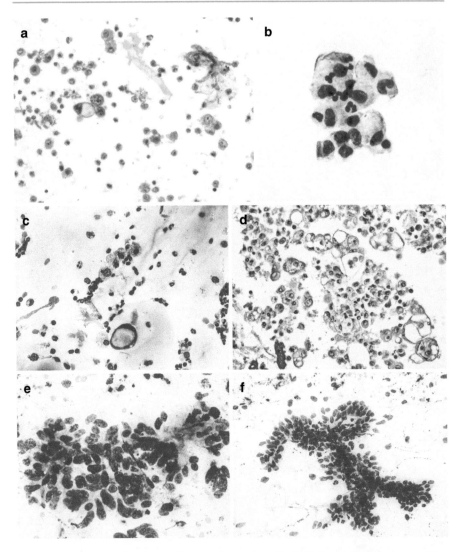

Fig. 9.20 (a) Mucinous carcinoma (high-grade, ovarian). Single highly atypical mucinous epithelial cells with pleomorphic nuclei, high N/C ratio, intracellular mucin, and coarse chromatin. Cytospin, Papanicolaou stain. (b) Mucinous carcinoma (high-grade, ovarian). Single highly atypical epithelial cells with pleomorphic nuclei, abundant intracellular mucin, and coarse chromatin. Cytospin, modified Giemsa stain. (c) Mucinous carcinoma (high-grade, ovarian). Background acellular mucin with single highly atypical mucinous epithelial cells, one with compression of the nucleus by the cytoplasmic vacuole. Cytospin, modified Giemsa stain. (d) Mucinous carcinoma (high-grade, ovarian). Single and small clusters of highly atypical mucinous epithelial cells with pleomorphic nuclei, intracellular mucin, coarse chromatin, and prominent nucleoli. Cell block, H&E stain. (e) Metastatic mucinous carcinoma (colorectal origin). Highly atypical tall columnar cells with pleomorphic nuclei, scant cytoplasm, coarse chromatin, and multiple nucleoli. Cytospin, modified Giemsa stain. (f) Metastatic mucinous carcinoma (colorectal origin). "Picket fence" columnar nuclear arrangement of pleomorphic nuclei with high N/C ratio and coarse chromatin. Cytospin, modified Giemsa stain

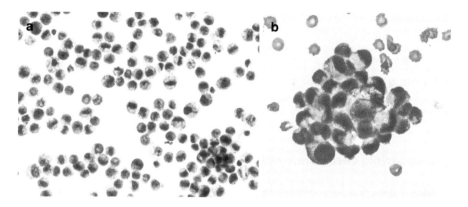

Fig. 9.21 (**a**) Metastatic gastric adenocarcinoma. Cellular specimen shows numerous discohesive, single atypical epithelial cells with variable nuclei, high N/C ratio, and coarse chromatin. Cytospin, Papanicolaou stain. (**b**) Metastatic gastric adenocarcinoma. A cluster showing pushed together single cells with discernable cytoplasmic borders, pleomorphic nuclei, coarse chromatin, and prominent nucleoli. Cytospin, modified Giemsa stain

- Presence of abundant background mucin (see "acellular mucin") that suggests *pseudomyxoma peritonei*
- Nuclear pleomorphism, irregular nuclear membranes, and coarse, irregular chromatin
- Prominent nucleoli or macronucleoli, single or multiple
- Mitoses

Additional Criteria

- Signet ring cells (cells with nuclei compressed by intracytoplasmic mucin vacuoles) suggest gastric or appendiceal origin.
- "Dirty" background suggests colorectal origin.
- Small, monomorphic, mildly pleomorphic cells with small intracytoplasmic mucin-positive vacuoles suggest breast origin.

Explanatory Notes

A panel of immunochemistries may help define cellular origin, along with PAS with diastase (PASD) and/or mucicarmine to confirm mucin production. Vacuolated cells should not be assumed to produce mucin since vacuoles are a feature of cellular degeneration in fluids. Mucinous ovarian carcinoma is positive for CK7; PAX8, ER, and PR may be negative in more than half of mucinous carcinomas. Most cases will be negative or only focally positive for CK20. Mucinous tumors from the lower gastrointestinal tract and appendix are positive for CK20 and SATB2 but negative for PAX8, CK7, and ER. Pancreaticobiliary and stomach mucin-producing carcinomas are positive for CK7, but negative for PAX8, CK20, and ER. Among these, only pancreaticobiliary tumors have loss of expression of DPC4 [88].

Pseudomyxoma peritonei (intraperitoneal mucin) associated with high-grade neoplastic cells is usually from the gallbladder or other areas within the gastro-intestinal tract. These tumors often have formed implants within the peritoneal cavity (*peritoneal mucinous carcinomatosis*), and these patients have a worse prognosis [89, 90].

Endometrioid Carcinoma (EC)

Uterine endometrioid carcinoma arises from endometrial hyperplasia in a background of long-term unopposed estrogen stimulation and is the most common histologic sub-type of endometrial cancers. High-grade (FIGO 3) tumors are not as common as low-grade but are more likely to deeply invade the myometrium and involve the peritoneum. While pelvic washings are no longer included in staging, they are still collected as part of initial surgery. One study has demonstrated that positive peritoneal washings rarely upstaged endometrial carcinomas and, where upstaging occurred, patient outcome was not impacted [10]. However, a larger study performed by FIGO recommended the continued collection of pelvic washings in the setting of endometrial carcinoma after finding that a positive cytology was associated with decreased survival of women with Stage I/II endometrial carcinoma. In these patients, treatment with adjuvant chemo-therapy was associated with increased survival [91]. Prognosis is related to stage of disease but is usually excellent when confined to the uterus.

Cytologic Criteria

- Cohesive clusters with focal acinar or papillary formations
- Pleomorphic single cells
- Greater variation in size than lower-grade endometrioid carcinomas
- Nuclear enlargement, overlapping, and crowding
- Intermediate to high nuclear-to-cytoplasmic ratio
- Round to elongated nuclei with variable chromatin
- Finely to coarsely vacuolated cytoplasm
- Mild to moderate nuclear membrane irregularitiesgv
- Prominent nucleoli
- Squamous metaplastic cells; in sheets, clusters (morules), or single cells
- Mitotic figures and necrotic debris

Explanatory Notes

Only rare cases of EC have been described in the literature, mostly by fine needle aspiration, and the cytomorphologic features are expected to be similar to those

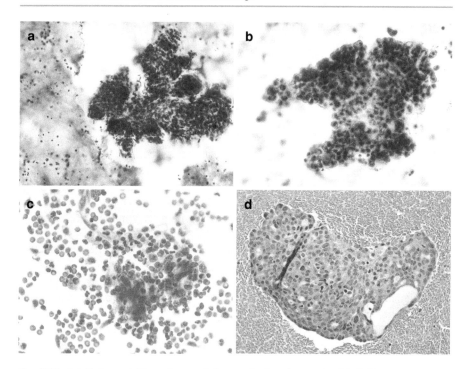

Fig. 9.22 (**a**) Endometrioid carcinoma. A large cohesive cluster of epithelioid cells with short columnar nuclei and focal papillary formation. Cytospin, Papanicolaou stain. (**b**) Endometrioid carcinoma. This large cohesive cluster shows short columnar cells along the edges, nuclear over-lapping, and crowding. Cytospin, Papanicolaou stain. (**c**) Endometrioid carcinoma. The elongated shape of variable-sized nuclei is evident along with coarsely stipulated chromatin and indistinct nucleoli. Cytospin, Papanicolaou stain. (**d**) Endometrioid carcinoma. A large cluster of epithelioid cells with pleomorphic hyperchromatic nuclei, distinct single nucleoli, and a mitotic figure. Note the squamoid appearance of the cytoplasm. Cell block, H&E stain

seen in uterine high-grade endometrioid carcinoma [92, 93]. Both tumors show fewer endometrioid features when higher grade and are easily confused with HGSC and other high-grade neoplasms (Fig. 9.22). EC may cytologically mimic patterns of serous and clear cell carcinoma (CCC) [94] and may be positive for p53, WT1, and p16. They may produce peritoneal keratin granulomas and thus be associated with histiocytes, squamous cells, and giant cells.

Clear Cell Carcinoma

Ovarian clear cell carcinoma (OCCC) is one of the two epithelial ovarian cancer subtypes strongly associated with endometriosis and is theorized to arise from pro-genitor cells in this lesion [95]. OCCC is usually unilateral and more commonly diagnosed at an early stage compared to other histologic subtypes. It is relatively chemotherapy-resistant with a 5-year survival of approximately 66% for all stages [96]. Metastatic disease, as indicated by a positive peritoneal washing, confers a poor prognosis. Endometrial clear cell carcinoma (ECCC) is uncommon, occurs primarily in postmenopausal women, and is usually detected as Stage I or II carcinomas. Peritoneal spread is uncommon [47].

Cytologic Criteria

- Large spherules of cells surrounding densely eosinophilic, hyaline cores ("raspberry bodies"); single cells may appear to skate across the surface of the spherules.
- Small, tight spherules with hobnail protruding cells from a central hyaline core.
- Cellular cohesiveness (compared to yolk sac tumors).
- Occasional papillary structures with well-defined cell borders.
- Monomorphic to pleomorphic cell population with mild to moderate variation in cell size.
- Peripheral, enlarged nuclei with uniformly thickened nuclear membranes and fine vesicular chromatin.
- Prominent nucleoli, usually single.
- Polygonal cells with abundant, pale, granular, or champagne-bubble vacuolated cytoplasm.
- Cytoplasmic clearing with condensation along the cytoplasmic membrane, imparting a watery or clear appearance to the cytoplasm.
- Mitotic figures.
- No psammoma bodies.

Explanatory Notes

The presence of densely eosinophilic, acellular matrix that forms raspberrylike structures is highly characteristic of OCCC and occurs in 80% of involved peritoneal fluids [97–99]. The cellular features of clear cell carcinoma (CCC) from the ovary [100, 101], endometrium, or kidney are essentially identical and with the exception of the prominence of raspberry bodies in OCCC (Fig. 9.23). IC is likewise similar, except for CD10, CAIX (positive in papillary and some clear cell renal cell carcinomas), and CK7 (positive in ovarian and endometrial clear cell carcinoma). OCCC is positive for HNF1 and napsin A, which appear to be relatively specific and sensitive markers to distinguish CCC from other ovarian malignancies. In contrast to HGSC, OCCC demonstrates wild-type p53 expression and is negative for WT1 and ER. Endometrioid carcinoma is positive for ER and negative for napsin A and HNF1 [102, 103]. Clear cell cytoplasm contains glycogen which is PAS positive and digested with diastase.

Malignant Brenner Tumor (Transitional Cell Carcinoma)

Malignant Brenner tumor/transitional cell carcinoma of the ovary is rare, occurring in women over age 50, and is usually Stage I at discovery. It may occur in

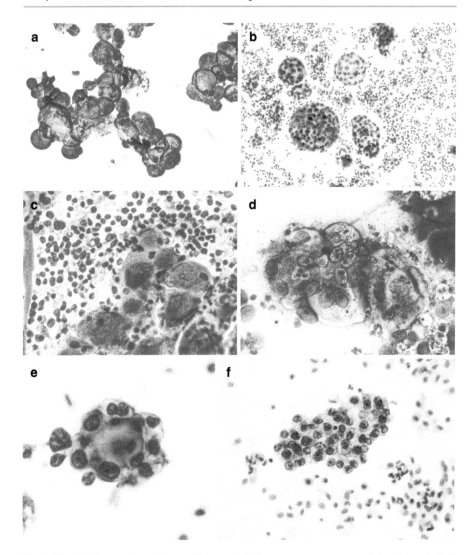

Fig. 9.23 (**a**) Clear cell carcinoma. Characteristic low-power appearance of "raspberry balls," pleomorphic cells tightly clustered around hyaline cores. Cytospin, modified Giemsa stain. (**b**) Clear cell carcinoma. Small tight spherules with hobnail protruding cells from a central hyaline core. Cytospin, Papanicolaou stain. (**c**) Clear cell carcinoma. Large cells with abundant, pale, granular cytoplasm and pleomorphic nuclei. The hyaline core stains bright magenta. Cytospin, modified Giemsa stain. (**d**) Clear cell carcinoma. Variable-sized polygonal cells with abundant, pale, granular, or "champagne-bubble" vacuolated cytoplasm. Cytospin, modified Giemsa stain. (**e**) Clear cell carcinoma. A small tight spherule with hobnail clear cells protruding from a central hyaline core. Cytospin, modified Giemsa stain. (**f**) Clear cell carcinoma. A cluster of polygonal cells with abundant champagne-bubble vacuolated to cleared cytoplasm. Cytospin, Papanicolaou stain

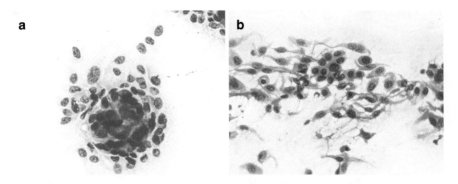

Fig. 9.24 (**a**) Transitional cell carcinoma. Whorled cluster of squamoid epithelial cells with markedly enlarged, hyperchromatic, irregular nuclei and abundant dense waxy cytoplasm. Cytospin, modified Giemsa stain. (**b**) Transitional cell carcinoma. Squamoid and "tadpole" epithelial cells with markedly enlarged, hyperchromatic, irregular nuclei and abundant dense waxy pink cytoplasm. Cell block, H&E stain

conjunction with benign and borderline Brenner tumors, benign teratoma, struma ovarii, carcinoid tumor, or serous carcinoma. It is comprised of urothelial and/or squamous epithelium, with occasional mucinous metaplasia (Fig. 9.24) [47].

Cytologic Criteria

- Variable cellularity; possibly hypercellular.
- Papillary structures and clusters of squamous and/or transitional cells.
- Polygonal squamous cells with small, irregular nuclei, abundant dense, waxy cytoplasm in irregular, sometimes bizarre shapes.
- Round-to-oval transitional cells with moderate cytoplasm.
- Markedly enlarged, hyperchromatic, irregular nuclei; binucleation.
- Presence of cells with nuclear grooves in transitional cells suggests origin.
- Background lymphocytes.

Explanatory Notes

Peritoneal involvement by malignant Brenner tumor has rarely has been described but has been reported in up to 10% of cases [104, 105]. It should be considered when atypical squamous cells are present with another malignant component. The squamous component may predominate and be mistaken for squamous cell carcinoma, which is rare in the ovary. The IC profile is similar to HGSC: positive for PAX8, WT1, CK7, and ER, often p53 and p16 positive, and negative for CK20. Uroplakin and thrombomodulin are negative, making these useful markers to differentiate it from metastatic urothelial carcinoma of bladder origin, but a small percent is positive for GATA3, similar to urothelial carcinoma [106].

Sample Reports

Example 1

Pelvic washings:
- Satisfactory for evaluation.
- High-grade serous carcinoma (see note).
- Category: Malignant.

Note: The specimen is hypercellular and contains fragments of enlarged, hyperchromatic malignant cells with prominent nucleoli and cytoplasmic vacuolization. The cells demonstrate similar morphology to that seen on the patient's concurrent surgical specimen. The presence of malignant cells in a pelvic washing specimen is strongly correlated with the presence of peritoneal implants.

or

Note: The specimen is hypercellular and contains fragments of enlarged, hyperchromatic malignant cells with prominent nucleoli and cytoplasmic vacuolization. Immunohistochemical studies were performed on corresponding cell block material, and the malignant cells are diffusely positive for PAX8, ER, p16, and p53. These findings are compatible with involvement by the patient's reported high-grade serous ovarian carcinoma.

Example 2

Peritoneal washings:
- Satisfactory for evaluation.
- High-grade mucinous neoplasm (see note).
- Category: Malignant.

Example 3

Peritoneal washings:
- Interpretation limited by processing artifact.
- Features suggestive of clear cell carcinoma (see note).
- Category: Suspicious for malignancy.

Note: A corresponding surgical specimen was not available for comparison with this case. The specimen shows marked cellular degeneration that hinders interpretation. There are numerous atypical groups of cells with focally clear cytoplasm that are reactive for napsin A, HNF1, PAX8, and CD10 but nonreactive for calretinin, WT1, CK7, and ER, with a wild-type p53 pattern. These findings suggest clear cell carcinoma of ovarian origin, but endometrial or renal origins cannot be entirely excluded.

Unusual and Uncommon Gynecologic Tumors

Ovarian Sex Cord Stromal Tumors

The most common sex cord stromal tumor is the benign fibroma-thecoma, which does not shed cells. Granulosa cell tumor is the only sex cord stromal tumor that occurs with any frequency in fluids. Sertoli-Leydig cell tumors are very rare but have been described in fluid [107, 108].

Granulosa Cell Tumor

The most common malignant ovarian sex cord stromal tumor is granulosa cell tumor, and it is the most common to involve peritoneal washings. It separated into adult (AGCT) and juvenile (JGCT) types based on histologic features. The most common is the AGCT, which is often associated with hyperestrogenemia, resulting in endometrial hyperplasia or carcinoma, vaginal bleeding, or isosexual pseudoprecocity. Less commonly, excessive progesterone/androgen may result in masculinization. These tumors are unilateral, large, and mostly solid with cystic spaces. Although the prognosis is good for Stage I tumors, they tend to show late local recurrence, sometimes decades later [47]. AGCT is considered chemotherapy-resistant, but survival is excellent due to the indolent nature of tumor growth. JGCT occur primarily in children and adolescents, are also Stage I tumors, and have a better prognosis than AGCT. Their cytologic features are markedly different (see explanatory notes).

Cytologic Criteria (AGCT)

- Typically hypercellular
- Three-dimensional spherules and papillae of uniform cells with smooth peripheral borders
- Loosely cohesive cells in variably sized groups
- Monotonous, uniform, round to slightly oval nuclei
- High nuclear-to-cytoplasmic ratio
- Powdery fine chromatin, single small conspicuous nucleoli, longitudinal nuclear grooves
- Focally vesicular nuclei with rare mild nuclear atypia
- Scant, indistinct, diaphanous cytoplasm without distinct borders between cells
- Rare acinar-like cell arrangement around eosinophilic hyaline globules (Call-Exner bodies)
- Numerous background single tumor cells
- Rarely, small cytoplasmic vacuoles and/or prominent nucleoli
- No mitoses or necrosis

Explanatory Notes

Because most of these tumors present as Stage I disease without rupture, they are rarely present in peritoneal fluid and have been infrequently described [109, 110]. The presence of nuclear grooves is an important clue, and although these are also

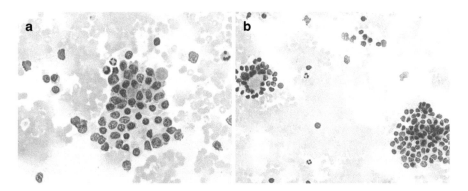

Fig. 9.25 (**a**) Granulosa cell tumor. A loosely cohesive sheet of cells with oval-shaped, "coffee bean" nuclei and minimal nuclear size variation. Two pink spherical globules (Call-Exner bodies) are present. Smear preparation, modified Giemsa stain. (**b**) Granulosa cell tumor. Two sheets of cells are present with dispersed single tumor cells in the background. The cells are arranged around a pink core (Call-Exner body) on the left-hand side of the field. Smear preparation, modified Giemsa stain

present with Brenner tumors and mesothelial cells, each of those has distinct cell borders (Figs. 9.25 and 9.26) [111, 112]. GCT cells are positive for calretinin (a mesothelial marker), but negative for uroplakin, which is positive in urothelium, and show variable expression of keratin. Fortunately, AGCTs have distinct morphology, and familiarity with these features should lead to suspicion for AGCT even if the patient's distant history of AGCT is unknown. Inhibin and CD99 have been shown to be relatively sensitive and specific markers for AGCT [110, 113–118]. Recurrence can be detected by evaluation of peritoneal or pleural fluid.

JGCT cells have more abundant cytoplasm with finely vacuolated cytoplasm and do not have nuclear longitudinal grooves. Clusters are loosely cohesive and comprised of 2–4 cells, small smooth-edged clusters, or large, irregular monolayered sheets. Nuclei are larger, round with slight to moderate anisonucleosis and occasional bizarre nuclei. Chromatin is fine, uniformly distributed and nucleoli are indistinct. Mitoses and necrosis are more common on fine needle aspiration but may not be visible in fluids [113]. They have the same IHC profile as AGCT. JGCT is more likely to be interpreted as a malignant germ cell neoplasm than its adult counterpart [119].

Germ Cell Tumors

Germ cell tumors rarely involve the pelvic cavity and have been described in case reports. Of these, dysgerminoma is the most commonly found in serous cavity specimens [120]. Most of the cytologic features of these unusual tumors have been described from ovarian fine needle aspiration cytology [51, 121]. Specific features in fluids for the more common mature and immature teratoma, dysgerminoma, and yolk sac tumor (YST) are included in the criteria below.

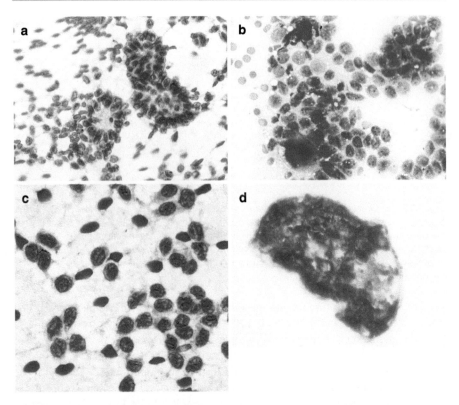

Fig. 9.26 (**a**) Granulosa cell tumor, adult type. The neoplastic cells are elongated with prominent nuclear grooves ("coffee beans"); these features are reminiscent of those seen in papillary thyroid carcinoma. Cell block, H&E stain. (**b**) Granulosa cell tumor, adult type. Although rare, the neoplastic cells may form Call-Exner bodies (cells forming rosettes around central matrix). The cells have elongated nuclei and a bland chromatin pattern. Smear preparation, modified Giemsa stain. (**c**) Granulosa cell tumor, adult type. At high magnification, numerous nuclear grooves are apparent. These grooves, together with the elongated nuclei, provide a "coffee bean" appearance. Cell block, H&E stain. (**d**) Granulosa cell tumor. While the morphologic features are distinctive of granulosa cell tumor, immunostains can help confirm a diagnosis. The tumor cells in this cell block preparation are diffusely reactive for inhibin. Cell block, inhibin immunostain

Teratoma: Mature and Immature

Teratomas (benign and malignant) are composed of epithelium representing all three germ layers: ectodermal, endodermal, and mesodermal. They arise in the mediastinum and ovary in women or testicle in men. Mature (cystic) teratoma is the most common ovarian and germ cell tumor, and it is benign (Fig. 9.27). It occurs primarily in reproductive women and may be bilateral. Immature teratoma is a malignant counterpart, accounting for 2% of ovarian cancer, occurs primarily in children and young adults, and is defined by the presence of embryonic-appearing neuroectodermal tissue in combination with other immature elements (Fig. 9.28). The prognosis is excellent with surgery and chemotherapy [47].

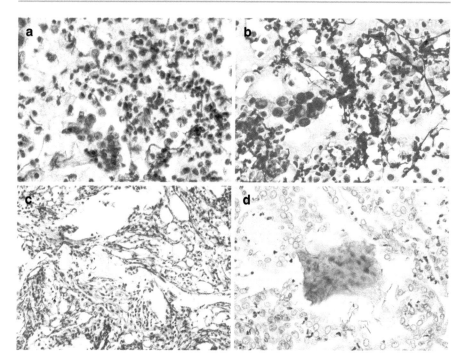

Fig. 9.27 (**a**) Mature teratoma. Anucleated and nucleated benign squamous cells mixed with lymphocytes. Cytospin, Papanicolaou stain. (**b**) Mature teratoma. Benign glandular cells mixed with anucleate squamous debris and lymphocytes. Cytospin, modified Giemsa stain. (**c**) Mature teratoma. Refractile keratin debris, squamous cells, and histiocytes. Cell block, H&E stain. (**d**) Anucleated and nucleated benign squamous cells. Cell block, H&E stain

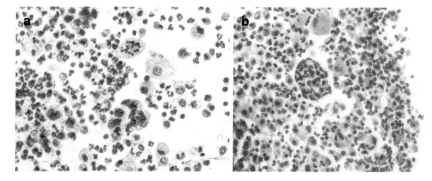

Fig. 9.28 (**a**) Immature teratoma. A cluster of small round blue cells is seen adjacent to a group of larger atypical cells and a squamous cell. The background is cellular with inflammatory cells. The patient was found to have an immature teratoma containing a yolk sac tumor. Cytospin, Papanicolaou stain. (**b**) Immature teratoma. Small hyperchromatic cells in a three-dimensional cluster. The cells have a high N/C ratio, round-to-oval nuclei with fine, evenly dispersed chromatin. The patient had a primitive neuroendocrine tumor in an immature teratoma. Cell block, H&E stain

Cytologic Criteria (Mature Teratoma)

- Variable mixture of benign squamous, glandular, and/or transitional cells in clusters or sheets
- Flat, translucent anucleate and nucleated squamous cells; may be surrounded by histiocytes and neutrophils (if associated with hair)
- Hair shafts surrounded by histiocytes and scant neutrophils (unique to teratoma)
- Squamoid metaplastic cells
- Keratinized squamous cells with benign features
- Cholesterol clefts; amorphous material
- Histiocytes, giant cells; may be surrounding keratin debris
- Columnar cells with cilia possible
- Fat cells

Cytologic Criteria (Immature Teratoma)

- Components of mature teratoma may be present (see above)
- Variety of disordered, overlapping, immature-appearing cells with a high N/C ratio
- Tight clusters of small cells
- High nuclear-to-cytoplasmic ratio
- Round-to-oval nuclei with fine, evenly dispersed chromatin
- 1–2 small, distinct nucleoli
- Small, hyperchromatic cells in small three-dimensional tubules
- Rosette/pseudorosette formation
- Immature glial cells with hyperchromatic, oval nuclei and spindled cytoplasm

Explanatory Notes

Mature teratomatous elements are found primarily due to intraoperative rupture and are rarely described in the literature. Hair shafts and benign squamous cells with associated inflammation may occur with or without rupture and are characteristics of mature teratoma [122]. Peritoneal keratin granulomas may also occur and be associated with anucleate keratin debris, "ghost" squamous cells, and granulomatous inflammation [123]. Immature teratoma is more likely to involve the peritoneum than mature teratoma, but its cytology is not well-characterized [124, 125]. Peritoneal implants are primarily comprised of the immature neural elements. Neuroepithelium is strongly positive for glial cell line-derived neurotrophic factor α-1 (GFR α-1) and depending on its grade, OCT4, PAX6, and CD56 [47].

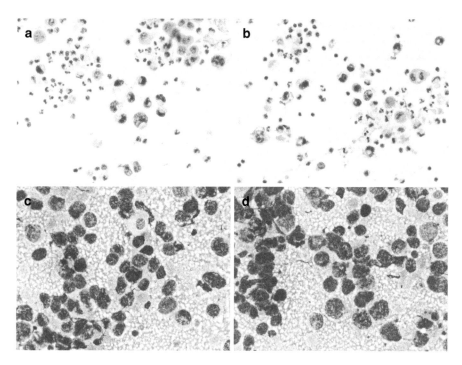

Fig. 9.29 (**a**) Dysgerminoma. Large, pleomorphic, loosely cohesive tumor cells are seen in a background of mixed inflammation. The nuclei are hyperchromatic with coarse chromatin and single, round, large nucleoli. Cytospin, Papanicolaou stain. (**b**) Dysgerminoma. The tumor cells are large and discohesive and contain large, dark nuclei with irregular nuclear contours. Intermixed lymphocytes, a characteristic component seen in histologic sections, are often reduced in the cytologic preparation of fluid specimens. Cytospin, Papanicolaou stain. (**c**) Dysgerminoma. Large tumor cells with prominent nuclei are intermixed with lymphocytes in a bubbly, "tigroid" background. This background is characteristically seen on touch preparations and usually absent in preparations of serous fluid specimens. Smear preparation, modified Giemsa stain. (**d**) Dysgerminoma. The malignant cells crowd together but do not form true tissue fragments. The large size and marked pleomorphism suggest a germ cell tumor. Smear preparation, modified Giemsa stain

Dysgerminoma

Dysgerminoma (Fig. 9.29) is the ovarian equivalent to testicular seminoma and one of the most common malignant germ cell tumors. It occurs in the first three decades of life and has spread to the peritoneum or other organs in about a third of the cases at presentation [47].

Cytologic Criteria

- Dissociated, loose sheetlike groups and single cells
- Large, uniform, monomorphic polygonal cells
- Characteristic vesicular nucleus with a single large, smooth, central nucleolus
- Nucleus centrally placed with prominent nuclear membrane irregularities
- Coarsely clumped chromatin
- Fragile, well-delineated pale granular, or vaguely vacuolated cytoplasm
- Frequent mitotic figures and apoptotic bodies
- No tigroid background present in fluid
- Lymphocytes, giant cells, and histiocytes possible (less frequent than FNA)

Explanatory Notes

Dysgerminoma is well described in fine needle aspiration cytology [121, 126], but there are rare reports involving fluid, where association with lymphocytes, granulomas, and syncytiotrophoblastic giant cells is less frequent [107, 127]. The malignant cells are positive for OCT3/4, CD117 (c-kit), and PLAP and usually express SALL4 [128, 129]. Unlike embryonal carcinoma, dysgerminoma is CD30 negative.

Yolk Sac Tumor (Endodermal Sinus Tumor)

Yolk sac tumor (YST) is a malignant germ cell tumor that is also more common in the pediatric age group. Patients experience abdominal pain, have a large abdominal mass, and usually have an elevated serum alpha-fetoprotein (AFP). At the time of discovery, tumor has often spread to the peritoneum and retroperitoneal lymph nodes [47].

Cytologic Features

- Moderate to highly cellular.
- Loosely cohesive, three-dimensional clusters with smooth borders and overlapping nuclei.
- Irregular, papillary, or glandular clusters; tight spherules may have smooth margins.
- Papilla may be contorted or twisted (snake-like) with fibrovascular cores.
- Prominent, sharply defined cytoplasmic vacuoles of variable sizes.
- Enlarged, eccentric, hyperchromatic nuclei with large 1–2 nucleoli, often multiple nucleoli, and vesicular, coarse chromatin.

- Distinct nuclear membranes but indistinct cytoplasmic borders (syncytial-like).
- High nuclear-to-cytoplasmic ratio.
- Marked nuclear pleomorphism; sizes up to 5–8X of a red blood cell in conjunction with monomorphous, uniform cells.
- Round, eosinophilic hyaline globules in and around tumor cells; may fuse (positive with AFP and PAS with diastase).
- Mitoses, apoptoses.
- Schiller-Duvall bodies are rare in fluid.
- Histiocytes possible.

Explanatory Notes

YST is rarely described in peritoneal fluid [107, 113, 130, 131]. The tumor cells are often mistaken for adenocarcinoma, but in a young person, YST should be considered first [132]. YST is known for its plethora of histologic patterns, but the cells are typically monomorphic. The presence of hyaline globules is distinctive but not specific. YST is positive for glypican3 (more sensitive), AFP, and SALL4, but negative for CD117 and OCT4, to differentiate it from dysgerminoma.

Sample Reports

Example 1
Pelvis, left gutter, washing:
- Satisfactory for evaluation.
- Benign squamous cells, hair shafts, inflammation, and keratin debris consistent with mature teratoma.
- Category: Atypia of undetermined significance.

Example 2
Peritoneal washing:
- Satisfactory for evaluation.
- Mature and immature epithelial elements suggestive of immature teratoma (see note).
- Category: Suspicious for malignancy.
  Note: Although there are numerous benign-appearing epithelial groups, rare clusters show immature, possibly neural, features. A cell block was noncontributory. The presence of immature elements, particularly neuroepithelium, raises suspicion for an immature teratoma. Correlation with the surgical specimen is desirable.

Example 3
Pelvic washing:
- Satisfactory for evaluation.

- Features consistent with dysgerminoma.
- Category: Malignant.

Note: The immunochemical profile and morphologic features are concordant with the patient's prior history of dysgerminoma. Cells are positive for OCT4, SALL4, PLAP, and CD117, supporting this interpretation.

Mesenchymal Neoplasms/Mixed Epithelial and Mesenchymal Neoplasms

Sarcomas rarely involve serous cavities, and the patient typically has a known history once involvement is identified. Leiomyosarcoma [133] (Fig. 9.30) and

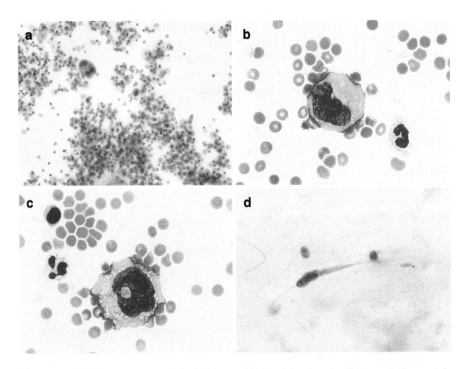

Fig. 9.30 (a) Leiomyosarcoma. A single large atypical multinucleated cell is seen in the top left-hand corner of the field. Serous fluid specimens involved by sarcomas often only demonstrate rare malignant cells that tend to round up in fluids. Cytospin, Papanicolaou stain. (b) Leiomyosarcoma. A single large cell contains a large nucleus with irregular nuclear contours and a coarse chromatin pattern. Sarcomas that produce spindle-shaped cells on histologic sections may "round up" and appear more epithelioid in fluid specimens. Cytospin, modified Giemsa stain. (c) Leiomyosarcoma. This single, overtly malignant cell has a large nucleus and an intranuclear pseudoinclusion. While the differential diagnosis is broad, this pattern is typical of aggressive sarcoma. Cytospin, modified Giemsa stain. (d) Leiomyosarcoma. Unlike the previous examples, this leiomyosarcoma cell maintained its spindle shape. The nucleus is dark and has irregular chromatin and nuclear contours. Smear preparation, Papanicolaou stain

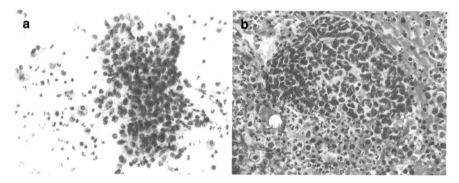

Fig. 9.31 (**a**) Endometrial stromal sarcoma, high grade. The sarcoma cells form a cohesive fragment and have oval-shaped nuclei and syncytial cytoplasm. This fragment could easily be mistaken for an adenocarcinoma. Cytospin, Papanicolaou stain. (**b**) Endometrial stromal sarcoma. This fragment contains many dark, crowded nuclei in cells with scant cytoplasm. Some nuclei are epithelioid, while others are more elongated, which may suggest a mesenchymal rather than epithelial origin. Cell block, H&E

endometrioid stromal sarcoma (Fig. 9.31) [134, 135] are most commonly present in peritoneal washings, owing to their increased frequency in the pelvic cavity. Carcinosarcoma (malignant Müllerian mixed tumor (MMMT)) is a biphasic malignant neoplasm, usually originating in the uterus, containing carcinomatous as well as sarcomatous components. The carcinomatous component is more likely to metastasize to the peritoneum without the sarcomatous component; rarely, both components may be present [136–138]. Discussion of these, and other rare findings in washings, is beyond the scope of this text.

Lymphoma

Peritoneal washing is not typically performed for lymphoproliferative diseases, which are more commonly diagnosed on ascites fluid or pleural effusion specimens (Fig. 9.32). However, lymphoma ranks foremost among uncommon peritoneal neoplastic effusions [73], although effusion is not usually the presenting feature. Children are more likely to have leukemia or lymphoma involving peritoneal fluid than adenocarcinoma or other small round blue cell tumors [139, 140]. Non-Hodgkin lymphoma is more frequent than Hodgkin lymphoma in both populations [141]. It is rare that peritoneal fluid is involved with primary lymphoma, which typically involves the pleura [142]. Plasmablastic myeloma has also been described in peritoneal fluid [143]. If concern exists that a peritoneal washing specimen is involved by lymphoma, examination of the specimen should follow the guidelines presented in Chap. 7, "Malignant-Secondary (Metastatic)." Lymphoma/leukemia is suspected when cells lack cohesion, are relatively small and monotonous, and contain scant cytoplasm. Chromatin is usually finely granular and nucleoli smooth, small, and round, except in high-grade neoplasms.

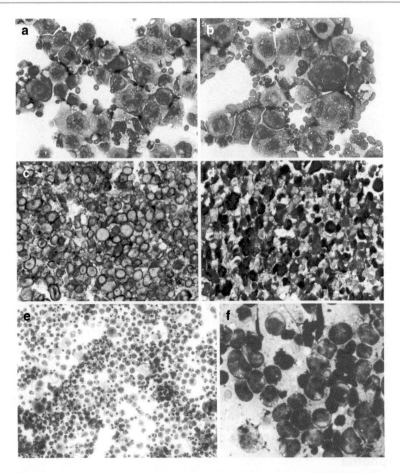

Fig. 9.32 (**a**) Anaplastic large cell lymphoma. Large single malignant cells pushed together into loose groups. The cells have large, pleomorphic nuclei and blue, finely vacuolated cytoplasm. Lymphoglandular bodies are not usually evident in fluid specimens. Cytospin, modified Giemsa stain. (**b**) Anaplastic large cell lymphoma. The lymphoma cells have highly convoluted nuclei as well as multinucleation and multiple, irregular nucleoli. Cytospin, modified Giemsa stain. (**c**) Anaplastic large cell lymphoma. The lymphoma cells are diffusely positive for CD30, a cytomembranous stain. Cell block, CD30 immunostain. (**d**) Anaplastic large cell lymphomas. A large subset of ALCLs express ALK, as demonstrated by positive nuclear and cytoplasmic staining in these cells. ALK-negative ALCLs have a worse prognosis. Cell block, ALK immunostain. (**e**) Burkitt lymphoma. The background contains a cellular, monotonous population of medium-sized dispersed cells with coarse chromatin. While this finding is suspicious for lymphoma, ancillary studies should be used to confirm clonality. Cytospin, Papanicolaou stain. (**f**) Burkitt lymphoma. The lymphoid cells have blue cytoplasm with tiny cytoplasmic vacuoles. The nuclei are large with irregular nuclear contours. Cytospin, modified Giemsa stain. (**g**) Plasma cell neoplasm. An abundance of plasma cells is an unusual finding in fluid specimens and should raise suspicion for a plasma cell neoplasm. The cells have eccentrically placed nuclei, and chromatin is clumped along the cell's nuclear membrane. Cytospin, Papanicolaou stain. (**h**) Plasma cell neoplasm. Perinuclear hofs can be more clearly seen on this H&E-stained cell block preparation. Several cells show binucleation. Cell block, H&E stain

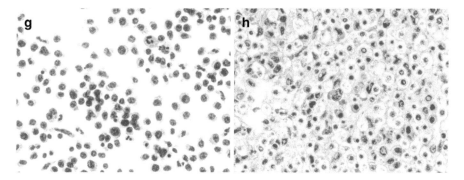

Fig. 9.32 (continued)

Metastatic Carcinoma

The most common tumors to metastasize to the peritoneum are adenocarcinomas: ovarian epithelial tumors in women and gastrointestinal or pancreaticobiliary tumors in men. Even though prostatic carcinoma (men) and breast carcinoma (women) are the most frequent tumors in the United States [144], neither is common in peritoneal washings (Fig. 9.33). Peritoneal fluid cytology is highly sensitive in confirming the presence of peritoneal carcinomatosis, regardless of the tumor origin [80]. Pancreatic and gastric carcinomas are not uncommon and are important to recognize in peritoneal fluid because of the impact on prognosis and treatment. Metastatic carcinoma is discussed more fully in Chap. 7, "Malignant-Secondary (Metastatic)."

Cervical Carcinoma: Squamous Cell Carcinoma and Endocervical Adenocarcinoma

Most cervical carcinomas arise from infection with high-risk HPV subtypes. They include cervical squamous cell carcinoma (SCC) (Fig. 9.34) and endocervical adenocarcinoma (ECA) (Fig. 9.35); both entities infrequently involve the peritoneal cavity and thus are rarely considered in the differential diagnosis. Involvement by endocervical adenocarcinoma has been reported more frequently than involvement by squamous cell carcinoma, and it presents as a high- or low-grade mucinous tumor. Features concordant with ECA are described earlier in this chapter.

Cytologic Criteria (Squamous Cell Carcinoma)

- Usually highly cellular specimens.
- Tissue fragments lacking glandular formation with irregular borders as well as single dispersed cells in the background.

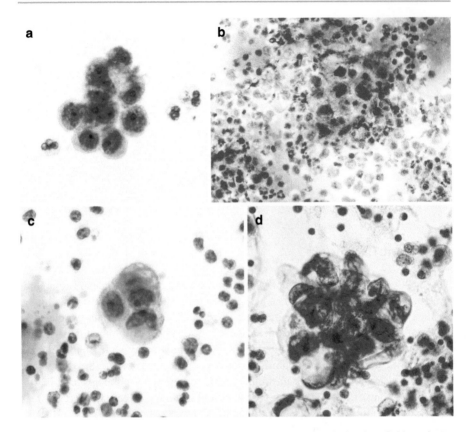

Fig. 9.33 (a) Prostate adenocarcinoma. Prostate adenocarcinoma rarely involves fluid specimens but is suggested by cells with foamy cytoplasm, round nuclei, and prominent single nucleoli. Patients usually have a known history of prostatic adenocarcinoma. Cytospin, Papanicolaou stain. (b) Pancreatic adenocarcinoma. Pleomorphic malignant cells are seen in a background of granular debris, likely necrosis. The nuclei are enlarged and have irregular contours and coarse chromatin. The features are compatible with but not specific for a pancreatic origin. Cytospin, modified Giemsa stain. (c) Pancreatic adenocarcinoma. This group of three malignant cells has enlarged nuclei with irregular borders and prominent nucleoli. Their size can be compared to the smaller lymphocytes in the background. Cytospin, Papanicolaou stain. (d) Breast adenocarcinoma. A three-dimensional cluster of malignant cells with anisonucleosis, hyperchromasia, and irregular nuclear contours. Some of the cells have vacuolated cytoplasm. The patient had a history of breast ductal carcinoma, and this was a biopsy-proven metastases to the peritoneum. Cytospin, Papanicolaou stain

- Cells with dense cytoplasm and centrally located nuclei, in contrast to the eccentrically located nuclei often seen in adenocarcinomas.
- Anisonucleosis and irregular nuclear contours.
- Basaloid morphology includes cells with enlarged, dark nuclei and highly elevated N/C ratio.
- Keratinized cells have orangeophilic cytoplasm.

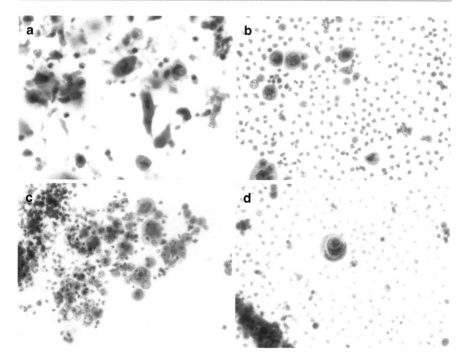

Fig. 9.34 (**a**) Squamous cell carcinoma. Squamous cell carcinoma rarely involves serous fluid specimens but may represent involvement by a cervical squamous cell carcinoma. Some of the malignant cells are hyperkeratinized and have irregular, rigid cytoplasmic projections. Cytospin, Papanicolaou stain. (**b**) Squamous cell carcinoma. Several round malignant cells are seen with centrally placed pyknotic nuclei and dense cytoplasm. The background contains acute inflammatory cells and degenerated cells, associated with the necrosis often seen in squamous cell carcinoma. Cytospin, Papanicolaou stain. (**c**) Squamous cell carcinoma. While these cells do not contain the pink cytoplasm of keratinizing squamous cell carcinoma cells, the dense and waxy cytoplasm is suggestive of squamous cell carcinoma. Immunostains may be necessary to prove squamous differentiation in patients without an established history. Cytospin, Papanicolaou stain. (**d**) Squamous cell carcinoma. An unusual cell-in-cell-in-cell pattern in which malignant cells have been engulfed (wrapped or overlain) by other malignant cells, a feature common in this neoplasm. The malignant cells are typically huge and have large, compressed, dark nuclei. Cytospin, Papanicolaou stain. (**e**) Squamous cell carcinoma, cervical origin. Poorly differentiated malignant cells with high nuclear-to-cytoplasmic ratios and dark, coarse chromatin. The cytomorphologic features are nonspecific and could represent other poorly differentiated malignancies as well. Cytospin, modified Giemsa stain. (**f**) Squamous cell carcinoma, cervical origin. These malignant cells are enlarged and have large nuclei with irregular nuclear contours and coarse chromatin. This patient had a poorly differentiated squamous cell carcinoma of the cervix. Cytospin, Papanicolaou stain. (**g**) Squamous cell carcinoma, cervical origin. Non-keratinizing squamous cell carcinoma with enlarged nuclei and frequent prominent nucleoli from the same patient. Cell block, H&E. (**h**) Squamous cell carcinoma. This cell block preparation contains spindle-shaped keratinizing squamous cell carcinoma cells, with irregular, pink cytoplasmic projections and coal-black pyknotic nuclei. Cell block, H&E

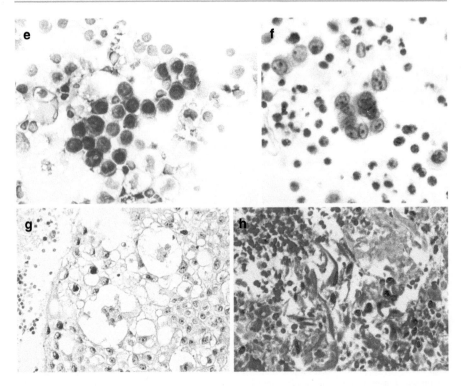

Fig. 9.34 (continued)

- Keratinized cells may have abundant, irregularly shaped cytoplasm and pyknotic nuclei, resulting in paradoxically low N/C ratios.
- Fragments of irregularly shaped keratin without discernible nuclei.

Explanatory Notes

Squamous cell carcinoma (SCC) shows the spectrum of changes characteristic of its appearance in other sites and reflects the tumor grade. Squamous differentiation can be seen in non-cervical adenocarcinomas such as endometrioid carcinoma, mature and immature teratoma, Brenner tumors, carcinosarcoma, and metastatic squamous cell carcinomas from other sites, such as the lung. Patients with metastatic or locally invasive pelvic cervical carcinoma usually have a known history. Squamous cell carcinoma, as well as cells with squamous differentiation arising from adenocarcinoma, will be positive for squamous markers: p40 and p63 are nuclear stains used to demonstrate squamous differentiation. HPV studies can also help confirm a cervical origin.

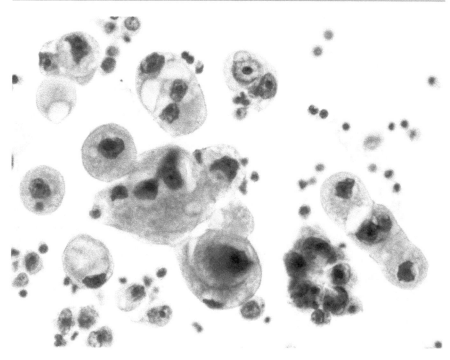

Fig. 9.35 Endocervical adenocarcinoma. Numerous enlarged malignant cells with abundant, vacuolated cytoplasm and enlarged nuclei with prominent nucleoli. The features are consistent with adenocarcinoma but not specific to a site of origin. Cytospin, Papanicolaou stain

Immunochemistry in Peritoneal Fluid

Immunochemistry (IC) is essential for differentiating tumors, particularly given the propensity of cells to take a spherical shape and form vacuoles in fluids. As with all IC, the initial panel should be developed based upon the patient's clinical history and cell morphology to determine the most likely primary sites. Table 9.4 outlines useful or distinctive morphologic features, and Table 9.5 demonstrates typical IC staining patterns for some of the tumors discussed in this chapter.

Epithelial neoplasms are usually first confirmed with an epithelial marker (such as MOC 31, Ber4, or claudin 4) and the lack of staining with a mesothelial marker (calretinin or D2-40). PAX8 and WT1 can be useful in confirming an ovarian origin. WT1 is superior to PAX8 for detecting serous carcinoma, but WT1 is also reactive in benign and malignant mesothelial cells. Initial staining with a WT1/pankeratin cocktail together with claudin 4 has also been reported [145]. Serous neoplasms are usually negative for the mesothelial markers D2-40 and calretinin. PAX8 is useful in identifying epithelial ovarian tumors other than mucinous tumors, including clear cell carcinoma and mixed cell types [146]. A major pitfall in the usage of markers positive in serous neoplasms (such as PAX8) is that they are also positive in benign processes, such as endosalpingiosis and endometriosis, as well as borderline tumors.

Table 9.4 Morphologic features distinguishing serous benign/borderline ovarian tumors from malignant tumors

Features	SBT	LGSC	MPSC	HGSC
Fluid cellularity	Low	Low to high	Low to high	High
Single atypical cells	Rare	Occasional	Rare to variable	Frequent
Cluster contours	Smooth, cohesive, uniform	Hobnailed, scalloped, uniform	Hobnail to peripheral palisading	Irregular, frayed
Cluster branching	Medium to large; infrequent cores	Large; uniform, hierarchical branching	Fibrovascular core, minimal short branches ("knobs")	Variable sizes; nonuniform hierarchical branching
Psammoma bodies	Occasional	Frequent	Frequent	Rare
Enlarged nuclei (>2X)	Absent	Present	Present	Present
Nuclear pleomorphism; nuclear size > 4X	Absent	Absent	Rare	Present
Nuclear-to-cytoplasmic (N/C) ratio	Medium to high	Low	Medium to high	High
Nuclear chromatin	Fine, uniform	Fine to variable	Fine, uniform	Coarse, clumped
Nuclei	Round to oval	Mildly irregular	Round to oval; mildly irregular	Pleomorphic
Nucleoli	Indistinct, single	Small, single	Small, multiple	Macronucleoli; multiple
Cytoplasmic vacuoles	Rare	Occasional, small	Occasional, small	Common; "soap bubble"
Mitoses	Rare	Infrequent	Infrequent	Frequent

References:
Sadeghi and Ylagan [41]
Katabuchi et al. [62]

Therefore, immunoreactivity does not in itself indicate the presence of a malignant or even neoplastic process.

Gastrointestinal carcinomas may be positive for CDX2, SATB2, and/or CK20 (Fig. 9.36); while these markers are more frequently expressed in lower gastrointestinal tract carcinomas as compared to upper gastrointestinal tract carcinomas, CDX2 is the least specific and can often be found expressed in upper gastrointestinal tract carcinomas, pancreatobiliary carcinomas, and a third of ovarian mucinous carcinomas. Approximately half of all pancreatobiliary carcinomas will lose expression of DPC4, which can be helpful in distinguishing them from an upper gastrointestinal tract primary.

Table 9.5 Useful immunochemistry for indeterminate cells in peritoneal washings

Entity	Positive markers	Negative markers	Notes
Endometriosis	ER, PR, BerEP4, MOC 31, claudin 4, PAX8	Calretinin, D2-40, WT1	
Endosalpingiosis	ER, PR, BerEP4, MOC 31, claudin 4, PAX8, WT1	Calretinin, D2-40	WT1 is positive in endosalpingiosis, which can distinguish it from endometriosis
Serous cystadenoma	ER, PR, BerEP4, MOC 31, MOC 31, PAX8, WT1	Calretinin, D2-40	
Borderline serous tumor	ER, PR, BerEP4, MOC 31, MOC 31, PAX8, WT1	Wild-type p53[a]; Calretinin, D2-40	Diffuse, strong p16 expression suggests HGSC
Low-grade serous carcinoma (LGSC)	ER, PR, BerEP4, MOC 31, MOC 31, PAX8, WT1	Wild-type p53[a]; Calretinin, D2-40, WT1	Diffuse p16 expression suggests HGSC
High-grade serous carcinoma (HGSC)	ER, PR, BerEP4, MOC 31, MOC 31, PAX8, WT1, p53 (aberrant)[a], p16 (diffuse)	Calretinin, D2-40	
Granulosa cell tumor	Calretinin, inhibin, CD99, SF1	SALL4	
Dysgerminoma	SALL4, OCT3/4, CD117 (c-kit), PLAP	CD30	
Yolk sac tumor	Glypican3, AFP, SALL4	CD117, OCT3/4	
Endometrioid carcinoma	ER, PR, BerEP4, PAX8	WT1, wild-type p53[a]	Grade 3 may show aberrant p53[a] pattern
Clear cell carcinoma (CCC)	HNF1β, napsin A	WT1, ER, PR	Aberrant[a] p53 and/or diffuse p16 suggests HGSC; CCC may have aberrant p53
Low-grade mucinous neoplasm	Variable	Variable	Depends on site of origin; most arise from the gastrointestinal tract and express CK20, CDX2, and SATB2 and are negative for PAX8
Borderline mucinous tumor/ ovarian mucinous carcinoma	CK7, ER (+/−), PR (+/−), PAX8 (+/−), CK20(−/+), CDX2(−/+)	SATB2	CK20 usually negative or focal; CDX2 positive in ~1/3 of mucinous carcinomas, but mostly focal or weak if ovarian. More than half of primary ovarian mucinous tumors are negative for ER, PR, and PAX8

(continued)

Table 9.5 (continued)

Entity	Positive markers	Negative markers	Notes
Mesothelioma and mesothelial proliferations	Calretinin, D2-40, HBME1, WT1	BerEP4, MOC 31, MOC 31, claudin 4	May be positive for PAX8; nuclear loss of BAP-1 differentiates mesothelioma from benign mesothelial proliferations
Leiomyosarcoma	Desmin, h-caldesmon	CD10	
Endometrial stromal sarcoma	CD10	Desmin, h-caldesmon	

[a]A "wild-type" p53 pattern shows diffuse but patchy nuclear staining of differing intensities and is a finding in both normal tissues and most tumors. An aberrant p53 pattern is either null (no nuclear staining in the cells of interest) or strong and diffuse nuclear staining (either aberrant pattern is considered "positive")

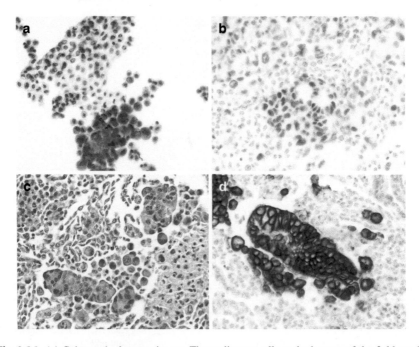

Fig. 9.36 (**a**) Colorectal adenocarcinoma. The malignant cells at the bottom of the field can be contrasted with the benign mesothelial cells present in a sheet at the top of the field. The malignant cells are larger and have enlarged nuclei, high N/C ratios, coarse chromatin, and irregularly shaped nuclei. ThinPrep, Papanicolaou stain. (**b**) Colorectal adenocarcinoma. This fragment demonstrates cytomorphologic features suggestive of a colorectal origin – columnar cells with elongated nuclei that are reactive with SATB2, a marker for colorectal carcinoma. SATB2 immunostain. (**c**) Colorectal adenocarcinoma. Malignant cells may occur as fragments or singly dispersed and, in less differentiated tumors, may not appear columnar. These nuclei are rounded, of varied size and shape, with prominent nucleoli. Cell block, H&E. (**d**) Colorectal adenocarcinoma. Adenocarcinomas are typically positive for epithelial markers such as MOC-31 (cytomembranous staining; seen here), BerEP4 (cytomembranous staining), and claudin-4 (cytomembranous staining). Reactive and malignant mesothelial cells typically do not express these markers. Cell block, MOC-31 immunostain

Summary

The cytomorphology of malignant cells found in peritoneal fluids, as well as the results of any ancillary studies, should be compatible with the patient's known history or concurrently resected neoplasm. Inconsistencies should prompt a workup for a possible secondary neoplasm.

References

1. Amin MB, Edge S, Greene F, et al., editors. AJCC cancer staging handbook: from the AJCC cancer staging manual. 8th ed. New York: Springer; 2017.
2. Armstrong DK, Alvarez RD, Bakkum-Gamez JN, et al. Ovarian cancer- including fallopian tube cancer and primary peritoneal cancer (Version 1.2019; dated March 8, 2019). National Comprehensive Cancer Network. https://www.nccn.org/professionals/physician_gls/pdf/ovarian.pdf.
3. Davidson W, Madan R, O'Neil M, Tawfik OW, Fan F. Utility of peritoneal washing cytology in staging and prognosis of ovarian and fallopian tube neoplasms: a 10-year retrospective analysis. Ann Diagn Pathol. 2016;22:54–7.
4. Zuna RE, Behrens A. Peritoneal washing cytology in gynecologic cancers: long-term follow-up of 355 patients. J Natl Cancer Inst. 1996;88(14):980–7.
5. Bakkum-Gamez JN, Richardson DL, Seamon LG, Aletti GD, Powless CA, Keeney GL, O'Malley DM, Cliby WA. Influence of intraoperative capsule rupture on outcomes in stage I epithelial ovarian cancer. Obstet Gynecol. 2009;113(1):11–7.
6. Montavon Sartorius C, Mirza U, Schotzau A, et al. Impact of the new FIGO 2013 classification on prognosis of stage I epithelial ovarian cancers. Cancer Manag Res. 2018;10:4709–18.
7. Abu-Rustum NR, Yashar CM, Bean S, et al. Uterine Neoplasms (Version 3.2019; dated February 11, 2019). National Comprehensive Cancer Network. https://www.nccn.org/professionals/physician_gls/pdf/uterine.pdf.
8. Creasman WT, Morrow CP, Bundy BN, Homesley HD, Graham JE, Heller PB. Surgical pathologic spread patterns of endometrial cancer: a Gynecologic Oncology Group study. Cancer. 1987;60:2035–41.
9. Tebeu PM, Popowski Y, Verkooijen HM, et al. Positive peritoneal cytology in early-stage endometrial cancer does not influence prognosis. Br J Cancer. 2004;91:720–4.
10. Fadare O, Mariappan MR, Hileeto D, Wang S, McAlpine JN, Rimm DL. Upstaging based solely on positive peritoneal washing does not affect outcome in endometrial cancer. Mod Pathol. 2005;18:673–80.
11. Dede M, Yenen MC, Goktolga U, et al. Is adjuvant therapy necessary for peritoneal cytology-positive surgical-pathologic stage I endometrial cancer? Preliminary results. Eur J Gynaecol Oncol. 2004;25:591–3.
12. Ayhan A, Taskiran C, Celik C, Aksu T, Yuce K. Surgical stage III endometrial cancer: analysis of treatment outcomes, prognostic factors and failure patterns. Eur J Gynaecol Oncol. 2002;23:553–6.
13. Obermair A, Geramou M, Tripcony L, Nicklin JL, Perrin L, Crandon AJ. Peritoneal cytology: impact on disease-free survival in clinical stage I endometrioid adenocarcinoma of the uterus. Cancer Lett. 2001;164:105–10.
14. Havrilesky LJ, Cragun JM, Calingaert B, et al. The prognostic significance of positive peritoneal cytology and adnexal/serosal metastasis in stage IIIA endometrial cancer. Gynecol Oncol. 2007;104:401–5.
15. Takeshima N, Katase K, Hirai Y, Yamawaki T, Yamauchi K, Hasumi K. Prognostic value of peritoneal cytology in patients with carcinoma of the uterine cervix. Gynecol Oncol. 1997;64:136–40.

16. Ditto A, Martinelli F, Carcangiu M, Lorusso D, Raspagliesi F. Peritoneal cytology as prognostic factor in cervical cancer. Diagn Cytopathol. 2015;43:705–9.
17. Roberts WS, Bryson SC, Cavanagh D, Roberts VC, Lyman GH. Peritoneal cytology and invasive carcinoma of the cervix. Gynecol Oncol. 1986;24:331–6.
18. Landon G, Stewart J, Deavers M, Lu K, Sneige N. Peritoneal washing cytology in patients with BRCA1 or BRCA2 mutations undergoing risk-reducing salpingo-oophorectomies: a 10-year experience and reappraisal of its clinical utility. Gynecol Oncol. 2012;125:683–6.
19. Blok F, Roes EM, van Leenders GJ, van Beekhuizen HJ. The lack of clinical value of peritoneal washing cytology in high risk patients undergoing risk-reducing salpingo-oophorectomy: a retrospective study and review. BMC Cancer. 2016;16:18.
20. Ohwada M, Suzuki M, Suzuki T, et al. Problems with peritoneal cytology in second-look laparotomy performed in patients with epithelial ovarian cancer. Cancer. 2001;93(6):376–80.
21. Nakagawa S, Nashimoto A, Yabusaki H. Role of staging laparoscopy with peritoneal lavage cytology in the treatment of locally advanced gastric cancer. Gastric Cancer. 2007;10(10):29–34.
22. Assaly M, Bongiovanni M, Kumar N, et al. Cytology of benign multicystic peritoneal mesothelioma in peritoneal washings. Cytopathology. 2008;19:224–8.
23. Wojcik EM, Naylor B. "Collagen balls" in peritoneal washings: prevalence, morphology, origin and significance. Acta Cytol. 1992;36(4):466–70.
24. Prentice L, Stewart A, Mohiuddin S, Johnson NP. What is endosalpingiosis? Fertil Steril. 2012;98(4):942–7.
25. Heinig J, Gottschalk I, Cirkel U, Diallo R. Endosalpingiosis- an underestimated cause of chronic pelvic pain or an accidental finding? A retrospective study of 16 cases. Eur J Obstet Gynecol Reprod Biol. 2002;103(1):75–8.
26. Zuna RE, Mitchell ML, Mulick KA, Weijchert WM. Cytohistologic correlation of peritoneal washing cytology in gynecologic disease. Acta Cytol. 1989;33(3):327–36.
27. Sneige N, Dawlett MA, Kologinczak TL, Guo M. Endosalpingiosis in peritoneal washings in women with benign gynecologic conditions: thirty-eight cases confirmed with paired box-8 immunohistochemical staining and correlation with surgical biopsy findings. Cancer Cytopathol. 2013;121(10):582–90.
28. Seguin RE, Ingram K. Cervicovaginal psammoma bodies in endosalpingiosis. A case report. J Reprod Med. 2000;45(6):526–8.
29. Vila M, Thompson K, Erdem G. Mobile ciliary microorganisms in peritoneal fluid. Diagn Cytopathol. 2011;39(8):606–7.
30. van Baal JO, van de Vijver KK, Nieuwland R, et al. The histophysiology and pathophysiology of the peritoneum. Tissue Cell. 2017;49(1):95–105.
31. Salzer WL. Peritoneal dialysis-related peritonitis: challenges and solutions. Int J Nephrol Renovasc Dis. 2018;11:173–86.
32. Gupta RK, Johnston PS, Naran S, Lallu S, Fauck R. Cytological findings in a sample of peritoneal aspirate from a case of bile peritonitis. Diagn Cytopathol. 2005;32(1):35–7.
33. Stowell SB, Wiley CM, Perez-Reyes N, Powers CN. Cytologic diagnosis of peritoneal fluids: applicability to the laparoscopic diagnosis of endometriosis. Acta Cytol. 1997;41(3):817–22.
34. Cantley RL, Yoxtheimer L, Molnar S. The role of peritoneal washings in the diagnosis of endometriosis. Diagn Cytopathol. 2018;46(5):447–51.
35. Shield P. Peritoneal washing cytology. Cytopathology. 2004;15:131–41.
36. Barkan GA, Naylor B, Gattuso P, Küllü S, Galan K, Wojcik EM. Morphologic features of endometriosis in various types of cytologic specimens. Diagn Cytopathol. 2013;41(11):936–42.
37. Fanning J, Markuly SN, Hindman TL, Galle PC, McRae MA, Visnesky PM, Hilgers RD. False positive malignant peritoneal cytology and psammoma bodies in benign gynecologic disease. J Reprod Med. 1996;41(7):504–8.
38. DeMay RM. The art & science of cytopathology. 2nd ed: American Society of Clinical. Hong Kong: Pathology Press; 2012.
39. Alli PM, Ali SZ. Micropapillary serous carcinoma of the ovary: cytomorphologic characteristics in peritoneal/pelvic washings. Cancer. 2002;96(3):135–9.

40. Parwani AV, Chan TY, Ali SZ. Significance of psammoma bodies in serous cavity fluid: a cytopathologic analysis. Cancer. 2004;102(2):87–91.
41. Sadeghi S, Ylagan LR. Pelvic washing cytology in serous borderline tumors of the ovary using ThinPrep: are there cytologic clues to detecting tumor cells? Diagn Cytopathol. 2004;30(5):313–9.
42. Gilks CB, Bell DA, Scully RE. Serous psammocarcinoma of the ovary and peritoneum. Int J Gynecol Pathol. 1990;9(2):110–21.
43. Riboni F, Giana M, Piantanida P, Vigone A, Surico N, Boldorini R. Peritoneal psammocarcinoma diagnosed by a Papanicolaou smear: a case report. Acta Cytol. 2010;54(3):311–3.
44. Carr NJ, Cecil TD, Mohamed F, et al. Peritoneal Surface Oncology Group International. A consensus for classification and pathologic reporting of pseudomyxoma peritonei and associated appendiceal neoplasia: the results of the Peritoneal Surface Oncology Group International (PSOGI) modified Delphi process. Am J Surg Pathol. 2016;40(1):14–26.
45. Quinn G, Hales S, Hamid B, Meara N. Comparison of mucoid-mimic artefact with true mucin in peritoneal cytology samples. Cytopathology. 2015;26:194–6.
46. Owens SD, Gossett R, McElhaney MR, Christopher MM, Shelly SM. Three cases of canine bile peritonitis with mucinous material in abdominal fluid as the prominent cytologic finding. Vet Clin Pathol. 2003;32(3):114–20.
47. Clement PB, Young RH. Atlas of gynecologic surgical pathology. 3rd ed. London: Saunders Elsevier; 2014.
48. Malpica A, Sant'Ambrogio S, Deavers MT, Silva EG. Well-differentiated papillary mesothelioma of the female peritoneum: a clinicopathologic study of 26 cases. Am J Surg Pathol. 2012;36(1):117–27.
49. Ikeda K, Suzuki T, Tate G, Mitsuya T. Cytomorphologic features of well-differentiated papillary mesothelioma in peritoneal effusion: a case report. Diagn Cytopathol. 2008;36(7):512–5.
50. Wheeler YY, Burroughs F, Li QK. Fine-needle aspiration of a well-differentiated papillary mesothelioma in the inguinal hernia sac: a case report and review of literature. Diagn Cytopathol. 2009;37(10):748–54.
51. Wojcik EM, Selvaggi SM. Fine-needle aspiration cytology of cystic ovarian lesions. Diagn Cytopathol. 1994;11(1):9–14.
52. Özkara SK. Significance of peritoneal washing cytopathology in ovarian carcinomas and tumors of low malignant potential: a quality control study with literature review. Acta Cytol. 2011;55(1):57–68.
53. Ventura KC, Yang GC, Levine PH. Atypical papillary proliferation in gynecologic patients: a study of 32 pelvic washes. Diagn Cytopathol. 2005;32(2):76–81.
54. De Cecio R, Cantile M, Collina F, et al. Borderline Brenner tumor of the ovary: a case report with immunohistochemical and molecular study. J Ovarian Res. 2014;7:101–5.
55. Cheng L, Wolf NG, Rose PG, Rodriguez M, Abdul-Karim FW. Peritoneal washing cytology of ovarian tumors of low malignant potential: correlation with surface ovarian involvement and peritoneal implants. Acta Cytol. 1998;42(5):1091–4.
56. Sneige N, Thomison JB, Malpica A, Gong Y, Ensor J, Silva EG. Peritoneal washing cytologic analysis of ovarian serous tumors of low malignant potential to detect peritoneal implants and predict clinical outcome. Cancer Cytopathol. 2012;120(4):238–44.
57. Lu D, Davila RM, Pinto KR, Lu DW. ThinPrep evaluation of fluid samples aspirated from cystic ovarian masses. Diagn Cytopathol. 2004;30(5):320–4.
58. Moh M, Krings G, Ates D, Aysai A, Kim GE, Rabban JT. SATB2 expression distinguishes ovarian metastases for colorectal and appendiceal origin from primary ovarian tumors of mucinous or endometrioid type. Am J Surg Pathol. 2016;40(3):419–32.
59. Vang R, Gown AM, Barry TS, Wheeler DT, Ronnett BM. Ovarian atypical proliferative (borderline) mucinous tumors: gastrointestinal and seromucinous (endocervical like) types ware immunophenotypically distinctive. Int J Gynecol Pathol. 2006;25(1):83–9.
60. Bell KA, Kurman RJ. A clinicopathologic analysis of atypical proliferative (borderline) tumors and well-differentiated endometrioid adenocarcinomas of the ovary. Am J Surg Pathol. 2000;24(11):1465–79.

61. Jetley S, Khetrapal S, Ahmad A, Jairajpuri ZS. Atypical proliferative endometrioid tumor of ovary: report of a rare case. J Postgrad Med. 2016;62(2):129–32.
62. Katabuchi H, Tashiro H, Cho KR, Kurman RJ, Hedrick EL. Micropapillary serous carcinoma of the ovary: an immunohistochemical and mutational analysis of p53. Int J Gynecol Pathol. 1998;17:54–60.
63. Kaldawy A, Segev Y, Lavie O, Auslender R, Sopik V, Narod SA. Low-grade serous ovarian cancer: a review. Gynecol Oncol. 2016;143:433–8.
64. Razack R, Van der Merwe H, Schubert P. Fine needle aspiration cytology of a nodal low-grade serous neoplasm: a case report of low-grade serous carcinoma arising from a serous borderline tumour with cyto-histological correlation. Cytopathology. 2017;28(4):333–6.
65. Cetinkaya K, Atalay F. Peritoneal cytology in endometrial cancer. Tumori. 2015;101(6):697–700.
66. Schulte JJ, Lastra RR. Abdominopelvic washings in gynecologic pathology: a comprehensive review. Diagn Cytopathol. 2016;44(12):1039–57.
67. Obermair A, Geramou M, Gucer F, et al. Does hysteroscopy facilitate tumor cell dissemination? Incidence of peritoneal cytology from patients with early stage endometrial carcinoma following dilatation and curettage (D & C) versus hysteroscopy and D & C. Cancer. 2000;88:139–43.
68. Cicinelli E, Tinelli R, Colafiglio G, et al. Risk of long-term pelvic recurrences after fluid minihysteroscopy in women with endometrial carcinoma: a controlled randomized study. Menopause. 2012;17(3):511–5.
69. Shinohara S, Sakamoto I, Numata M, Ikegami A, Teramoto K. Risk of spilling cancer cells during total laparoscopic hysterectomy in low-risk endometrial cancer. Gynecol Minim Invasive Ther. 2017;6(3):113–5.
70. Sonoda Y, Zerbe M, Smith A, Lin O, Barakat RR, Hoskins WJ. High incidence of positive peritoneal cytology in low-risk endometrial cancer treated by laparoscopically assisted vaginal hysterectomy. Gynecol Oncol. 2001;80:378–82.
71. Rivasi F, Palicelli A. Peritoneal keratin granulomas: cytohistological correlation in a case of endometrial adenocarcinoma with squamous differentiation. Cytopathology. 2012;23(5):342–4.
72. Badyal RK, Khairwa A, Rajwanshi A, et al. Significance of epithelial cell clusters in pseudomyxoma peritonei. Cytopathology. 2016;27(6):418–26.
73. Gupta S, Sodhani P, Jain S. Cytomorphological profile of neoplastic effusions: an audit of 10 years with emphasis on uncommonly encountered malignancies. J Cancer Res Ther. 2012;8(4):602–9.
74. Runyon BA. Malignancy-related ascites. UpToDate, published 11 June 2019. https://www.uptodate.com.
75. La Torre M, Rossi Del Monte S, Ferrir M, Cosenza G, Mercantini P, Ziparo V. Peritoneal washing cytology in gastric cancer. How, when and who will get a benefit? A review. Minerva Gastroenterol Dietol. 2011;57(1):43–51.
76. Virgillo E, Giarnieri E, Giovagnoli MR, et al. Gastric cancer cells in peritoneal lavage fluid: a systematic review comparing cytological with molecular detection for diagnosis of peritoneal metastases and prediction of peritoneal recurrences. Anticancer Res. 2018;38(3):1255–62.
77. Pulluri B, Kathait A, Tsai JL, et al. The significance of ascites in patients with pancreatic cancer: a case-control study. J Clin Oncol. 2015;33(Suppl 3):445.
78. Makary MA, Warshaw AL, Centeno BA, et al. Implications of peritoneal cytology for pancreatic cancer management. Arch Surg. 1998;133(4):361–5.
79. Merchant NB, Conlon KC, Saigo P, Dougherty E, Brennan MF. Positive peritoneal cytology predicts unresectability of pancreatic adenocarcinoma. J Am Coll Surg. 1999;188(4):421–6.
80. Runyon BA, Hoefs JC, Morgan TR. Ascitic fluid analysis in malignancy-related ascites. Hepatology. 1988;8(5):1104–9.
81. Huang CC, Attele A, Michael CW. Cytomorphologic features of metastatic urothelial carcinoma in serous effusions. Diagn Cytopathol. 2013;41(7):569–74.

82. Bodurka DC, Deavers MT, Tian C, et al. Reclassification of serous ovarian carcinoma by a 2-tier system: a Gynecologic Oncology Group Study. Cancer. 2012;118:3087–94.
83. Nik NN, Vang R, Shih Ie M, Kurman RJ. Origin and pathogenesis of pelvic (ovarian, tubal, and primary peritoneal) serous carcinoma. Annu Rev Pathol. 2014;9:27–45.
84. Lheureux S, Gourley C, Vergote I, Oza AM. Epithelial ovarian cancer. Lancet. 2019;393:1240–53.
85. Kurman RJ, Shih IM. The dualistic model of ovarian carcinogenesis: revisited, revised, and expanded. Am J Pathol. 2016;186:733–47.
86. Xiang M, English DP, Kidd EA. National patterns of care and cancer-specific outcomes of adjuvant treatment in patients with serous and clear cell endometrial carcinoma. Gynecol Oncol. 2019;152:599–604.
87. Kashimura M, Matsukuma K, Kamura T, Matsuyama T, Tsukamoto N. Cytologic findings in peritoneal fluids from patients with ovarian serous adenocarcinoma. Diagn Cytopathol. 1986;2(1):13–6.
88. Ramalingam P. Morphologic, immunophenotypic, and molecular features of epithelial ovarian cancer. Oncology. 2016;30(2):166–76.
89. Ronnett BM, Zahn CM, Kurman RJ, Kass ME, Sugarbaker PH, Shmookler BM. Disseminated peritoneal adenomucinosis and peritoneal mucinous carcinomatosis. A clinicopathologic analysis of 109 cases with emphasis on distinguishing pathologic features, site of origin, prognosis, and relationship to "pseudomyxoma peritonei". Am J Surg Pathol. 1995;19:1390–408.
90. Ronnett BM, Yan H, Kurman RJ, Shmookler BM, Wu L, Sugarbaker PH. Patients with pseudomyxoma peritonei associated with disseminated peritoneal adenomucinosis have a significantly more favorable prognosis than patients with peritoneal mucinous carcinomatosis. Cancer. 2001;92:85–91.
91. Seagle BL, Alexander AL, Lantsman T, Shahabi S. Prognosis and treatment of positive peritoneal cytology in early endometrial cancer: matched cohort analyses from the National Cancer Database. Am J Obstet Gynecol. 2018;218:e321–9.
92. Matsui N, Kajiwara H, Morishita A, et al. Cytologic study of grade 3 endometrioid adenocarcinoma of endometrial origin: cytoarchitecture and features of cell clusters assessed with endometrial brushing cytology- focusing on a comparison with endometrioid adenocarcinoma grade 1,2. Tokai J Exp Clin Med. 2015;40(3):29–35.
93. Johnson DN, Barroeta JE, Antic T, Lastra RR. Cytomorphologic features of metastatic endometrioid carcinoma by fine needle aspiration. Diagn Cytopathol. 2018;46(2):105–10.
94. Fulciniti F, Losito NS, Botti G, et al. Fine-needle cytology of metastatic endometrioid neoplasms: experience with eight cases. Diagn Cytopathol. 2009;37(5):347–52.
95. Fadare O, Parkash V. Pathology of endometrioid and clear cell carcinoma of the ovary. Surg Pathol Clin. 2019;12:529–64.
96. Torre LA, Trabert B, DeSantis CE, et al. Ovarian cancer statistics, 2018. CA Cancer J Clin. 2018;68:284–96.
97. Ito H, Hirasawa T, Yasuda M, Osamura RY, Tsutsumi Y. Excessive formation of basement membrane substance in clear-cell carcinoma of the ovary: diagnostic value of the "raspberry body" in ascites cytology. Diagn Cytopathol. 1997;16:500–4.
98. Khunamornpong S, Thorner PS, Suprasert P, Siriaunkgul S. Clear-cell adenocarcinoma of the female genital tract: presence of hyaline stroma and tigroid background in various types of cytologic specimens. Diagn Cytopathol. 2005;32(6):336–40.
99. Damiani D, Suciu V, Genestie C, Vielh P. Cytomorphology of ovarian clear cell carcinomas in peritoneal effusions. Cytopathology. 2016;27:427–32.
100. Kuwashima Y, Uehara T, Kurosumi M, et al. Cytological distinction between clear cell carcinoma and yolk sac tumor of the ovary. Eur J Gynaecol Oncol. 1996;17(5):345–50.
101. Sangoi AR, Soslow RA, Teng NN, Longacre TA. Ovarian clear cell carcinoma with papillary features: a potential mimic of serous tumor of low malignant potential. Am J Surg Pathol. 2008;32(2):269–74.
102. Kato N, Sasou S, Motoyama T. Expression of hepatocyte nuclear factor-1beta (HNF-1beta) in clear cell tumors and endometriosis of the ovary. Mod Pathol. 2006;19:83–9.

103. Yamashita Y, Nagasaka T, Naiki-Ito A, et al. Napsin A is a specific marker for ovarian clear cell adenocarcinoma. Mod Pathol. 2015;28:111–7.
104. Driss M, Mrad K, Dhouib R, Doghri R, Abbes I, Ben Romdhane K. Ascitic fluid cytology in malignant Brenner tumor: a case report. Acta Cytol. 2010;54:598–600.
105. Ahr A, Arnold G, Göhring UJ, Costa S, Scharl A, Gauwerky JF. Cytology of ascitic fluid in a patient with metastasizing malignant Brenner tumor of the ovary. A case report. Acta Cytol. 1997;41(4 Suppl):1299–304.
106. Esheba GE, Longacre TA, Atkins KA, et al. Expression of urothelial differentiation markers GATA3 and placental S100 (S100P) in female genital tract transitional cell proliferations. Am J Surg Pathol. 2009;33:347–453.
107. Valente PT, Schantz HD, Edmonds PR, Hanjani P. Peritoneal cytology of uncommon ovarian tumors. Diagn Cytopathol. 1992;8:98–106.
108. Guo M, Lim JC, Wojcik EM. Pelvic washing cytology of ovarian Sertoli-Leydig-cell tumor with retiform pattern: a case report. Diagn Cytopathol. 2003;29:28–30.
109. Gupta N, Rajwanshi A, Dey P, Suri V. Adult granulosa cell tumor presenting as metastases to the pleura and peritoneal cavity. Diagn Cytopathol. 2012;40:912–5.
110. Atilgan AO, Tepeoglu M, Ozen O, Bilezikc IB. Peritoneal washing cytology in an adult granulosa cell tumor: a case report and review of literature. J Cytol. 2013;30:74–7.
111. Omari M, Kondo T, Yuminamochi T, et al. Cytologic features of ovarian granulosa cell tumors in pleural and ascitic fluids. Diagn Cytopathol. 2015;43(7):581–4.
112. Harbhajanka A, Bitterman P, Reddy VB, Park JW, Gattuso P. Cytomorphology and clinicopathologic correlation of the recurrent and metastatic adult granulosa cell tumor of the ovary: a retrospective review. Diagn Cytopathol. 2016;44(12):1058–63.
113. Murugan P, Siddaraju N, Sridhar E, Soundararaghavan J, Habeebullah S. Unusual ovarian malignancies in ascitic fluid: a report of 2 cases. Acta Cytol. 2010;54:611–7.
114. Gordon MD, Corless C, Renshaw AA, Beckstead J. CD99, keratin, and vimentin staining of sex cord-stromal tumors, normal ovary, and testis. Mod Pathol. 1998;11:769–73.
115. Movahedi-Lankarani S, Kurman RJ. Calretinin, a more sensitive but less specific marker than alpha-inhibin for ovarian sex cord-stromal neoplasms: an immunohistochemical study of 215 cases. Am J Surg Pathol. 2002;26:1477–83.
116. Otis CN, Powell JL, Barbuto D, Carcangiu ML. Intermediate filamentous proteins in adult granulosa cell tumors. An immunohistochemical study of 25 cases. Am J Surg Pathol. 1992;16:962–8.
117. Ali S, Gattuso P, Howard A, Mosunjac MB, Siddiqui MT. Adult granulosa cell tumor of the ovary: fine-needle-aspiration cytology of 10 cases and review of literature. Diagn Cytopathol. 2008;36:297–302.
118. Kavuri S, Kulkarni R, Reid-Nicholson M. Granulosa cell tumor of the ovary: cytologic findings. Acta Cytol. 2010;54:551–9.
119. Sunil CS, Prayaga A, Uppin MS, Uppin SG. Juvenile granulosa cell tumour: a pitfall in cytologic diagnosis. Cytopathology. 2015;26(4):261–2.
120. Ajao M, Vachon T, Snyder P. Ovarian dysgerminoma: a case report and literature review. Mil Med. 2013;178:e954–5.
121. Gupta R, Mathur SR, Arora VK, Sharma SG. Cytologic features of extragonadal germ cell tumors: a study of 88 cases with aspiration cytology. Cancer Cytopathol. 2008;144(6):504–11.
122. Miyake Y, Hirokawa M, Kanahara T, Fujiwara K, Koike H, Manabe T. Diagnostic value of hair shafts and squamous cells in peritoneal washing cytology. Acta Cytol. 2000;44(3):357–60.
123. Sevestre H, Ikoli JF, Al Thakfi W. Histopathology and cytology of supposedly benign tumors of the ovary. J Gynecol Obstet Biol Reprod (Paris). 2013;42(8):715–21.
124. Selvaggi SM, Guidos BJ. Immature teratoma of the ovary on fluid cytology. Diagn Cytopathol. 2001;25:411–4.
125. Ikeda K, Tate G, Suzuki T, Mitsuya T. Cytomorphologic features of immature ovarian teratoma in peritoneal effusion: a case report. Diagn Cytopathol. 2005;33:39–42.

126. Collins KA, Geisinger KR, Wakely PE Jr, Olympio G, Silverman JF. Extragonadal germ cell tumours: a fine needle aspiration biopsy study. Diagn Cytopathol. 1995;12:223–9.
127. Kashimura M, Tsukamoto N, Matsuyama T, Kashimura Y, Sugimori H, Taki I. Cytologic findings of ascites from patients with ovarian dysgerminoma. Acta Cytol. 1983;27(1):59–62.
128. Naz S, Hashmi AA, Ali R, et al. Role of peritoneal washing cytology in ovarian malignancies: correlation with histopathological parameters. World J Surg Oncol. 2015;13:315.
129. Cao D, Guo S, Allan RW, Molberg KH, Peng Y. SALL4 is a novel sensitive and specific marker of ovarian primitive germ cell tumors and is particularly useful in distinguishing yolk sac tumor from clear cell carcinoma. Am J Surg Pathol. 2009;33:894–904.
130. Petrakakou E, Grapsa D, Stergiou ME, et al. Ascitic fluid cytology of yolk sac tumor of the ovary: a case report. Acta Cytol. 2008;53(6):701–3.
131. Roncalli M, Gribaudi G, Simoncelli D, Servide E. Cytology of yolk sac tumor of the ovary in ascitic fluid: report of a case. Acta Cytol. 1988;32:113–6.
132. Cho K, Myong N, Jang J. Effusion cytology of endodermal sinus tumor of colon: report of a case. Acta Cytol. 1991;35:207–9.
133. Ng WK, Lui PC, Ma L. Peritoneal washing cytology findings of disseminated myxoid leiomyosarcoma of uterus: report of a case with emphasis on possible differential diagnosis. Diagn Cytopathol. 2002;27:47–52.
134. Lim BJ, Choi SY, Kang DY, Suh KS. Peritoneal washing cytology of disseminated low grade endometrial stromal sarcoma: a case report. Acta Cytol. 2009;53:587–90.
135. Policarpio-Nicolas ML, Cathro HP, Kerr SE, Stelow EB. Cytomorphologic features of low-grade endometrial stromal sarcoma. Am J Clin Pathol. 2007;128:265–71.
136. Kanbour AI, Buchsbaum HJ, Hall A, Kanbour AI. Peritoneal cytology in malignant mixed müllerian tumors of the uterus. Gynecol Oncol. 1989;33(1):91–5.
137. Silverman JF, Gardner J, Larkin EW, Finley JL, Norris HT. Ascitic fluid cytology in a case of metastatic malignant mixed mesodermal tumor of the ovary. Acta Cytol. 1986;30(2):173–6.
138. Kato N, Motoyama T. Ascitic fluid cytology of a malignant mixed Müllerian tumor of the peritoneum: a report of two cases with special reference to p53 status. Diagn Cytopathol. 2009;37(4):281–5.
139. Hallman JR, Geisinger KR. Cytology of fluids from pleural, peritoneal and pericardial cavities in children. A comprehensive survey. Acta Cytol. 1994;38(2):209–17.
140. Wong JW, Pitlik D, Abdul-Karim FW. Cytology of pleural, peritoneal and pericardial fluids in children. A 40-year summary. Acta Cytol. 1997;41(2):467–73.
141. Das DK. Serous effusions in malignant lymphomas: a review. Diagn Cytopathol. 2006;34(5):335–47.
142. Jones D, Weinberg DS, Pinkus GS, Renshaw AA. Cytologic diagnosis of primary serous lymphoma. Am J Clin Pathol. 1996;106(3):359–64.
143. Mettler TN, Holman CJ, McKenna RW, Pambuccian SE. Plasmablastic myeloma in ascitic fluid. Diagn Cytopathol. 2011;40(9):806–9.
144. Cancer facts and figures 2019: leading sites of new cancer cases and deaths-2019 estimates. American Cancer Society, https://www.cancer.org/content/dam/cancer-org/research/cancer-facts-and-statistics/annual-cancer-facts-and-figures/2019/leading-sites-of-new-cancer-cases-and-deaths-2019-estimates.pdf.
145. Sundling K, Cibas E. Ancillary studies in pleural, pericardial, and peritoneal effusion cytology. Cancer Cytoapthol. 2018;126:590–8.
146. Zhao L, Guo M, Sneige N, Gong Y. Value of PAX8 and WT1 immunostaining in confirming the ovarian origin of metastatic carcinoma in serous effusion specimens. Am J Clin Pathol. 2012;137:304–9.
147. Prat J. FIGO Committee on Gynecologic Oncology. FIGO's staging classification for cancer of the ovary, fallopian tube, and peritoneum: abridged republication. Int J Gynecol Cancer. 2015;26(2):487–9.

Cytopreparatory Techniques

10

Donna K. Russell and Deepali Jain

Background

Diagnostic interpretation is not possible without optimal specimen preparation. The standard staining methods used are Papanicolaou stain for alcohol-fixed smears and preparations, modified Giemsa stain for air-dried smears and preparations, and hematoxylin and eosin stain (H&E) for formalin-fixed, paraffin embedded (FFPE) specimens. Ancillary tests can be performed on most cytology preparations. In an international survey on existing non-gynecologic cytology practices [1] (personal communication), most respondents indicated that direct smears (DS), cytocentrifugation (CF), and touch preparations (TP) were the most commonly used preparations in addition to cell blocks (CB), the preferred preparation (54.3%; 303/558) for most ancillary studies. Most respondents (73.84%; 271/367) agreed that both Papanicolaou and modified Giemsa stains should be used as a standard on all serous fluid cytology.

Collection and Storage

Serous effusion cytology is transported to the cytology laboratory immediately after collection. Refrigeration at 4 °C is required if the laboratory is closed or if transportation is delayed. All fluid obtained should be sent to the laboratory for testing. Refrigeration of the specimen is all that is needed and will preserve the specimen for several days [2].

D. K. Russell (✉)
University of Rochester, Rochester, NY, USA
e-mail: donna_russell@urmc.rochester.edu

D. Jain
Department of Pathology, All India Institute of Medical Sciences, New Delhi, India

© Springer Nature Switzerland AG 2020   239
A. Chandra et al. (eds.), *The International System for Serous Fluid Cytopathology*, https://doi.org/10.1007/978-3-030-53908-5_10

If the specimen is being transferred from a distance, a preservative may be added to ensure a quality sample for preparation. CytoLyt® is used for ThinPrep® samples and CytoRich™ is used for SurePath™ samples. Samples received in this manner will not be appropriate for modified Giemsa staining and may interfere with some immunohistochemical stains due to the alcohol fixation.

Gross examination of the fluid is noted upon receipt in the cytopathology laboratory. The method of cytopreparation may be selected on the basis of the physical properties of the specimen and the patient's clinical history. For example, highly viscous specimens may require a smear technique or mucolytic agents, and bloody specimens will benefit from methods that segregate larger epithelial cells from red blood cells. Highly cellular specimens are ideal for smeared preparations, whereas sparsely cellular specimens will require multiple centrifugation steps and special cell concentration methods.

Preparation Methods

Sample preparation for immunochemical (IC) studies (which include immunohisto-chemistry and immunocytochemistry), microbiology evaluation, and histochemical special stains can be prepared at the same time as the cytologic specimen preparation. A variety of options are available for serous fluid preparation.

Physical features such as volume of sample, color, clarity, opalescence, and viscosity should be documented in the cytopathology report [3]. If the cell sample is low in volume, clear in appearance, and contains only a few cells, the method of preparation should include cytocentrifugation or a liquid-based preparation method. Cell block preparation methods may include agar/gelatin, plasma-thrombin, collodion bag, Cellient®, or Thermo Scientific™ Shandon™ Cytoblock™ cell block. These methods work well with hypocellular samples.

If the sample is cloudy and has a cell pellet after centrifugation, preparation methods may include direct smears and/or liquid-based preparations. Cell block methods that work well with pellets include the traditional sediment, plasma-thrombin, gelatin, collodion bag or Cytoblock™ cell block. If the cell sample is bloody, direct smears and liquid based preparations are appropriate once the sample has been centrifuged with a lysing fixative. A common lysing agent used is glacial acetic acid and commercial products are available. Additional washings with a lysing fixative may be required in extremely bloody samples [4].

Samples received in the cytopathology laboratory should be processed according to the laboratory operating procedure manual. A protocol for serous effusions should be included in the laboratory procedure manual. There are a variety of preparation types that are available for preparation of serous fluid cytology. These include direct smears and cytocentrifugation spins, either Papanicolaou and/or modified Giemsa stained or ThinPrep® and SurePath™. Cell block preparations can be made from serous effusions. These are embedded in formalin, sectioned in histopathology and stained with hematoxylin and eosin (H&E).

Cell blocks can be stained with histochemical stains [e.g., mucicarmine, Kreyberg, Grocott methenamine silver (GMS), acid fast bacillus (AFB), periodic acid-Schiff (PAS)] and immunochemical stains to determine metastatic sites.

Direct Smear Preparations

Centrifugation of the serous effusion sample is performed after gross description and electronic accessioning is performed. The specimen is given a unique specimen number. Each specimen is unique and prepared differently depending upon the quantity of fluid received. Samples are poured into conical tubes and capped. Up to two 50 mL conical tubes are spun for each sample in the centrifuge. Exact amounts are poured to balance the centrifuge.

Conical tubes are placed in the centrifuge and spun for 2500 rpm for 5 minutes. Tubes are removed from the centrifuge and the supernatant is decanted. Two slides are labeled with the patient's last name, accession number and type of fluid. A pipette is used to take sediment remaining in the conical tube. A few drops are placed on a labeled slide and the second slide is used to smear the preparation. One slide is placed immediately in 95% ethanol fixative for Papanicolaou staining, while the other is air dried for modified Giemsa staining (Figs. 10.1 and 10.2).

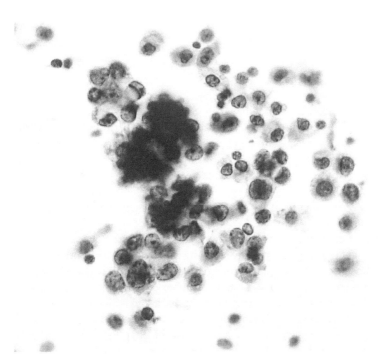

Fig. 10.1 Metastatic ovarian adenocarcinoma. (Peritoneal fluid, DS, Papanicolaou stain, high magnification)

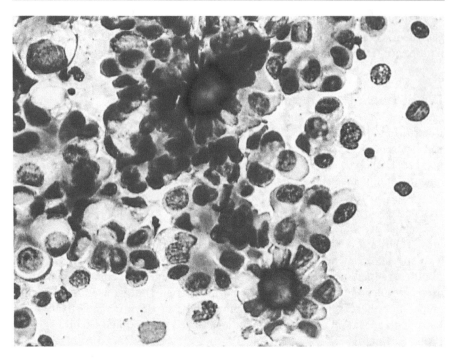

Fig. 10.2 Metastatic ovarian adenocarcinoma, (Peritoneal fluid, DS, Modified Giemsa stain, high magnification)

Cytocentrifugation

Thermo Scientific™ Cytospin™ Cytocentrifuge

(Thermo Fisher Scientific, Waltham, MA, USA)

Centrifugation (CF) of the serous effusion sample is performed after gross description and electronic accessioning is performed. Up to two 50 mL conical tubes are spun for each sample in the centrifuge. Samples are poured into conical tubes and capped. Exact amounts are poured to balance the centrifuge. Conical tubes are placed in the centrifuge and spun for 2500 rpm for 5 minutes. Tubes are removed from the centrifuge and the supernatant is decanted. A pipette is used to re-suspend the sediment.

Cytocentrifugation with the cytospin allows for the cells to be placed onto a vertical slide, while the fluid suspension is absorbed by the surrounding absorbent paper. The cytospin slide clips are used placing a slide (label at the top) in the clip with an absorbent paper on top and the plastic funnel chamber on top of both. The cytospin clip is closed by swinging the wire toward the clip back and hooking it closed. The circle of the funnel and the slide must match up exactly. Slide clips are placed exactly opposite one another for balancing, and specimen is added to the chamber. Five to eight drops are placed in the chamber for clear fluid and one to two drops for cloudy fluids. The sample chambers are capped and the cytocentrifuge unit covered (Fig. 10.3). Specimens are spin at 800 rpm for 5 minutes on low acceleration.

The program will begin when "start" is selected and the unit will chime when complete. Once complete, the top of cytocentrifuge is removed, the slide clip unit opened, and the paper and slide are removed. One slide is placed in 95% alcohol and the other slide set aside to air-dry. The air-dried slide is stained with modified Giemsa stain and the wet fixed (95% alcohol) slide with Papanicolaou stain (Figs. 10.4 and 10.5). (For exact details, refer to manufacturer's procedure manual.) [5]

Fig. 10.3 Thermo-Scientific CytoSpin® Processor. CytoSpin® ThermoScientific instrument

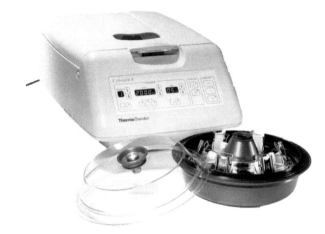

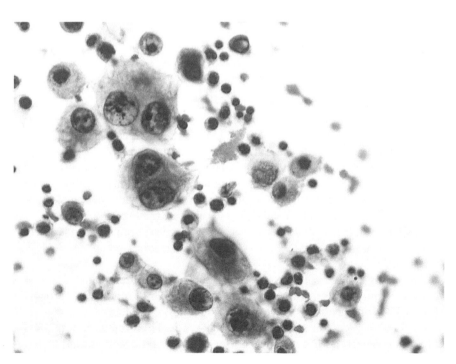

Fig. 10.4 Metastatic adenocarcinoma, CytoSpin®. (Peritoneal fluid, CS, Papanicolaou stain, high magnification)

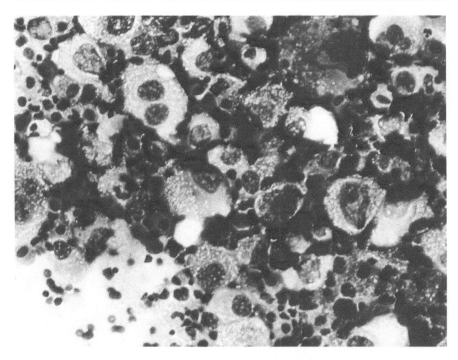

Fig. 10.5 Metastatic adenocarcinoma, CytoSpin®. (Peritoneal fluid, CS, Modified Giemsa stain, high magnification)

ThinPrep

ThinPrep® Liquid Based Preparation
   (Hologic, Inc., Marlborough, MA, USA)
   Centrifugation of the serous effusion sample is performed after gross description and electronic accessioning is performed. Up to two 50 mL conical tubes are spun for each sample in the centrifuge. Samples are poured into conical tubes and capped. Exact amounts are poured to balance the centrifuge. Conical tubes are placed in the centrifuge and spun for 2500 rpm for 5 minutes. If the specimen is bloody, 30 mL of CytoLyt™ solution can be added after initial spinning, and the sample can be rerun at 2500 rpms for 5 additional minutes. Tubes are removed from the centrifuge and the supernatant is decanted. A pipette is used to re-suspend the sediment. Three to five drops are added to the PreservCyt™ manufacturer's non-gynecologic vial (Fig. 10.6).
   The vial is labeled with the specimen number and patient name. The cap is removed from the vial and it is placed on the ThinPrep® 2000 processor (Fig. 10.7) for specimen processing, producing a liquid based preparation ready for Papanicolaou staining (Fig. 10.8). The ThinPrep® 5000 processor (Fig. 10.9) received FDA approval for non-gynecologic samples and delivers a fully automated slide preparation option for non-gynecologic serous fluid

Fig. 10.6 ThinPrep®
Process. ThinPrep
non-gynecologic
preparation

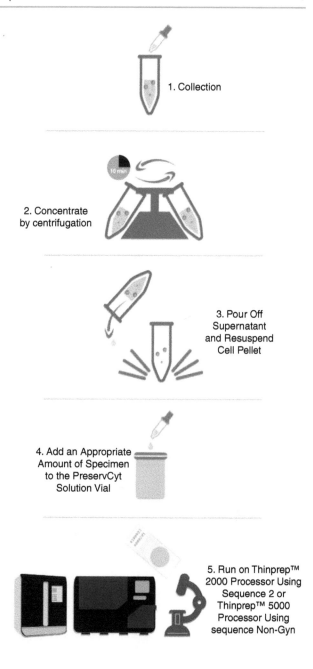

1. Collection

2. Concentrate
by centrifugation

3. Pour Off
Supernatant
and Resuspend
Cell Pellet

4. Add an Appropriate
Amount of Specimen
to the PreservCyt
Solution Vial

5. Run on Thinprep™
2000 Processor Using
Sequence 2 or
Thinprep™ 5000
Processor Using
sequence Non-Gyn

samples. It is a continuous hands-free processor and prepares up to 20 samples per batch, which allows 45 minutes of free walk-away time for the cytopreparatory technologist. (For exact details, refer to manufacturer's procedure manual.) [6, 7]

Fig. 10.7 Hologic
ThinPrep® Processor.
ThinPrep® 2000 processor

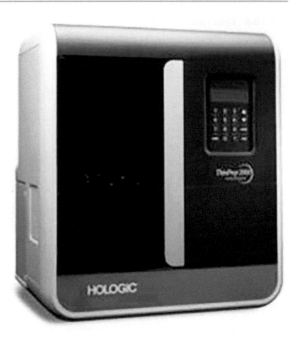

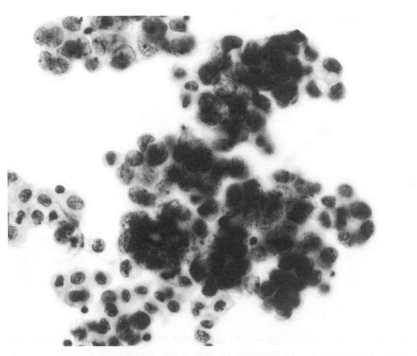

Fig. 10.8 Metastatic ovarian adenocarcinoma, ThinPrep®. (Peritoneal fluid, ThinPrep®, Papanicolaou stain, high magnification)

Fig. 10.9 Hologic
ThinPrep® Processor.
ThinPrep® 5000 processor

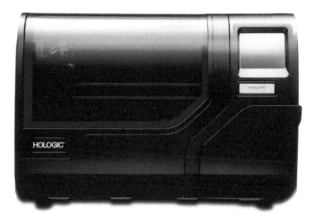

SlidePrep

BD Totalys™ Multiprocessor and BD Totalys™ SlidePrep
   (Becton Dickinson and Company, Sparks, MD, USA)
   BD Totalys™ SlidePrep prepares and stains non-gynecologic samples. It is a fully automated slide preparation and staining system when used with the BD Totalys™ Multiprocessor (Fig. 10.10). The multiprocessor is an automated sample transfer, centrifugation, aspiration, and decanting system for cytology. It minimizes the hands-on time for preparation. The laboratory integration system (LIS) provides sample identification to prepare for diagnostic systems. It features an optional aliquot system that transfers specimen to secondary vials for ancillary testing. The tubes are loaded onto the BD Totalys™ SlidePrep (Fig. 10.11).

   The system provides a full chain of custody by automatically scanning each slide and matching it to the associated specimen. The system has flexibility; it allows for both liquid based Pap tests and non-gynecologic samples on the same system. A graphical interface with touch screen takes users through each step and offers random loading to reduce manual steps. It offers consistent results and stains individual chambers using fresh reagents for each specimen and reduces the risk of contamination while ensuring sample match and chain of custody through automatic slide barcode scanning (Fig. 10.12). A single run of 48 slides can be processed in 68 minutes and is completely automated. It reduces cytopreparatory staff time to allow performance of additional tasks in the laboratory. A Papanicolaou-stained liquid based slide is produced (Fig. 10.13). (For exact details, refer to manufacturer's procedure manual.) [8, 9]

Techniques for Molecular Testing

Molecular pathology has experienced vast changes due to the development of new prognostic and predictive biomarkers for targeted therapies. Cytology specimens have proven to be excellent sources for molecular testing, yielding maximum information

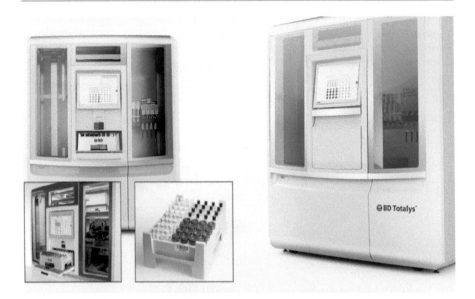

Fig. 10.10 BD BD Totalys® Sample Prep Instrument. Totalys® sample Multiprocessor

Fig. 10.11 BD Totalys®
SlidePrep Instrument.
Totalys® multiple slide
preparation processor

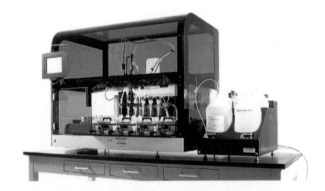

with minimally invasive techniques [10]. Cytopathology professionals have the opportunity to play a critical role in personalized medicine. Rapid on-site assessment (ROSE) of minimally invasive fine needle aspiration (FNA) specimens provides diagnoses and appropriate triage of tissue for ancillary studies. According to the College of American Pathologists (CAP) 2015 non-gynecologic survey, more than half of the laboratories that participated in the survey performed ROSE of touch imprints of needle core biopsies (NCB) to ensure high quality collection of tissue samples [11].

Fresh specimens from FNAs and serous effusion cytology are ideal for molecular analysis. Cytology samples at some institutions are fully integrated into the molecular testing pipeline and are considered equivalent or superior to small biopsies for molecular testing [12, 13]. Mutational testing has been reported to be successful in

Fig. 10.12 BD Totalys®
Preparation. Non-
gynecologic
preparation scheme

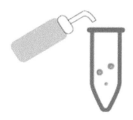

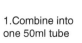
1.Combine into
one 50ml tube

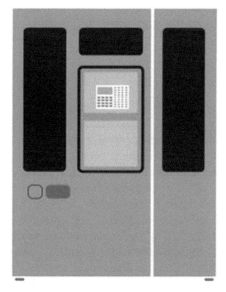

2. Automated sample transfer,
centrifugation, aspiration and
decanting for cytology preparation.

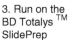
3. Run on the
BD Totalys ^{TM}
SlidePrep

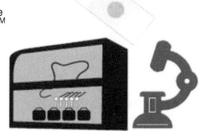

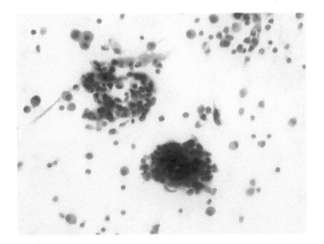

Fig. 10.13 Metastatic small cell carcinoma. (Peritoneal fluid, SurePath®, Papanicolaou stain, high magnification)

most cytologic samples, even from cases referred from different countries with considerable variation in the acquisition, preparation, and processing of tumor samples due to different routine clinical procedures.

FNA or NCB can be used for molecular studies. The evaluation of prognostic and predictive biomarkers for the selection of patients for targeted therapy has made it necessary to ensure standardization so that molecular markers can be accessed accurately in the limited biologic specimens (cytology samples and NCB) usually obtained by minimally invasive procedures [14]. The versatility of cytology sample preparation and fixation offers some advantages over NCB and surgical biopsy specimens. Cytology specimens are fixed immediately and processed right after collection has occurred. This leads to well preserved nucleic acids. High-quality DNA can be harvested from fresh cells in cell suspension; but good quality DNA is also possible from formalin-fixed cell blocks, archival stained smears, unstained cytospin preparations, liquid-based samples, Flinders Technology Associate (FTA) cards, and cryopreserved cells.

The majority of ancillary tests have been validated on formalin-fixed tissue blocks and biomarker/clinical trials have been structured using formalin-fixed blocks. As a result, formalin-fixed cell blocks have been used and recommended for the vast majority of current molecular assays. Other cytology specimens are equally acceptable, but usually require additional validation processes prior to implementation, primarily due to differences in cell fixation.

Cell Block Preparations

Cell blocks (CB) have many advantages and play a pivotal role in cytology. Currently, the utility of CBs is recognized due to their role in ancillary testing, particularly in molecular diagnostics [15–19]. ROSE has improved the diagnostic cellular yield in CB samples. Additional dedicated passes for CB can be obtained during the procedure for improved cell block quality.

Fig. 10.14 Metastatic adenocarcinoma, (Peritoneal fluid, CB, H&E stain, high magnification)

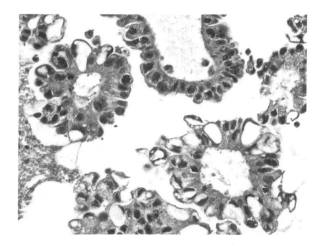

CBs can be made from aggregation of exfoliated cells from serous cavity fluids. Although the diagnostic sensitivity between DS/CF and CB is statistically insignificant, CBs increase diagnostic yield due to the provision of ancillary studies such as immunochemistry (IC) and molecular testing (MT). Cells are re-suspended in fluids by agitation immediately prior to processing the fluid to ensure homogeneous distribution of the cell types throughout the specimen. The architecture present in CB is similar to that seen in surgical pathology specimens (Fig. 10.14). Cell blocks can produce multiple sections for performing ancillary testing. Histochemical stains, IC, and MT can all be performed on CB material.

CB preparation methods vary among laboratories internationally. There is no consistent standardized collection media for CB. Formalin, saline, Roswell Park Memorial Institute (RPMI), and alcohol are common media used by laboratories for CB preparation. Saline solution provides flexibility to submit for microbial or fungal culture, flow cytometry, and liquid-based cytology, but cell integrity can be compromised if left in this media for long periods of time. Saline is isotonic but not necessarily physiologic. Formalin is used for collection of CBs by many laboratories and is validated for IC and MT. RPMI is the medium of choice for lymphoproliferative disorders. It is a cell culture medium that enhances cell growth and can be used in a flow cytometer. RPMI also can be used for CB collection, with the advantage that it contains no fixative and therefore does not require an additional validation step for ancillary studies that have been validated for formalin. Alcohol media is comparable, if not superior, for molecular testing [15]. Not all alcohol is equal: weaker IC staining with some antibodies [e.g., thyroid transcription factor-1 and p63] has been reported in cell blocks prepared with Cellient® cell block preparation method [20] due to the manufacturer's methanol fixation.

Centrifugation Sediment

Serous effusion samples are shaken to distribute cells and then poured into two 50 mL conical centrifuge tubes labeled with patient identification. The tubes are placed in the centrifuge and spun at 2400 rpm for 5 minutes to achieve a concentrated cell pellet. The supernatant is poured off. If the cell pellet is not cohesive, formalin can be added, and the sample is spun at 2400 rpm for an additional 5 minutes. The tube can sit for an additional 30–60 minutes to harden. The hardened button is removed with a metal spatula by loosening the edges so it breaks free of the tube. The cell pellet is placed on histology tissue paper moistened with neutral buffered formalin. Tissue paper is folded around the cell pellet and placed in a histology cassette labeled with patient identification (Fig. 10.15). Once all steps are

Fig. 10.15 Centrifugation sediment cell block technique

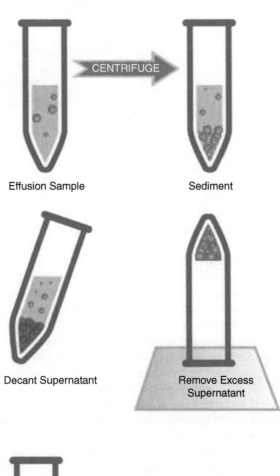

Effusion Sample   Sediment

Decant Supernatant   Remove Excess
                                         Supernatant

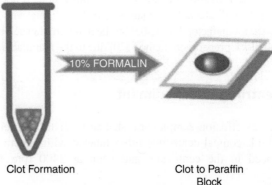

Clot Formation   Clot to Paraffin
                                         Block

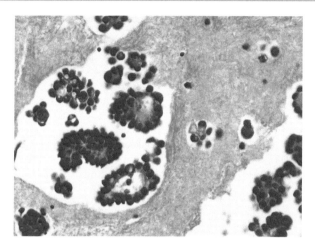

Fig. 10.16 Metastatic ovarian adenocarcinoma. (Peritoneal fluid, CB, H&E stain, high magnification)

complete, the tissue cassette is placed in a formalin filled cup for additional time in formalin. The time is noted on the requisition. Time in formalin should be at least 6 hours fixation for specific ancillary testing immunohistochemical protocols [21, 22]. A quality control sheet is signed by two laboratory technologists documenting correct patient identification and accession number, as well as any additional instructions, such as IC protocol. The specimen is then processed routinely in the histopathology laboratory and stained with H&E stain (Fig. 10.16). If the cell pellet is extremely small after spinning the sample, HistoGel™/agar, collodion, or Cellient® automated cell block preparation methods should be considered.

Plasma Thrombin (PT) or Thrombin Clot Method

While exudative effusions usually contain sufficient fibrin to produce an adhesive clot, in transudate effusions, pellet formation is enhanced by the addition of adjuvants. Plasma and thrombin are the most commonly used adjuvants added to centrifuged cell pellets to produce a firm clot. In principle, the fibrin clot traps all cells in the suspension, but single, smaller cells may be less adherent.

Following agitation of the fluid for resuspension, 10–20 mL of the total sample is centrifuged. The supernatant is poured off. A few drops of plasma are added to the cell pellet, followed by thrombin. Mixing allows a cell clot to form, which is subsequently placed in formalin for processing as a tissue biopsy (Fig. 10.17).

This is a simple and low-cost method and is performed at room temperature. One limitation of this method is uneven concentration of cells within the clot. Continuous agitation during the clot formation will enhance even dispersion of cells in the fibrin meshwork of clot. Another limitation is that use of expired patient plasma and commercially available thrombin introduces potential for contamination by extraneous cell-free DNA. With the availability of high-sensitivity molecular testing platforms such as next-generation sequencing (NGS), contamination by even a tiny amount of

Fig. 10.17 Plasma thrombin cell block technique

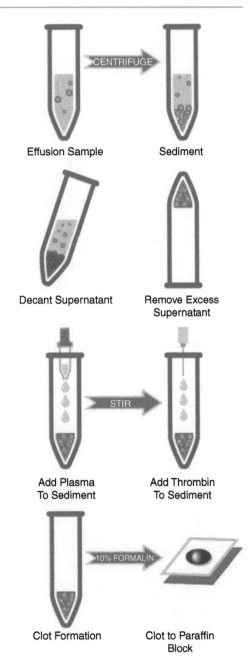

Effusion Sample   Sediment

Decant Supernatant   Remove Excess
                         Supernatant

Add Plasma   Add Thrombin
To Sediment   To Sediment

Clot Formation   Clot to Paraffin
                         Block

foreign DNA will affect results of molecular testing. CBs made from the plasma-thrombin (PT) method offer good morphology and better cellularity than simple sedimentation, HistoGel™ or albumin-based methods, and are compatible with immunochemistry and most molecular testing.

HistoGel™ Method

Richard-Allan Scientific™ HistoGel™ Specimen Processing Gel
   (Thermo Fisher Scientific, Waltham, MA, USA)
   In comparison to the PT method, HistoGel™ (HG) method is a more labor inten-sive procedure that involves heating and maintaining the liquid form of HG. HG is a modified agar added to the cell pellet to cause amalgamation. It is useful in situa-tions where no visible sediment is seen after initial centrifugation, since the gel permeates the cells and traps them in a solid matrix.
   After centrifuging the cell suspension, supernatant is poured off, and liquefied HistoGel™ is added to the pellet. Subsequently, the pellet is congealed on ice to solidify the HG-cellular complex (Fig. 10.18). Limitations include low cellularity, poor visualization of cellular material within the block, and technical processing challenges. For example, the HG solution must be maintained at a temperature above its gelling temperature. Modifications have been described for HG methods to optimize HG volumes and melting conditions. Although these modifications have been performed on aspirate samples, they can also be applied to serous effusion samples to improve cell capture. For immunochemistry and molecular testing, HG provides good cellular and architectural preservation.

Agar Method

Agar solidifies below 50° Celsius; this property of agar is used to form a solid cell pellet. It is more cost-effective when compared to automated methods. The process-ing steps mirror that of HG; agar also requires appropriate heat treatment protocols to ensure proper liquefaction of the agar during cell resuspension. On the other hand, excess heat will lead to heat-induced artifacts that alter cellular morphology. Similar to HG, agar CBs are optimum for immunochemistry and molecular testing (Fig.10.18).

Collodion Bag Method

Collodion is a commercially available liquid polymer that has a syrupy consistency. It is a nitrocellulose solution that is used to coat conical specimen tubes before cen-trifugation in order to capture the cell pellet. A conical centrifugation tube is filled

Fig. 10.18 HistoGel or
agar cell block technique

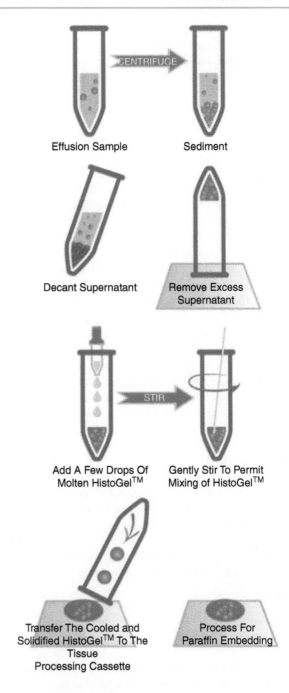

with the collodion solution and then poured out, leaving a thin layer of solution coating the test tube wall. This forms a membrane bag inside the tube once it is dried. Serous fluid is poured into the collodion-lined tube and centrifuged to form a cell pellet. The membrane bag containing the cell pellet is gently removed from the tube. The pellet end is tied off from the liquid end and excess bag and liquid cut off, leaving a pellet in a collodion bag that is embedded as a tissue biopsy (Fig. 10.19).

Collodion bag method is useful for specimens when low cellularity is anticipated. It is superior for cellular yield when compared to HG and PT methods [23, 24]. Limitations include the need for ether-based flammable solvents and their storage requirements. Preparation of collodion bags must be done under a laminar hood to protect employees from flammable and toxic fumes. Preparation of the bags is time-consuming and removal from the test tube requires technical skill. Tubes can be prepared in advance and kept in a refrigerator for up to 1 month.

Clot Technique

A cell block can be obtained by expressing the contents of an aspirated specimen, or from a centrifuged fluid specimen, directly onto a glass slide or precut tissue paper. The specimen aspirated with a FNA needle is deposited in a tight circular motion on the glass slide or paper to build up a cone-shaped coagulum of tissue and blood mixture. This allows for the specimen to dry or clot (Fig. 10.20). The material can then be scraped off the slide with a thin needle or expelled with a syringe of formalin into the formalin container labeled with the patient's identification (Fig. 10.21). A similar process can be used for fluids by aspirating centrifuged specimen from a tube following decantation. The sample is placed in a conical tube and centrifuged at 2400 rpm for 5 minutes. The tube is removed from the centrifuge and the supernatant is decanted. The pellet is then removed and placed in a tissue cassette. The specimen can be processed routinely in the histology laboratory and stained with hematoxylin and eosin stain and adjunct IC stains (Fig. 10.22).

Shandon Cytoblock™ Cell Block

Thermo Scientific™ Cytoblock™ Cell Block Preparation System
  (Thermo Fisher Scientific, Waltham, MA, USA)
This system is designed to facilitate the preparation of paraffin-embedded cell suspensions, cell aggregates, and tissue fragments [25]. The Cytoblock™ system simplifies the preparation of paraffin blocks from a kit and can be used to process cell blocks from FNA, NCB, serous fluids, and residual sediment from other cytologic samples. The Cytoblock™ kit (Fig. 10.23) consists of 50 Cytoblock™ cassettes with backing papers and board inserts, reagent 1 (clear) and reagent 2 (colored). Patient information is recorded on Cytoblock™. The specimen should be fixed prior to beginning Cytoblock™ preparation in the cytospin (Fig. 10.24). The fixed cells are concentrated by centrifugation and excess fluid is decanted. If the total amount of specimen is two drops or less, add four drops of reagent 1. A pipette

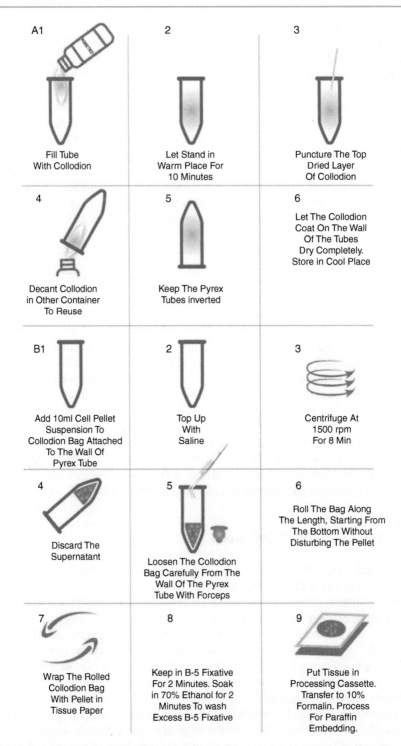

Fig. 10.19 Collodion bag cell block technique

Fig. 10.20 Clot cell block technique. Gross image of equipment and clot sample

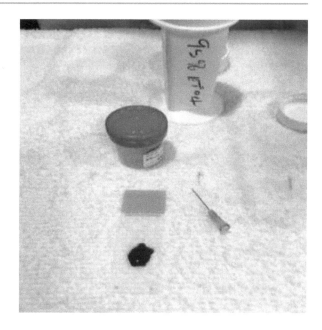

is used to vortex the sample. The Cytoblock™ cassette is then assembled in the Shandon Cytoclip™. Three drops of reagent 1 is placed in the center of the well. A cytofunnel disposable chamber is placed over the prepared Cytoblock™, and the metal clip is attached.

The assembled Cytoclip™ is placed into the Cytospin™ sealed head. The mixed cell suspension is placed in each Cytofunnel™. The Cytospin™ is set at 1500 rpm for 5 minutes. When the Cytospin™ stops, the funnel assembly is removed, and then the clip and funnel removed. The cell button should be in the well and not adherent to the funnel. One drop of reagent 1 is placed in the well on top of the cell button. The cassette is closed and placed in fixative for processing. Fixative should be unbuffered formalin. Cassettes are processed in a standard tissue processor. At embedding, the cassette is opened, the paper folded back, and the board insert is removed from the cassette. The cell button should easily dislodge and be placed back in the cassette. The cassette is closed and placed with the flat side up for addition of paraffin. The Cytoblock™ should be handed similar to any paraffin block. One must use caution when facing the block and sectioning: these are thin specimens and the block can be rapidly exhausted.

Cellient® Cell Block

Cellient® Automated Cell Block System
(Hologic, Inc. Medical Technology Company, Marlborough, MA, USA)

Fig. 10.21 Clot cell block technique

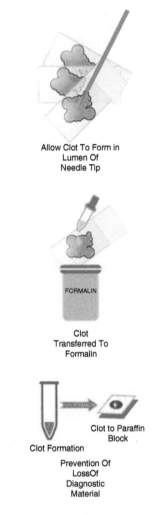

Allow Clot To Form in
Lumen Of
Needle Tip

Clot
Transferred To
Formalin

Clot Formation

Clot to Paraffin
Block

Prevention Of
LossOf
Diagnostic
Material

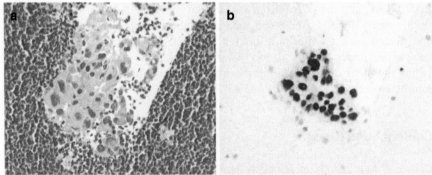

Fig. 10.22 Metastatic lung adenocarcinoma. (**a**) Microscopic image standard stain (Pleural fluid, CB, H&E stain, high magnification); (**b**) Microscopic image immunostain (Pleural fluid, CB, Thyroid transcription factor-1 (TTF-1) nuclear positivity, high magnification)

Fig. 10.23 Thermo-Scientific Cytoblock® cell block preparation system

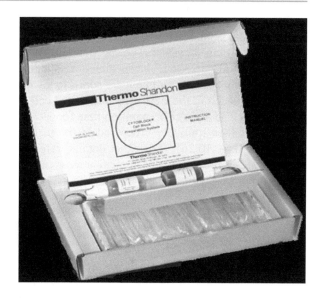

Fig. 10.24 Cytospin Instrument for Cytoblock® cell block preparation, ThermoScientific

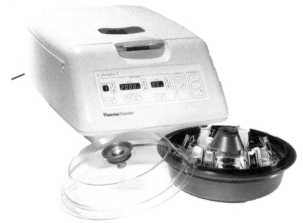

Fig. 10.25 Cellient® Instrument. Automated cell block system instrumentation

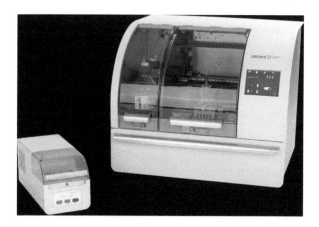

This technique is commonly used when the specimen consists of small tissue fragments and is made directly from a liquid based preparation vial. It is a fully automated cell block system. The specimen is centrifuged in a 60 mL tube for 5 minutes at 2400 rmp. Once the specimen is spun, the supernatant is poured off. Only three drops of cell sediment are added to the PreservCyt™ vial to be fixed. The vial is placed in the Cellient® automated cell block system for processing (Fig. 10.25). The average preparation time for each cell block is 45 minutes. The specimen is then routinely processed in the histology laboratory and stained with H&E (Fig. 10.26). (For exact details, refer to manufacturer's procedure manual.) [26] Immunohistochemical stains can be performed (Fig. 10.27).

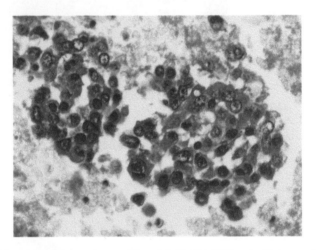

Fig. 10.26 Metastatic breast carcinoma. (Pleural fluid, CB, H&E stain, high magnification)

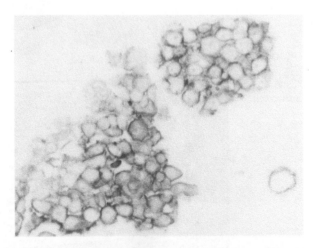

Fig. 10.27 Metastatic breast carcinoma, HER2. Positive HER2 immunostain in a case of breast carcinoma showing strong membranous reactivity. (Pleural fluid, CB, HER2 immunostain, high magnification)

Table 10.1 Cell block techniques: advantages and disadvantages

Cell block technique	Clot and scrape	Cell block pellet alcohol fixation	Cell block pellet formalin fixation	Plasma thrombin method	Collodion method	Cellient™ automated system	HistoGel™ or agar method	Thermo Shandon™ Cytoblock™
Advantages	Inexpensive, no additional equipment required	Inexpensive, easy and rapid method, good for FNAs of any type and fluids	Inexpensive, easy and rapid method, good for FNAs of any type and fluids	Simple, low cost, clean background for ancillary studies, suitable for FNAs of any type and fluids	Good cellular yield, great for specimens with scant cellularity	Great for small/scanty samples, crisp architecture, fully automated processing, consistent results, no cross contamination	Concentration of cells in HistoGel™ or agar for an adequate sample, good cellular preservation	Good cellular yield due to cell suspensions, good for small/scanty samples, eliminates the need for tissue wrapping and loss of scanty samples
Disadvantages	Does not work well with small samples, crush artifact is common, variable cellularity	Cellular yield variable, limited data on IC due to alcohol fixation	Cellular yield variable, optimal results for IC and molecular studies	Cross contamination from plasma and thrombin, uneven concentration of cells	Time consuming method of preparation, toxic ether fumes for storage	Time consuming method of preparation – 45 minutes for each cell block preparation, expensive, training of histology for cutting thin blocks, limited data on IC due to alcohol fixation	Tedious process as HistoGel™ or agar has to be converted to liquid state	Time consuming method of preparation, cost of kit for preparation of cell blocks

Validation of immunochemistry using this technique must be performed in the laboratory because it involves alcohol fixation prior to formalin fixation [27].

Processing of cell blocks is not standardized across laboratories. Cell block preparations are prepared from a variety of different fixations and processing techniques and make valid comparison difficult. However, they are a valuable adjunct to the case due to their versatility for ancillary testing. Advantages and disadvantages for the various cell block preparation are discussed in detail in Table 10.1, and excellent references are available that provide further details [28, 29].

References

1. Kurtycz DFI, Crothers BA, Schmitt F, Chandra A. International system for reporting serous fluid cytopathology: initial project survey. Acta Cytol. 2019;63(Suppl1):13. https://doi.org/10.1159/000500433.
2. Bibbo M, Draganova-Tacheva R, Naylor B. Pleural, peritoneal and pericardial effusions. In: Bibbo M, Wilbur DC, editors. Comprehensive Cytopathology. 4th ed. Philadelphia: Elsevier Saunders; 2015. p. 404.
3. Shidham VB, Epple J. Collection and processing of effusion fluids for cytopathologic evaluation. In: Cytopathologic diagnosis of serous fluids. Philadelphia: Elsevier; 2007. p. 207–35.
4. Weidmann JE, Keebler CM, Facik MS. Cytopreparatory techniques. In: Bibbo M, Wilbur DC, editors. Comprehensive Cytopathology. 4th ed. Philadelphia: Elsevier Saunders; 2015. p. 851–2.
5. Thermo Scientific™. Cytospin® preparation system: instructions for use, 2015. www.thermoscientic.com/pathology.
6. Hologic, Inc. ThinPrep® 2000 processor: instructions for use, 2017. https://www.hologic.com/sites/default/files/package-insert/MAN-02624-001_005_002.pdf.
7. Hologic, Inc. ThinPrep® 5000 processor: operator's manual, 2017. https://www.hologic.com/sites/default/files/package-insert/MAN-02624-001_005_002.pdf.
8. Becton Dickinson and Company (BD). BD Totalys™ Multiprocessor, 2016. https://www.bd.com/en-us/offerings/capabilities/cervical-cancer-screening/cytology-instruments/totalys-system/totalys-multiprocessor.
9. Becton Dickinson and Company (BD). BD Totalys™ SlidePrep, 2016. https://www.bd.com/en-us/offerings/capabilities/cervical-cancer-screening/cytology-instruments/totalys-system/totalys-slideprep.
10. Aissner DL, Sams SB. The role of cytology specimens in molecular testing of solid tumors: techniques, limitations and opportunities. Diagn Cytopathol. 2012;40(6):511–24.
11. Padmanabhan V, Barkan G, Tabatabai L, Souers R, Nayar R, Crothers BA. Touch imprint (TI) cytology of needle core biopsies (NCB) in pathology laboratories: a practice survey of participants in the College of American Pathologists (CAP) Non Gynecologic Cytopathology (NGC) Education Program. Diagn Cytopathol. 2019;47(3):149–55.
12. Rekhtman N, Roy-Chowdhuri S. Cytology specimens: a goldmine for molecular testing. Arch Pathol Lab Med. 2016;140(11):1189–90.
13. Shi Y, Aus JS, Thongprasert S, et al. A prospective, molecular epidemiology study of EGFR mutations in Asian patients with advanced non-small cell lung cancer of adenocarcinoma histology (PIONEER). J Thorac Oncol. 2014;9(2):154–62.
14. da Cunha Santos G. Standardizing preanalytical variables for molecular cytopathology. Cancer Cytopathol. 2013;121(7):341–3.
15. Troncone G, Roy-Chowdhuri S. Key issues in molecular cytopathology. Arch Pathol Lab Med. 2018;142(3):289–90.
16. da Cunha Santos G, Saieg MA. Preanalytical specimen triage: smears, cell blocks, cytospin preparations, transplant media and cytobanking. Cancer Cytopathol. 2017;125(S6):455–64.

17. Michael CW, Davidson B. Pre-analytical issues in effusion cytology. Pleura Peritoneum. 2016;1(1):45–56.
18. Salim AA, Luthra R, Singh R, et al. Pre-analytical factors involved in the clinical analysis of a comprehensive next-generation sequencing panel. Lab Investig. 2016;96(1):504A.
19. da Cunha Santos G, Saieg MA, Troncone G, Zeppa P. Cytological preparations for molecular analysis: a review of technical procedures, advantages and limitations for referring samples for testing. Cytopathology. 2018;29(2):125–32.
20. Montgomery E, Gao C, DeLuca J, Bower J, Attwood K, Ylagan L. Validation of 31 of the most commonly used immunohistochemical antibodies in cytology prepared using the Cellient® automated cell block system. Diagn Cytopathol. 2014;42(12):1024–33.
21. Hammond ME, Hayes DF, Dowsett M, et al. American Society of Clinical Oncology/College of American Pathologists guideline recommendations for immunohistochemical testing of estrogen and progesterone receptors in breast cancer. Arch Pathol Lab Med. 2010;134(6):907–22.
22. Wolff AC, Hammond ME, Hicks DG, et al. Recommendations for human epidermal growth factor receptor 2 testing in breast cancer: American Society of Clinical Oncology/College of American Pathologists clinical practice guideline update. Arch Pathol Lab Med. 2014;138(2):241–56.
23. Balassanian R, Wool GD, Ono JC, et al. A superior method for cell block preparation for fine-needle aspiration biopsies. Cancer Cytopathol. 2016;124(7):508–18.
24. Wilgenbusch H, et al. It is all in the bag: collodion bag versus HistoGel cell block method. J Am Soc Cytopathol. 2020;9:20–25.
25. Thermo Scientific. 2015. Thermo Scientific Shandon Cytoblock Cell Block Preparation System Instructions for Use. https://tools.thermofisher.com/content/sfs/manuals/231803%20Cytoblok%20IFU.pdf/.
26. Hologic, Inc. 2015. Cellient® Automated Cell Block System: Operator's Manual. https://www.hologic.com/sites/default/files/package-insert/MAN-02078-001_003_02.pdf.
27. Fitzgibbons PL, Bradley LA, Fatheree LA, et al. Principles of analytic validation of immunohistochemical assays: guideline from the College of American Pathologists Pathology and Laboratory Quality Center. Arch Pathol Lab Med. 2014;138(11):1432–43.
28. Nambirajan A, Jain D. Cell blocks in cytopathology: an update. Cytopathology. 2018;29(6):505–24.
29. Jain D, Mathur SR, Iyer VK. Cell blocks in cytopathology: a review of preparative methods, utility in diagnosis and role in ancillary studies. Cytopathology. 2014;25(6):356–71.

Quality Management

11

Barbara Centeno, Paul Cross, Marilin Rosa,
and Rosario Granados

Introduction

The quality management (QM) of serous fluid cytopathology shares requirements with other clinical laboratory specimens. However, with the exception of gynecologic cytology, there is scant statistical data supporting specific practices for quality management for cytopathology specimens [1–6]. Guidelines for reporting non-gynecologic cytopathology specimens, to include effusion cytology, have been published. These meet the criteria of the College of American Pathologists' Laboratory Accreditation Program (CAP LAP) checklists [1]. The Code of Practice on exfoliative, non-gynecologic cytopathology produced by the British Society for Clinical Cytology [4] and the Royal College of Pathologists' Tissue Pathways for exfoliative cytology and fine needle aspiration cytology [7] also address standard practices on specimen procurement, preparation, and staining for the international community. The QM practices in this section represent expert recommendations that focus on identifying and preventing errors based on common practices and literature review, and suggests monitoring for practice improvement. The authors support standardization of QM activities to permitcomparison and statistical compilation across practices that will provide data for future recommendations [8].

B. Centeno (✉) · M. Rosa
Department of Pathology, H. Lee Moffitt Cancer Center and Research Institute,
Tampa, FL, USA
e-mail: Barbara.Centeno@moffitt.org

P. Cross
Department of Pathology, Queen Elizabeth Hospital, Gateshead, Tyne and Wear, UK

R. Granados
Pathology Department, Hospital Universitario Getafe, Madrid, Spain

© Springer Nature Switzerland AG 2020
A. Chandra et al. (eds.), *The International System for Serous Fluid Cytopathology*, https://doi.org/10.1007/978-3-030-53908-5_11

267

Background

Quality management includes all of the activities that contribute to quality outcomes. Quality assurance (QA) activities are proactive and investigate system processes with a focus on preventing errors, while quality control (QC) activities investigate the final product (a cytology report) or outcomes (implications to patient care) of the process to detect error. Quality improvement (QI) is a continuous process of analyzing data that ties QA and QC to corrective actions and follow-on monitoring to ensure that the desired outcome is achieved.

As one component of quality management, we recommend accreditation of cytology laboratories. This recognizes laboratory competence based on external evaluation of daily practice as a primary means of improving the quality of the cytology laboratory and enhancing patient safety. Accreditation is an obligatory step for clinical practice in some countries and may be government regulated [9]. External quality assurance (EQA) in pathology is an important step in the process of international accreditation [10]. EQA programs are available in many countries. Some of the most common providers include the College of American Pathologists (CAP), the United Kingdom National External Quality Assessment Service (UK NEQAS), the European Quality Assurance programs (EQA), and the Nordic Immunohistochemical Quality Control (NordicQC). However, EQA in international non-gynecological cytology is a recent event [5].

There are multiple organizations providing standards and recommendations for improving quality in clinical laboratories. Two organizations that provide international accreditation for pathology laboratories are the CAP [11], who base inspections on regulations imposed by the US Clinical Laboratory Improvement Amendments of 1988 (CLIA) [12], and the International Organization for Standardization (ISO) [13], who establish and promote international standardization of laboratory processes. ISO standard 15189 [14] addresses the requirements for quality and competence in medical laboratories and is largely used in non-US countries [9]. Most US cytopathology laboratories receive accreditation from the Centers for Medicare and Medicaid Services (CMS) through deemed inspection agencies such as CAP, the Joint Commission (TJC), [15] or state agencies. Although these accreditation standards vary among countries or continents, they all control the same phases of laboratory practice – *pre-analytic*, *analytic*, and *post-analytic* – in a rigorous manner and require evidence of performance and competence using the best standards of practice.

The entire laboratory staff must be committed to continuous improvement through the evaluation of daily practices to adhere to a quality program. The aim of all QI programs is to reduce errors and enhance quality to improve patient safety. There is no standardization for QI programs, nor should there be: QI programs should be designed to detect, monitor, correct, and prevent errors that are specific to the laboratory. What is desirable are consensus guidelines on general quality monitors and agreement on calculations derived from those monitors to allow for laboratory comparison. Thereafter, laboratories would have external benchmarks upon which to compare their performance. Consensus guidelines for quality monitors in gynecologic cytology have been widely implemented and employed [8], but none exist in non-gynecologic cytology. The authors propose implementing the successful relevant monitors of gynecologic cytology as monitors for serous fluid cytology.

It is well-known that most errors (over 50%) in a laboratory occur in the *pre-analytic phase* and include errors of patient identification, clinical information (or lack thereof) on requisition forms, specimen collection adequacy, and integrity, transport, and specimen labeling with unequivocal and unique patient identifiers [2, 16]. All of these are outside of the direct control of the laboratory. For accreditation purposes, the responsibility for pre-analytics falls on the pathologist, who must regulate adequate sample collection and management through communication with the providers [9].

The *analytic phase* includes processing, staining, interpretation, and reporting of the sample. Internal quality control checks of the technical aspects of processing, such as the quality of the fluid preparation, should be enforced. Cytotechnologists can play a pivotal role in quality improvement by reviewing peer interpretations, serving as internal consultants, and training and supervising technical staff. In Europe and other countries, there are wide variations in training, quality, and competency assessment of cytotechnologists and biomedical scientists practicing non-gynecologic cytology, so it is critical to apply initial competency assessments and provide continuous training to improve their performance [5]. Ancillary techniques applied to serous effusions should also be subject to quality assessment. Automated processing, staining, and reporting, preferably using laboratory information system (LIS) platforms that can trace the specimen, are important tools to help improve quality by forcing standardization and by providing statistical analysis of processes and outcomes, thereby reducing technical variability and human errors. Although most surgical pathology and cytology quality improvement programs have focused on monitoring the correct interpretation of the specimen, this area only accounts for an average of 1–5% of analytical errors in anatomic pathology [17, 18]. There are different methods to detect diagnostic errors, such as rescreening, post-interpretive review, internal and external consultation, and cytologic-histologic correlation. Performing a root cause analysis on detected errors can also improve quality [19].

The *post-analytic phase* defines the outcomes of cytology reporting and is essential for the quality of cytopathology. There is an ever-growing awareness of the importance of harmonizing global cytology reporting with common elements and language. Powsner et al. showed that surgeons misunderstand up to 30% of surgical pathology reports [20], and one can surmise that similar misunderstandings occur with cytology reports. Chandra et al. attributed 32% of their errors to the post-analytic phase [16]. The ISO 15189 standard provides recommendations for the post-interpretative reporting phase to improve quality of cytopathology laboratories [14]. Nomenclature is one of the most commonly required aspects still lacking standardization. To meet the ISO standard, specimen results should be unambiguous, concise, and reproducible. In cytology, a general diagnostic category and a descriptive nomenclature are widely used [1]. Reporting on ancillary tests, such as molecular techniques, is also evolving targets of standardization [21].

Elements of Quality Assurance

Specific quality assurance (QA) practices or monitors for serous fluid cytology have not been defined. An effective QA program for serous fluids should monitor pre-analytic, analytic, and post-analytic variables as applicable to cytopathology practice. Serous fluid specimens can be combined with other non-gynecologic specimens for statistical purposes or reported separately if perceived problems arise related to those specimens. In the USA and in many other countries, report turnaround time (TAT) and customer satisfaction are measured as part of the QI program but will not be addressed in this section. QA/QC monitors may be either perpetual (consistently measured due to regulatory guidelines or as a baseline monitor) or intermittent (measured because of a perceived problem or as a sample quality measurement when organizational, environmental, or personnel changes occur). Intermittent QA monitors can be changed over time. In principle, if a problem is fixed and subsequent measurements show a steady state, there may be no need for continued measurement. QA/QC monitors should measure technical and processing components as well as comparing individual cytologists' diagnostic results with their peers and overall cumulative laboratory results [22]. Charts, graphs, and tables that plot data over time are most conducive to longitudinal assessment. When comparing statistics of individuals with one another or clinics with each other, it is ideal to anonymize all participants using a numerical code or other substitute. While most participants want to know how they perform in relationship with others, most are not keen to be easily recognized as an outlier. Suggestions for ongoing monitoring/audit are outlined in Table 11.1 and are highlighted in some published guidance [7].

Table 11.1 Examples of quality monitors for serous fluid cytopathology

Pre-analytic phase	Analytic phase	Post-analytic phase
Patient and specimen identification	Rate of laboratory mislabeled cases, specimens, blocks, slides	Completeness of final report
Specimen adequacy (volume)	Staining quality	Adherence to laboratory reporting standards and standardized terminology
Specimen preservation	Adequacy of specimen preparation (air-drying, adequate fixation, and preservation)	Report receipt by clinical team
Appropriate clinical information	Percentage of cases with prospective secondary review	Documented notification of urgent or unexpected diagnoses
Time from sample procurement to sample receipt in the laboratory	Diagnostic category rates	Overall turn-around time of specimen and by analytical phase
	Cytology-histology correlation (CHC)	
	Error rates after peer review	
	Adequacy and appropriateness of ancillary studies	
	Utilization of ancillary studies	
	Corrected report rates	

Pre-analytic Phase Monitors

Pre-analytic variables can be easily monitored through a specimen rejection process. An adequate specimen volume is necessary to ensure that a "negative for malignancy" (NFM) result is truly representative. Serous fluids are best received fresh, and the entire specimen volume collected should be submitted to the laboratory. The laboratory should have specimen acceptance criteria, and specimens that do not reach the laboratory's criteria (based upon laboratory-established procedures and policies) should be rejected and feedback given to the contributor. Deficiencies of specimen submission should reflect the laboratory's submission directives and policies. The LIS can potentiate the collection of data by providing deficiency menus listing the reasons for rejection. For most serous fluids, delays in processing seldom interfere with analysis if the specimen is refrigerated or fixed, so specimens can be held until the deficiency is corrected. In hospital-based laboratories in the USA, pathologists often have access to the patient's medical record. However, in reference laboratories and those where the pathologist does not have access to the medical record, obtaining pertinent history from the clinical team is essential and can be a useful quality monitor. Computer-generated statistics can identify error-prone areas and providers or clinics with the highest errors so that laboratories can intervene with improvement suggestions. In the absence of computer programs to facilitate these efforts, laboratories must collect the data manually.

Analytic Phase Monitors

This phase includes all of the steps involved in analyzing the specimen once it is received in the laboratory. These include accessioning, gross examination, specimen preparation, staining, ancillary studies, microscopic evaluation, and diagnosis. For serous fluids, volume and color should be recorded as part of the specimen gross description. Specimen accessioning should include site and laterality (if applicable).

Good specimen preparation is essential to accurate interpretation. The samples should be adequately prepared, fixed, and stained (see Chap. 10, Cytopreparatory Techniques). Daily review of cytology preparations with feedback to the technical preparatory staff ensures consistency. If the preparation is not adequate, it should be repeated if there is sufficient remaining specimen volume. Ancillary studies must have adequate control specimens that mirror the fixation and processing of the specimen examined. Analytic monitors should measure the quality of staining and fixation. Mislabeling of specimens, blocks, and slides are additional monitors that may be tracked. Intralaboratory specimen labeling error rates are an important measure because mislabeling of specimens, slides, or blocks are just as significant as misidentification of the patient.

The pathologist's/cytologist's interpretation, the outcome of this phase, is formed based on the correlation of the microscopic and ancillary findings with clinical information. Analytic monitors assessing individual pathologist/cytologist performance and diagnostic accuracy include error rates detected after peer review, cytology-histology correlation, and corrected report rates. Assessment of pathologists'/cytologists' performance should also track diagnostic category rates against the laboratory as a whole. For example, tracking individual rates of atypia of undetermined significance (AUS) against the total laboratory rate can detect individual outliers or escalating laboratory AUS rates that might indicate submission or processing issues. Generally, AUS rates should be low; in other cytology terminology systems, atypical rates of 5–10% are deemed acceptable. Monitoring adherence to standardized terminology and reporting policies, as established by the individual laboratory, is also a good practice.

Peer review includes retrospective and prospective review. Retrospective review occurs after the case has been finalized and includes random review of a percentage of cases, focused peer review, case review for tumor boards or multidisciplinary conferences, unsolicited case reviews by an outside facility to which the patient was referred for a second opinion, correlation of original in-house diagnosis with solicited expert consultation, and results of cytology-histology correlation. Prospective peer review is a secondary review of a case before the report is finalized and occurs in consultation between pathologists or at a consensus conference.

Secondary review of surgical pathology and cytopathology cases detects diagnostic discrepancies. The CAP Pathology and Laboratory Quality Center in association with the Association of Directors of Anatomic and Surgical Pathology (ADASP), both US-based pathology organizations, published evidence-based guidelines with five recommendations for prospective peer review [23]. These guidelines state that anatomic pathologists should:

- Develop procedures for the review of selected pathology cases to detect disagreements and potential interpretive errors.
- Perform case reviews in a timely manner to avoid having a negative impact on patient care.
- Have documented case review procedures that are relevant to their practice setting.
- Continuously monitor and document the results of case reviews.
- Take steps to improve agreement, if pathology case reviews show poor agreement within a defined case type [23].

Pathologists frequently seek out a second opinion prior to finalizing a case when faced with a diagnostic challenge or diagnostic uncertainty. A Q-probes study performed by the CAP showed an aggregate rate of review of 8.2% for surgical pathology cases [24]. This rate has not been established for cytopathology. Review of the literature shows a median rate of discrepancy for cytopathology cases of 24.8% (range 17.4–38.8%) and a median rate of major discrepancies of 4.3% (2.8–7.5) [23]. Most of these articles focused on thyroid fine needle aspiration. One study of patients with mesothelioma in serous fluids found a false-negative rate of nearly 50% [25].

The laboratory should establish policies for retrospective and prospective review. Prospective peer review is preferred, when possible, because it prevents cases from being released with significant errors that may impact patient care and it appears to decrease the number of errors compared to retrospective review [26]. Laboratories with established, written policies have greater rates of secondary review prior to sign-out compared with those that do not [24]. Examples of cases that may require prospective second opinion include indeterminate cases, challenging diagnoses such as clinically suspected mesothelioma, and specimens with scant representative cells. Some laboratories require prospective review on all malignant cases. The appropriate rate of review is not known but is typically between 5% and 15% of cases. The case review should be documented in the report. Methods that may reduce interobserver disagreements and errors include consensus conferences, the use of a calibration slide set, and review of standardized criteria [23]. The use of consensus conferences significantly decreases the rate of disagreements [27].

Cytology-histology correlation (CHC) is an important part of a cytology laboratory QM program and is defined as the correlation of cytology and histology specimens from the same site to determine whether they are concordant or discordant [28]. CLIA 1988 mandates CHC for gynecological specimens [12]. The CAP cytopathology accreditation checklist requires CHC of non-gynecological specimens, but does not dictate the process [11]. CHC is not standardized. Each laboratory will need to establish its criteria for CHC of serous fluids, including the correlate histology sample to use, the look back period, and the grading scale for discrepancies. In patients with concurrent serous fluid specimens and biopsies of the serous surface, correlation can be performed prospectively. Positive serous fluids may be correlated with biopsies from other organs to confirm diagnosis (e.g., a lung mass biopsy with a pleural effusion). The laboratory should establish the follow-up time period for retrospective review. A short time interval may miss subsequent histology samples. Finally, the laboratory must decide what it will consider a significant discrepancy [28]. However, it must be acknowledged that serous fluid cytology may not always correlate with contemporaneous biopsies. This can reflect sampling issues but also the natural biology of tumors and disease processes.

A survey of CHC practices of 802 laboratories performed by the CAP Cytopathology Committee in 2019 (personal communication) showed that 89% performed CHC on non-gynecologic specimens and 76% correlated reports along with a review of both cytology and surgical pathology slides. Other trends practiced by over 50% of the surveyed laboratories included reviewing corresponding cytology slides at the time that the surgical specimen is reviewed, investigating why a discordance occurred, correlating specimens within a 6-month time frame, and addressing the reason for the discordance in a pathology report when current patient management would change due to the interpretive change. The most common reason for discordance between specimens was sampling issues (94%), followed by processing or preparation issues (2%). The only metric that was monitored by over half of the laboratories was the percent of cytology cases that correlated with the surgical specimen. About one-third of laboratories also monitored cytologists' interpretive/screening error rates and sampling discordances. The primary method used to improve patient care based on these results was through issuance of a QA document.

Corrected reports are an important metric of QM and an indicator of error rates. Rates of corrected reports for serous fluids should be maintained and monitored, with review of outliers. Each laboratory should also define its own list of urgent diagnoses and significant, unexpected diagnoses [11]. In serous fluids, this may include a diagnosis of malignancy in a patient with no known primary site or diagnosis of an unsuspected new primary malignancy. These results must be communicated to the clinical team and the communication documented in the report.

Post-analytic Phase Monitors

Post-analytic quality activities focus on quality control of the cytology report and patient outcomes. Important aspects of the post-analytic phase are the quality of the report and communication of critical or unexpected diagnosis to the clinical team [22, 29]. The final report should be formatted correctly to highlight the diagnosis and other important information [1]. Reports should not include unnecessary data. A complete cytopathology report should include patient demographics, unique patient identifiers, and specimen type, quantity, source, and method of collection. A gross description of the specimen received (color and turbidity; fixed or air-dried for smears) and the preparation method and stains (e.g., smears, automated liquid-based, cytocentrifugation, membrane filtration, cell-block) should also be provided. Due to specimen variability, a specific number and/or type of cells needed to render a specimen adequate has not been established across all specimen types and varies according to the clinical presentation and suspected underlying pathology. However, a statement regarding the adequacy should be included, especially if the interpretation is compromised due to low specimen volume, scant cellularity, obscuring factors, or poor fixation, among others [29]. When performed, immunohistochemical stains should be individually reported along with the preparation method used for immunohistochemistry (smears, cytospins, or cell-block) and the presence of adequate controls [30].

The final report should use up-to-date diagnostic terminology and provide possible differential diagnoses and explanatory notes as needed. It is of critical importance that the laboratory communicates final interpretations to the treating physician using clear and concise terms. While a certain degree of flexibility is necessary when using cytology diagnostic terminology, standardization is necessary to meet the needs of the clinical team as well as to guide further patient management. This is of utmost importance when dealing with uncertain diagnostic categories such as atypical and suspicious. In these cases, a statement including reasons for which a definitive diagnosis could not be provided is necessary.

Critical results are an important part of the laboratory accreditation process and have the most immediate impact on patient care. In anatomic pathology (AP), the terms urgent diagnoses and significant, unexpected findings are preferred, as the concept of a critical value does not have direct correlation with AP diagnoses. Urgent diagnoses are those that should be addressed as soon as possible. Significant, unexpected diagnoses are defined as clinically unusual or unforeseen and need to be addressed at some point in the patient's treatment [31]. The list of urgent and significant, unexpected diagnoses is established by each laboratory in agreement with the clinical team, taking into consideration their practice setting, clinical needs, and expectations. However, even when a policy is in place, cytologists should use their judgment and promptly communicate urgent diagnoses if patient safety is at risk [32]. The results should be communicated verbally and directly with physicians, but other forms of communication may be used. The communication should be documented, either in the report, as an addendum, in the electronic medical record, or by another mechanism. Documentation should include the person with whom the case was discussed, the time and date, and, when appropriate, the means of communication [31].

An effective method of monitoring report completeness and comprehension mirrors that of a specimen rejection process. Using a checklist of possible report deficiencies, a supervisor or QC pathologist can review a percent of completed reports for missing or incomprehensible information and tabulate the information over time for individuals and the laboratory as a whole. Some metrics that might be monitored include appropriate lead line for specimen type, presence of an adequacy statement, employment of standardized cytology terminology, notes or comments explaining uncertain findings, inclusion of or reference to ancillary study results affecting the interpretation, documentation of control specimens, and documentation of notification for urgent or unexpected results.

A final component of the post-analytic process is ongoing training and competency assessment. It is essential that all staff screening and/or reporting cytology is appropriately trained, qualified, and kept up to date. The statutory and legal requirements for this will vary from country to country and will also vary depending if the cytologist is medically qualified or not. While acquiring cytological interpretative and diagnostic skills is essential, so also is maintaining these skills. This can be done with ongoing regular education, such as cytology meetings, self-study for existing cases, multiheaded microscope group case review, web-based resources, EQA, case discussion with peers, and multidisciplinary meetings. It is essential to be able to objectively demonstrate maintenance of a skill but also that new skills are competency-based and objectively demonstrable. This is required as part of the total quality approach to laboratory quality but also for external quality assessments and as part of annual personnel appraisals.

References

1. Crothers BA, Tench WE, Schwartz MR, et al. Guidelines for the reporting of nongynecologic cytopathology specimens. Arch Pathol Lab Med. 2009;133(11):1743–56.
2. Hollensead SC, Lockwood WB, Elin RJ. Errors in pathology and laboratory medicine: consequences and prevention. J Surg Oncol. 2004;88(3):161–81.
3. Nodi L, Balassanian R, Sudilovsky D, Raab SS. Improving the quality of cytology diagnosis: root cause analysis for errors in bronchial washing and brushing specimens. Am J Clin Pathol. 2005;124(6):883–92.
4. Chandra A, Cross P, Denton K, et al. The BSCC code of practice-exfoliative cytopathology (excluding gynaecological cytopathology). Cytopathology. 2009;20(4):211–23.
5. Wilson A. The role of cytotechnologists in quality assurance and audit in non-gynaecological cytology. Cytopathology. 2015;26(2):75–8.
6. Cummings MC, Greaves J, Shukor RA, Perkins G, Ross J. Technical proficiency in cytopathology: assessment through external quality assurance. Cytopathology. 2017;28(2):149–56.

7. The Royal College of Pathologists. G086. Tissue Pathways for Diagnostic Cytopathology. 2019. https://www.rcpath.org/search-results.html?q=Tissue+pathways.
8. Tworek J, Nayar R, Savaloja L, Tabbara S, Thomas N, Winkler B, Howell LP. General quality practices in gynecologic cytopathology: findings from the College of American Pathologists Gynecologic Cytopathology Quality Consensus Conference Working Group 3. Arch Pathol Lab Med. 2013;137(2):190–8.
9. Tzankov A, Tornillo L. Hands-on experience: accreditation of pathology laboratories according to ISO 15189. Pathobiology. 2017;84(3):121–9.
10. Long-Mira E, Washetine K, Hofman P. Sense and nonsense in the process of accreditation of a pathology laboratory. Virchows Arch. 2016;468(1):43–9.
11. College of American Pathologists Laboratory Accreditation Program. 2019. https://www.cap.org/laboratory-improvement/accreditation/laboratory-accreditation-program.
12. Clinical Laboratory Improvement Amendments (CLIA). Standards and certifications: laboratory requirements (42 CFR 493) Electronic Code of Federal Regulations e-CFR. https://www.ecfr.gov/cgi-bin/text-idx?SID=1248e3189daSe5f9.
13. International Organizations of Standardization (ISO). https://www.iso.org.
14. ISO 15189:2012E 2012. https://www.iso.org/standard/56115.html.
15. The Joint Commission Laboratory Accreditation Program. https://www.jointcommission.org/accreditation/laboratory.aspx.
16. Chandra S, Chandra H, Kusum A, Gaur DS. Study of the pre-analytical phase of an ISO 15189: 2012-certified cytopathology laboratory: a 5-year institutional experience. Acta Cytol. 2019;63(1):56–62.
17. Raab SS. Improving patient safety by examining pathology errors. Clin Lab Med. 2004;24:849–63.
18. Raab SS, Nakhleh RE, Ruby SG. Patient safety in anatomic pathology: measuring discrepancy frequencies and causes. Arch Pathol Lab Med. 2005;129(4):459–66.
19. Raab SS, Grzybicki DM. Measuring quality in anatomic pathology. Clin Lab Med. 2008;28(2):245–59.
20. Powsner SM, Costa J, Homer RJ. Clinicians are from Mars and pathologists are from Venus: clinician interpretation of pathology reports. Arch Pathol Lab Med. 2000;124(7):1040–6.
21. Payne DA, Baluchova K, Russomando G, et al. Towards harmonization of clinical molecular diagnostic reports: findings of an international survey. Clin Chem Lab Med. 2018;57(1):78–88.
22. Nakhleh RE. Core components of a comprehensive quality assurance program in anatomic pathology. Adv Anat Pathol. 2009;16(6):418–23.
23. Nakhleh RE, Nose V, Colasacco C, et al. Interpretive diagnostic error reduction in surgical pathology and cytology: guideline from the College of American Pathologists Pathology and Laboratory Quality Center and the Association of Directors of Anatomic and Surgical Pathology. Arch Pathol Lab Med. 2016;140(1):29–40.
24. Nakhleh RE, Bekeris LG, Souers RJ, Meier FA, Tworek JA. Surgical pathology case reviews before sign-out: a College of American Pathologists Q-Probes study of 45 laboratories. Arch Pathol Lab Med. 2010;134(5):740–3.
25. Ascoli V, Bosco D, Carnoval Scalzo C. Cytologic re-evaluation of negative effusions from patients with malignant mesothelioma. Pathologica. 2011;103(6):318–24.
26. Renshaw AA, Gould EW. Measuring the value of review of pathology material by a second pathologist. Am J Clin Pathol. 2006;125(5):737–9.
27. Layfield LJ, Hammer RD, Frazier SR, et al. Impact of consensus conference review on diagnostic disagreements in the evaluation of cervical biopsy specimens. Am J Clin Pathol. 2017;147(5):473–6.
28. Raab SS, Grzybicki DM. Cytologic-histologic correlation. Cancer Cytopathol. 2011;199(5):293–309.
29. American Society of Cytopathology. Non-gynecological Cytology Practice Guideline, March 2, 2004. https://www.cytopathology.org/wp-content/dynamic_uploads/54.pdf.

30. Shidham VB, Epple J. Collection and processing of effusion fluids for cytopathology evaluation. In: Shidham VB, Atkinson BF, editors. Cytopathologic diagnosis of serous fluids. China: Saunders Elsevier, Inc.; 2007. p. 207–14.
31. Nakhleh RE, Myers JL, Allen TC, et al. Consensus statement on effective communication of urgent diagnoses and significant, unexpected diagnoses in surgical pathology and cytopathology from the College of American Pathologists and the Association of Directors of Anatomic and Surgical Pathology. Arch Pathol Lab Med. 2012;136(2):148–54.
32. Nakhleh RE. Quality in surgical pathology communication and reporting. Arch Pathol Lab Med. 2011;135(11):1394–7.

Serous Effusion Anatomy, Biology, and Pathophysiology

Stefan E. Pambuccian and Miguel Perez-Machado

Background

The serous membranes covering the lungs (pleurae), heart (pericardium), abdominal organs (peritoneum), and testis (tunica vaginalis testis) are derived from the embryonic mesoderm, specifically from the coelomic cavity. They were first described without the use of the microscope by the French pathologist Marie François Xavier Bichat (1771–1802), who used them to develop his theory of tissues [1]. However, it was not until 1890 that the American anatomist and embryologist Charles Sedgwick Minot (1852–1914) proposed the term "mesothelium" to reflect the epithelial-like nature of the cells lining mesodermally derived coelomic cavities [2]. His observation that the mesothelium is an epithelial differentiated tissue of mesodermal origin and as such shows both epithelial and mesenchymal characteristics has been confirmed by subsequent morphologic and molecular findings.

Anatomy, Embryology, and Histology of Serous Membranes

The mesoderm, which forms between the ectoderm and endoderm in the first week of gestation, differentiates into three plates: the paraxial (around the neural tube), intermediate, and lateral plates. In the third week of embryonic development, a cleft in the lateral plate of the mesoderm forms the coelomic cavity, which

S. E. Pambuccian (✉)
Department of Pathology, Loyola University Health Systems, Loyola University, Maywood, IL, USA
e-mail: spambuccian@lumc.edu

M. Perez-Machado
Royal Free London NHS Foundation Trust, London, UK
e-mail: miguel.perez-machado@nhs.net

© Springer Nature Switzerland AG 2020
A. Chandra et al. (eds.), *The International System for Serous Fluid Cytopathology*, https://doi.org/10.1007/978-3-030-53908-5_12

separates the parietal (somatic) mesoderm underlying the ectoderm from the visceral (splanchnic) mesoderm overlying the endoderm. The somatic mesoderm and immediately overlying ectoderm form the somatopleure, which will become the body wall and parietal mesothelium, while the visceral mesoderm and underlying endoderm will become the visceral mesothelium and the organs of the coelomic cavity. The initial single coelomic cavity will become the peritoneal cavity, the right and left pleural cavities (which normally do not communicate with each other), the pericardial cavity, and finally the tunica vaginalis testis, which forms as an outpouching of the peritoneum and transiently communicates with the peritoneal cavity. The peritoneum and ovaries both derive from the mesoderm, but while the peritoneum derives from the lateral plate, the ovaries derive from the intermediate plate. This similarity of embryologic derivation may help explain the similarity in the markers expressed by the peritoneal mesothelium and ovarian surface epithelium. Some authors also invoke the embryologic relatedness to explain the propensity of ovarian carcinomas to metastasize to the peritoneum [3], but this is controversial in view of the currently prevailing theory of ovarian carcinomas as originating from the fallopian tube.

Serous membranes are composed of a visceral layer, covering the lungs, the heart, some abdominopelvic organs, the testes, and a parietal layer attached to the wall of the cavity. The potential space (serous cavity) that is formed between the two serosal layers is normally very small and occupied by a few milliliters of serous fluid that forms a thin film and acts as a lubricant. The serous membranes have a similar structure with only minor differences based on anatomic location. They are lined by the mesothelium, which overlies two submesothelial connective tissue layers separated by a thin elastic layer and which contains lymphatics, capillaries, type I and type III collagen fibers, and elastin in a loose matrix. Despite their different embryologic derivations, the mesothelium and simple epithelia share the presence of junctional structures like tight junctions, gap junctions, and desmosomes and the presence of a basement membrane, apicobasal differentiation, and presence of microvilli as well as the expression of keratins.

The mesodermal origin of mesothelial cells may explain the fact that they show both epithelial and mesenchymal characteristics and the ability to undergo transitions from epithelial to mesenchymal phenotype. The epithelial characteristics of mesothelial cells are demonstrated by their expression of epithelial markers, including cytokeratins and cell adhesion molecules; their epithelial-like cell junctions; their polygonal shape and apicobasal polarization; presence of microvilli; and anchorage to a basal lamina. Their mesenchymal characteristics, which are most obvious in reactive mesothelial cells, include the expression of vimentin, desmin, and actin. Moreover, their mesenchymal-like characteristics may also explain the propensity of mesothelial cells to easily shift from an epithelial to a mesenchymal phenotype through epithelial to mesenchymal transition (EMT), more accurately referred to as "mesothelial-mesenchymal transition (MMT)" [4]. Through EMT, mesothelial cells can change phenotype, becoming spindle cells that lack polarity and intercellular junctions and have the capacity to migrate, invade, and resist apoptosis [5].

The mesothelial lining is normally formed of a monolayer of mesothelial cells, lying on a thin (100 nm) basal membrane composed of type IV collagen and laminin, which is produced by mesothelial cells and provides binding sites for mesothelial cells through hemidesmosomes. Histologically, mesothelial cells are large, flat, squamous-like cells measuring 20–40 μm in diameter and 1–4 μm in thickness. Depending on their location and functional state, the mesothelial cells lining these membranes may appear large and flattened (squamoid), similar to endothelial cells, or more cuboidal, similar to epithelial cells. The squamoid mesothelial cells are large, 20–25 μm in diameter, and contain few organelles. The cuboidal mesothelial cells appear smaller, measuring 8 μm in diameter. They have more microvilli, larger nuclei and nucleoli, and numerous cytoplasmic organelles, all denoting active metabolism. Cuboidal mesothelial cells are located preferentially in the mediastinal pleura, visceral pericardium, diaphragmatic peritoneum, and around milky spots. In contrast to the flattened mesothelial cells, the cuboidal mesothelial cells are rich in organelles, including mitochondria, rough endoplasmic reticulum, Golgi apparatus, and multilamellar bodies resembling those of type II pneumocytes and containing surfactant-like substances. These organelles may be involved in the mesothelial cells' absorption and phagocytosis functions. However, their most characteristic ultrastructural feature is the presence of long microvilli. These long, bushy microvilli, measuring 0.1 μm in diameter and 0.5–3 μm in length, unevenly cover the surface of the mesothelial cells. The density of the microvilli varies with the location of the mesothelial cells; the visceral pleurae and lower portions of the pleurae have denser microvilli than the parietal pleura and upper (apical) portions of the pleurae. Microvilli expand the mesothelial surface by about 20-fold and are covered by glycoproteins rich in hyaluronic acid. Although their function is incompletely understood, microvilli may serve as a scaffold and enmesh hyaluronan, providing support for the lubricating function of the mesothelial cells. Alternatively, the electrical charges on the oligolamellar surfactant molecules present on the surface of the microvilli of the parietal and visceral pleurae repulse each other, acting to reduce the friction between them. The same electrical changes make the mesothelial lining act like Teflon, repulsing microbes, cells, and particles. Adjacent mesothelial cells are connected by junctional complexes consisting of desmosomes, tight junctions (zonulae occludentes) located toward the apical side, adherens junctions, and finally gap junctions toward the basal side of the cells, with anchoring to the basal lamina with hemidesmosomes. The intercellular junctions of mesothelial cells contain E-, N-, and P-cadherin, but in contrast to the epithelium in which E-cadherin predominates, N-cadherin predominates in the mesothelium. Despite the presence of all these junctions, mesothelial cells are easily dislodged from the serous membranes by mechanical (frictional) forces and various injuries and can become free in the serous fluid. Free mesothelial cells change their shape from flat to spherical, become vacuolated, and acquire phagocytic properties akin to macrophages. Free mesothelial cells remain viable for a number of days and may reattach to areas of mesothelial damage, participating in their repair [6].

The mesothelial cells are normally long-lived and renew slowly. Mitoses are relatively uncommon, with only 0.16–0.5% of mesothelial cells undergoing mitosis at any one time. However, after injury mesothelial cells respond through proliferation, increasing their mitotic rate to 30–60% [7], and by chemotaxis to cover any areas of denuded extracellular matrix. The loose connective tissue underlying the mesothelium is rich in capillaries, which are involved in the formation of serosal fluids and freely intercommunicating lymphatics, which form a network of lymphatic capillaries involved in the absorption of the serous fluid. In contrast to the visceral serosae (pleurae, pericardium, peritoneum), which have lymphatics that are part of the underlying organ's lymphatic system, the parietal serosae (pleurae, pericardium, peritoneum) are innervated and have lymphatics that drain into regional lymph nodes. The parietal serosal lymphatics communicate with the serosal space through 2–10 μm round, oval, or slit-like stomata, which overlie cistern-like dilatations of the lymphatics called lacunae and act like a unidirectional valve system. Stomata are more numerous in the mediastinal, lower intercostal, and diaphragmatic portions of the parietal pleurae, pericardium, and peritoneum lining the omentum and mesentery. Milky spots, also termed Kampmeier foci, and serosa-associated lymphoid clusters (SALCs) are present in the proximity of the lymphatic stomata [8]. Histologically, they are aggregates of B and T lymphocytes, NK cells, plasma cells, and histiocytes centered on capillary blood vessels and surrounded by cuboidal mesothelial cells. They are considered to represent secondary lymphoid organs, part of the coelom-associated lymphoid tissue (CALT), the immune system of serous cavities. Milky spots are important in the early steps of serosal cancer metastasis and are involved in cancer cell homing and invasion and omental and serosal membrane colonization by tumor cells.

The primary function of the mesothelium is to provide a slippery surface, but it is also has multiple complex functions, such as selective fluid and cell transport, immune induction, modulation and inhibition, sensing and repairing tissue injuries, promoting angiogenesis, fighting infection, and transcellular migration.

Individual Serosal Cavity Anatomy and Fluid Dynamics

Peritoneum

The largest serous cavity is the peritoneal cavity, with a surface of 1.5–2.0 m², comparable to that of the skin, of which 30% is represented by parietal and 70% by visceral peritoneum.

The visceral peritoneum covers almost the entire liver, stomach, and intestines and contributes to the formation of the mesentery. Peritoneal folds (omenta) divide the peritoneal cavity into a lesser and greater sac, connected at the omental foramen. The parietal peritoneum lines the abdominopelvic cavity and reflects over the dome of the bladder and anterior rectal surface. In women it also covers the uterus, fallopian tubes, and ovaries, where it is continuous with the ovarian surface epithelium, which has similar (but not identical) morphologic, immunohistochemical, and molecular characteristics. In contrast to men, in whom the peritoneum is a closed sac, it is an open cavity in women, communicating through the fallopian tubes with the uterine cavity, cervix, vagina, and ultimately the external environment. This communication with the external environment potentially exposes the female peritoneum to microbial pathogens and particulate matter such as talc powder, with potential carcinogenic effects [9]. The protrusion of the vesical dome and uterus into the peritoneal cavity creates several virtual spaces: the rectovesical pouch in men and the vesicouterine and rectouterine pouch (Douglas pouch) in women.

The peritoneal cavity normally contains about 50 mL of fluid; about 1 L of fluid is produced daily and is reabsorbed into subperitoneal lymphatic channels, located mainly on the peritoneal surface of the diaphragm. Most peritoneal lymphatics drain into the thoracic duct and the right lymphatic duct.

Peritoneal fluid movement is governed by gravity, by the peritoneal and mesenteric anatomy, and by intraabdominal pressure gradients caused by the movements of the diaphragm. Gravity makes the peritoneal fluid flow into the decline regions of the peritoneal cavity, where it tends to pool. In the upright position, the lowest-lying parts of the peritoneal cavity are the rectovesical pouch in men and the vesicouterine and rectouterine pouch in women. In the supine position, the fluid tends to pool in the right and left paracolic gutters and pelvis. Intraabdominal pressure gradients explain the egress of the fluid from the decline positions: the intraperitoneal pressure in the upper abdominal cavity is subatmospheric and becomes even lower during inspiration. The diaphragm therefore acts like a pump moving the peritoneal fluid upward during inspiration; the fluid accumulated in the pelvis flows mostly along the right paracolic gutter toward the suprahepatic and right subphrenic spaces. The dynamics of the flow of peritoneal fluid explain the preferential location of peritoneal implants or metastases that are caused by the dissemination of tumor cells through the peritoneal fluid in the pelvis, pouch of Douglas, right lower quadrant, near the terminal ileum, and subdiaphragmatic space, which are locations where the peritoneal fluid pools or sites of maximal resorption.

Pleurae

The right and left pleural cavities are not connected to each other, which explains the frequent occurrence of unilateral pleural effusions. The parietal pleurae line the thoracic wall, from which it can be peeled off, and adhere to the pericardium and diaphragm. The visceral pleurae adhere tightly to the lung parenchyma starting at the pulmonary hila and line all major and minor fissures. The parietal pleurae contain the lymphatics responsible for the reabsorption of pleural fluid; the lymphatics from the costal region of the pleurae drain into parasternal nodes, while those from the diaphragmatic and mediastinal pleurae drain mostly into the mediastinal lymph nodes. The exact function of the pleural space is still uncertain; it is entirely absent in other mammals like the elephants, and its therapeutic obliteration (pleurodesis) is generally well-tolerated.

Pleural fluid is constantly produced, normally at a rate of 0.01 mL/kg/h, about 15 mL per day in an adult. There is normally a gravity-dependent downward flow of pleural fluid and a continuous redistribution through an upward flow along lobar margins. The production of pleural fluid is normally balanced by the reabsorption of fluid. The reabsorption capacity is much larger, up to 30 times the normal production rate; the accumulation of fluid in the pleural cavities only occurs when this absorption capacity is overwhelmed by increased production or when the reabsorption capacity is diminished by blockage of the lymphatics. The obstruction of the lymphatic stomata, which are exclusively present on the parietal pleurae, markedly decreases the resorption capacity and leads to the accumulation of pleural fluid. The mediastinal pleurae contain most of these stomata from which the fluid drains in the mediastinal lymph nodes, which explains the fact that pleural effusions frequently accompany metastatic involvement of mediastinal lymph nodes. It may also explain why malignancies that preferentially metastasize to the mediastinal nodes, especially pulmonary, breast, gastric, and ovarian carcinomas, are also the most common causes of malignant pleural effusions. Conversely, sarcomas, which only rarely metastasize to lymph nodes, also rarely cause of pleural effusions [10].

Pericardium

The pericardial consists of an external sac, the fibrous pericardium, and an internal sac, the serous pericardium, which lines the internal surface of the fibrous pericardium (parietal pericardium) and the heart (visceral pericardium or epicardium). The pericardial cavity is formed between the visceral and parietal pericardium.

Although the pericardium is not essential for survival and can be removed without serious adverse consequences, it has a number of subtle functions. Among other functions, the pericardium allows frictionless movement of the cardiac surfaces, stabilizes the heart's anatomic position and isolates it from the adjacent structures, thereby preventing the spread of infections, and equalizes gravitational, hydrostatic, and inertial forces that act on the heart, thereby neutralizing the effects of respiration and postural changes on the heart.

The pericardial fluid is mainly drained by the lymphatics in the parietal pericardium. Additional fluid drainage occurs on the epicardial surface of the heart and may also occur through anastomoses with other lymphatics in the epipericardial fat, mediastinal pleura, and diaphragm. The lymphatic vessels drain to the mediastinal, peribronchial, and tracheobronchial lymph nodes. The pattern of lymphatic drainage of the pericardium is similar to that of the pleurae, which may also explain the similarity in the etiology of malignant pleural and pericardial effusions.

Physiology and Pathophysiology of Serosal Fluid Formation and Resorption

Normally there is a balance between the secretion and reabsorption of fluid: the amount of fluid that is produced as an ultrafiltrate from parietal pleural capillaries is matched by the amount of fluid flowing out through lymphatics. Water can be reabsorbed into the blood capillaries by Starling forces across the visceral pleura and by mesothelial cell-mediated solute-coupled liquid absorption and endocytosis, while larger molecules are mainly reabsorbed through lymphatics.

An imbalance between secretion and reabsorption of fluid results in accumulation of fluid within the serous cavity, which, depending on the serosal cavity affected, is referred to as peritoneal effusion (ascites), pleural and pericardial effusion, and hydrocele. The control of volume and composition of the pleural liquid is affected by a number of mechanisms removing from the pleural space the liquid, small solutes, and protein filtered from the parietal pleura. These mechanisms include Starling forces that act through the mesothelium and underlying capillaries, the lymphatic drainage through the parietal serosal stomata, and the participation of mesothelial cells.

The Starling equation for fluid filtration was formulated in 1896 by the British physiologist Ernest Henry Starling (1866–1927) [11], who was also responsible for the introduction of the word hormone in 1905 and formulating Starling's law or Frank-Starling law of the heart. It states that in the capillary the water is forced out by the hydrostatic pressure and the interstitial protein osmotic pressure but is kept in by the oncotic pressure (the osmotic pressure of plasma proteins) and interstitial pressure. The balance between these opposing forces, the hydrostatic and oncotic forces, also called "Starling forces," determine the rate of transendothelial filtration, which can be expressed as a mathematical equation. In 1927 Kurt von Neergaard (1887–1947), a Swiss physiologist, used Starling's osmotic hypothesis to explain pleural fluid dynamics as an interplay between hydraulic and colloid osmotic pressure [12].

Serosal liquid originates from submesothelial capillaries through microvascular filtration. The transport of water, solutes, and protein occurs across two barriers, the capillary endothelium and the serosal membrane, both of which have similar permeability. Proteins and larger particles over about 5 nm in size do not pass the serosal membrane and are cleared from the serosal space by transcytosis, by phagocytosis, or through lymphatics. However, fluid and electrolytes pass freely between capillary endothelial cells and serosal mesothelial cells, taking the paracellular pathway or transcellularly, through aquaporin pores. According to the Starling equation, the filtration rate across the capillary endothelial barrier is a function of the hydrostatic and colloid osmotic pressure difference between capillary blood and serosal cavity liquid.

Increased amounts of serosal cavity fluids (effusions) occur when there is either increased fluid production or decreased fluid absorption. Effusions with low protein content are referred to as *transudates*, those rich in proteins are called *exudates*, while those rich in lipids are called *chylous* effusions. Starling's equation explains several mechanisms by which the fluid volume within a serosal cavity can expand, of which the most common are:

1. Changes in the transserosal pressure balance
   - Increased hydrostatic pressure, arterial and venous hypertension can cause excessive flow through the serosal membrane. This results in transudative effusions that are mainly caused by congestive heart failure, pulmonary

hypertension, superior vena cava syndrome, portal hypertension, and pulmonary hypertension.
- Reduced intravascular colloid osmotic pressure, due to a reduction in albumin. This results in transudative effusions that are mainly caused by hypoalbuminemia as a result of reduced production in liver diseases and severe malnutrition, increased metabolism in malignancy, or increased loss of albumin in renal diseases (nephrotic syndrome).
2. Reduced or impaired lymphatic drainage, due to obstruction of lymphatic vessels or lymph nodes by malignancy. This is an important cause of exudative effusions.
3. Increases in capillary endothelial and mesothelial permeability:
   - Increased capillary permeability, which can be caused by various injuries, including infections and inflammatory conditions. This usually results in exudative effusions.
   - Altered permeability of the serosal membranes, especially as a consequence of a heart failure, with fluid accumulating from the visceral serosa. The effusion is typically a transudate.
4. Malignant effusions

Malignancies are a common cause of effusions; their mechanism may involve mesothelial irritation with a local inflammatory response caused by tumor cell invasion, resulting in increased capillary permeability. Another potential mechanism of effusion formation in malignancies is the blockage of the efflux of the serosal fluid through lymphatics either by the obstruction of the stomata or by neoplastic replacement of the draining lymph nodes. Obstruction of the thoracic duct, as may occur in lymphomas, can result in chylothorax, the accumulation of milky fluid in the pleurae. However, by itself, blockage of the lymphatic outflow may not be the most important mechanism of effusion formation, since many malignant effusions accumulate more rapidly than would be predicted by the complete blockage of the serosal cavity's lymphatic drainage alone.

The serous effusion occurring in malignancies' fluid may or may not contain tumor cells. The latter condition is referred to as "paramalignant effusion" and represents an effusion which is secondary to malignancy but without direct extension or involvement of the serosal membrane by the malignancy. Paramalignant effusions are most commonly caused by obstruction of lymphatic outflow but may be caused by other mechanisms, like hypoproteinemia, impaired cardiac function, pulmonary emboli, and infections caused by obstruction of a duct or bronchus by tumor. However, most of these paramalignant effusions occur as a side-effect of radiation therapy or chemotherapy (methotrexate, procarbazine, cyclophosphamide, and bleomycin) [13].

The absence of tumor cells in a malignancy-related effusion may also occur in malignancies that do involve the serosal membrane, causing its irritation or obstruction of lymphatics, but do not easily shed cells, as in the case of sarcomas, in which the cells are tightly embedded in the matrix and some carcinomas, possibly related to the desmoplastic reaction that they elicit or to the fact that the metastatic deposit is covered by an intact mesothelial lining and does not communicate with the serosal space. Alternatively, for some tumors showing metastatic serosal deposits, the absence of tumor cells in the fluid may relate to survival time of the exfoliated tumor cells within the fluid. Some tumor cells survive and even thrive in the protein-rich liquid medium created by the exudative serous effusion forming spherical multicellular aggregates, like the "cannonballs" seen in metastatic breast cancer, which are similar to the "spheroids" obtained in tissue cultures. Other malignant tumor cells, however, may not survive in the serosal fluid for an extended period, decreasing the likelihood of encountering them in cytologic serous fluid preparations.

Interestingly, involvement of serosal membranes by tumor cell deposits does not always cause effusions; in fact in an older autopsy series of 52 cases with nodular pleural metastases originating mostly from carcinomas of the lungs, breast, and gastrointestinal tract, effusions were only present in 60%, and tumor cells were identified in the pleural fluid in only 11 of the 14 patients (79%) who had the pleural fluid examined cytologically during life [10]. This was also confirmed by studies correlating pleural fluid cytology to pleural metastatic involvement documented by thoracoscopically obtained biopsies, which found that cytology has a relatively low sensitivity (33–72%) [14]. The likelihood that pleural fluid cytology shows malignant cells is strongly dependent on the metastatic tumor type. Pleural metastases from adenocarcinomas from the breast, pancreas, ovary, lung, and urothelial carcinomas shed malignant cells into the fluid in 80–90% of cases [15]. At the other extreme, pleural metastases from sarcomas, head and neck and pulmonary squamous cell carcinomas, and renal cell carcinomas show tumor cells in only 20–40% of cases [15]. Pleural metastases from other primary sites (prostate, skin melanoma, colorectum, esophagus, cervix, liver, stomach, endometrium, and thyroid) show malignant cells in the pleural fluid between these extremes, i.e., 40–80% [15]. Another potential determinant of pleural fluid positivity in the presence of pleural metastases is visceral pleural invasion, while parietal pleural invasion, which is much more common, does not appear to correlate with pleural fluid cytology positivity [14].

Pathophysiology of Metastases to Serosal Membranes

Malignant cells can reach serosal membranes by direct extension and by lymphatic, transcoelomic, and hematogenous routes. Direct extension can, for instance, occur in lung cancer extending to the pleural or pericardial membranes or in intraabdominal malignancies with visceral peritoneal invasion. Obstruction of the lymph nodes by metastatic deposits may cause backflow of lymph and tumor cells into the serosal cavity and attachment to the serosal membrane. Hematogenous metastases to the parietal serosal membranes can also occur and may be the most common mechanism of spread of bronchogenic carcinomas to the pleurae. The transcoelomic route of serosal membrane metastasis is the main mechanism of ovarian cancer spread, which involves shedding of tumor cells into the peritoneal fluid, transit of the tumor cells throughout the peritoneal cavity, and colonization of the peritoneum with formation of micrometastases that may evolve into macroscopic tumor deposits [8].

The likelihood of any particular malignancy to metastasize to serosal membranes and be found in serous effusions depends on their anatomic location, i.e., proximity to a serosal membrane, the frequency and anatomic locations of their lymph node metastases, and to other tumor and serosal membrane factors that can be explained by the "seed and soil" hypothesis [16] proposed in 1899 by the English surgeon Stephen Paget (1855–1926), the son of the famous surgeon and pathologist Sir James Paget (1814–1899). According to this theory, the nonrandom distribution of metastases ("organotropism") is caused by both the properties of the tumor cells ("seed") and of the specific microenvironment of the organ receiving the metastasis ("soil"). In order to seed a serosal membrane, tumor cells must have certain characteristics that allow them to survive the metastatic cascade steps and have to implant onto a congenial soil, in this case the mesothelium. In the current understanding of the seed and soil hypothesis, the primary tumor may prime the soil by forming premetastatic niches that change the microenvironment of the soil to suit the implantation and growth of metastases. The serosal fluid is one of the premetastatic niches and malignant cells present in serosal fluid have been shown to release exosomes, soluble growth factors, adhesion molecules, and chemokines that create a permissive immune environment, allowing them to home to the mesothelium and activating pro-metastatic processes [17].

The ability of the malignant cells to form serosal metastatic deposits and nodules appears to be related to various factors, but the initiation of the metastatic process appears to be mainly related to their ability to undergo epithelial to mesenchymal transition. This may explain why serosal metastases almost always show gene expression patterns related to EMT, although their corresponding primary tumors may not show this expression pattern [18]. EMT involves "cadherin-switching," in which the expression of E-cadherin is downregulated and the expression of N-cadherin and P-cadherin concomitantly increases. E-cadherin is a glycoprotein that is present in desmosomes and, in addition to binding cells to each other, also suppresses cell motility and invasion and therefore suppresses metastasis. After undergoing EMT, the tumor cell loss of epithelial properties like adhesion and acquisition of mesenchymal properties plays an important role in the departure of tumor cells from the primary tumor and their transserosal migration into the serosal cavity. EMT is also closely associated with the stem-cell-like properties of cancer cells, including their ability to evade apoptosis.

After falling into the serosal fluid, such "homeless" cells are referred to as free cancer cells.

The presence of free cancer cells within serosal fluids and serosal cavity washings obtained intraoperatively does not always lead to the formation of serosal metastatic deposits, because they may either be unable to survive in the fluid or are unable to adhere and colonize the mesothelial membrane. Once in the serosal fluid, the detached malignant cells have to evade anoikis and survive flotation in a fluid milieu. In addition, malignant cells have to evade immune surveillance, since serosal fluids contain a variable number of other cells, including neutrophils, lymphocytes, and macrophages, as well as exfoliated mesothelial cells that have acquired phagocytic capacity, all of which could destroy the malignant cells that have reached the serosal fluid.

Anoikis (from Greek, meaning "the state of being without a home") [19] is a form of programmed cell death (apoptosis) suffered by anchorage-dependent cells when they lose contact with the extracellular matrix. One of the mechanisms that help free cancer cells to evade anoikis is their spontaneous aggregation into clumps or "spheroids," which may be facilitated by P-cadherin. These multicellular hetero-spheroids are formed with the participation of recruited cancer-associated fibro-blasts (CAFs) derived from fibroblasts, endothelial cells, and mesothelial cells that have undergone EMT in response to cytokines, including TNF-β1, that are secreted by the malignant cells and exosomes, which transfer miRNA and proteins from the malignant cells to the mesothelial cells. Within these spheroids, cancer cells maintain an epithelial phenotype, with expression of E-cadherin and EpCAM, and secrete cytokines that modify the serosal membrane microenvironment to favor their adhesion to the mesothelial lining. The formation of spheroids not only helps cancer cells escape anoikis but also facilitates their adherence to the mesothelial surface. Within the fluid milieu, cancer cells also undergo metabolic changes including a glycolytic switch from aerobic mitochondrial respiration to cytosolic glycolysis, which is less efficient but more rapid, with resultant lactate production and extracellular acidification, which helps the cancer cells' evasion of immunosurveillance [20]. The EMT-related acquisition of stem-cell-like properties by free cancer cells also confers them resistance to anoikis; these stem-cell-like properties are expressed by a higher percentage of cancer cells that are present singly as compared to those that are present in clusters.

Metastatic colonization, or the attachment of free cancer cells to the serosal membrane, is the least efficient step of the metastatic process. The intact continuous mesothelial lining with its intercellular attachments acts as a barrier to the invasion of the serosal membranes by cancer cells. The glycocalyx covering the mesothelial cells acts to repulse tumor cells, offering some protection from attachment. In addition, most free cancer cells that successfully attach to mesothelial cells die off due to the poor nutrient milieu. However, some of the cancer cells succeed by loosely attaching via adhesion molecules like CD44 that interacts with the hyaluronan on the surface of mesothelial cells. Attachment can also occur in areas of damaged mesothelium or in senescent mesothelium. After attachment, malignant cells secrete cytokines that lead to the exfoliation or contraction of mesothelial cells, leaving gaps of exposed basement membrane in between, to which cancer cells attach by way of integrins. This mechanism is referred to as "transmesothelial" serosal dissemination. Another mechanism that free cancer cells use to attach to the serosal membrane involves attachment to milky spots, which are soft spots for metastatic dissemination. Free cancer cells migrate to the lymphatic sinus of the milky spot and proliferate and induce neovascularization. Since this mechanism, referred to as translymphatic serosal dissemination, involves fewer steps, it leads to metastatic seeding of serosal membranes earlier than the more complicated transmesothelial mechanism.

After attachment to the basement membrane, malignant cells revert to their epithelial phenotype and invade the submesothelial tissue using motility factors and matrix metalloproteinases. To produce larger tumor deposits, tumor cells induce vascular neogenesis and lymphangiogenesis through secretion of vascular endothelial growth factor (VEGF) and basic fibroblast growth factor (bFGF). They also recruit cells to form tumor-associated stroma or "activated stroma," the major components of which are CAF, macrophages, lymphocytes, and endothelial cells, all of which play a major role in tumor progression.

The details of this complex metastatic cascade that leads to the formation of serosal membrane metastases are the result of extensive research into the mechanisms of pleural, pericardial, and especially peritoneal metastases. The elucidation of the essential steps of this metastatic cascade and the identification of a number of molecules that are involved in them will hopefully lead to targeted therapies aimed at reducing serosal membrane metastases, which are one of the main causes of morbidity and mortality in a number of cancers that have a predilection to metastasize to serosal membranes.

References

1. Bichat X. Traité des membranes en général et de diverses membranes en particulier. Nouv. éd. / revue et augm. de notes par M. Magendie. Paris: Méquignon-Marvis; 1827.
2. Minot CS. The mesoderm and the coelom of vertebrates. Am Nat. 1890;24:877–98.
3. Pereira A, Mendizabal E, de Leon J, et al. Peritoneal carcinomatosis: a malignant disease with an embryological origin? Surg Oncol. 2015;24(3):305–11.
4. Krausz T, McGregor SM. The mesothelium. Embryology, anatomy, and biology. In: Marchevsky AM, Husain AN, Galateau-Sallé F, editors. Practical pathology of serous membranes. Cambridge: Cambridge University Press; 2019. p. 1–9.
5. van Baal JO, Van de Vijver KK, Nieuwland R, et al. The histophysiology and pathophysiology of the peritoneum. Tissue Cell. 2017;49(1):95–105.
6. Kienzle A, Servais AB, Ysasi AB, et al. Free-floating mesothelial cells in pleural fluid after lung surgery. Frontiers in Med. 2018;5:89.
7. Mutsaers SE. The mesothelial cell. Int J Biochem Cell Biol. 2004;36(1):9–16.
8. van Baal J, van Noorden CJF, Nieuwland R, et al. Development of peritoneal carcinomatosis in epithelial ovarian cancer: a review. J Histochem Cytochem. 2018;66(2):67–83.
9. Penninkilampi R, Eslick GD. Perineal talc use and ovarian cancer: a systematic review and meta-analysis. Epidemiology. 2018;29(1):41–9.
10. Meyer PC. Metastatic carcinoma of the pleura. Thorax. 1966;21(5):437–43.
11. Starling EH, Tubby AH. On absorption from and secretion into the serous cavities. J Physiol. 1894;16:140–55.
12. Neergaard K. Zur Frage des Druckes im Pleuraspalt. Beitr Klin Tuberk Spezif Tuberkuloseforsch. 1927;65(4):476–85.
13. Vakil E, Ost D, Vial MR, et al. Non-specific pleuritis in patients with active malignancy. Respirology. 2018;23(2):213–9.
14. Froudarakis ME, Plojoux J, Kaspi E, et al. Positive pleural cytology is an indicator for visceral pleural invasion in metastatic pleural effusions. Clin Respir J. 2018;12(3):1011–6.
15. Grosu HB, Kazzaz F, Vakil E, Molina S, Ost D. Sensitivity of initial thoracentesis for malignant pleural effusion stratified by tumor type in patients with strong evidence of metastatic disease. Respiration. 2018;96(4):363–9.

16. Paget S. The distribution of secondary growths in cancer of the breast. Lancet. 1889;133(3421):571–3.
17. Mikula-Pietrasik J, Uruski P, Tykarski A, Ksiazek K. The peritoneal "soil" for a cancerous "seed": a comprehensive review of the pathogenesis of intraperitoneal cancer metastases. Cell Mol Life Sci. 2018;75(3):509–25.
18. Shelygin YA, Pospekhova NI, Shubin VP, et al. Epithelial-mesenchymal transition and somatic alteration in colorectal cancer with and without peritoneal carcinomatosis. Biomed Res Int. 2014;2014:629496.
19. Frisch SM, Francis H. Disruption of epithelial cell-matrix interactions induces apoptosis. J Cell Biol. 1994;124(4):619–26.
20. Wilson RB, Solass W, Archid R, Weinreich F-J, Königsrainer A, Reymond MA. Resistance to anoikis in transcoelomic shedding: the role of glycolytic enzymes. Pleura and Peritoneum. 2019;4(1):1–14.

Index

A

Abdominal fluid, paracentesis, 38
Acellular mucin, 183, 184
Acinar formation, 102
Actinomyces, 37
Acute inflammation, 10
Adenocarcinoma (ADC), 78, 101, 102, 104
 cannonballs, 102
 cytological criteria, 102
 psammoma bodies, 102
 pseudomyxoma peritonei, 103
Adenomatoid tumor, 64
Adult granulosa cell tumor, 124
ADx Amplification Refractory Mutation
    System (ADx-ARMS), 150
Agar cell block technique, 255, 256
ALK, *see* Anaplastic lymphoma kinase (AKL)
Anaplastic large cell lymphoma (ALCL),
    119, 222
Anaplastic lymphoma kinase (ALK), 133,
    134, 145
Ancillary studies for serous fluids, 129
 cell-based research, 154, 155
 cell free DNA, 154
 digital PCR (dPCR), 151, 152
 DNA testing
  methylation, 151
  next generation sequencing, 150, 151
  predictive DNA mutation analysis in
    effusions, 147
  Sanger sequencing, 150
  tumor cell enrichment, 148–150
 FISH analysis, 140
  diagnostic testing in
    mesothelioma, 141–143
  diagnostic testing in other tumor
    types, 143
  gene amplifications, 144, 147
  gene rearrangements, 144
  predictive testing, 143

technical aspects, 140, 141
 microRNAs, 153, 154
 predictive immunocytochemistry, 130, 131
  ALK, 133, 134
  ARID1A, 139
  estrogen receptor/progesteron
    receptor, 137
  MSI, 139
  Pan-TRK, 136, 137
  PD-L1, 131, 132
  ROS1, 134, 135
 RNA quantity and quality evaluation, 152
 RNA testing, in effusions, 152, 153
 testing predictive mutations, 147–148
Ancillary studies for serous fluids alterations
    in malignant effusions, 147–148
Anucleated and nucleated benign squamous
    cells, 215
Asbestos exposure, 73
Asbestos (ferruginous) body, 33
Ascitic fluid, 13
Aspergillus in fluid cytology, 36
AT-rich interaction domain 1A (*ARID1A*), 139
Atypia of undetermined significance (AUS),
    42, 54, 272
 cell clusters, atypical, 45, 48
 cells of undetermined origin, atypical, 47
 criteria, 42, 44
 definition of, 42
 diagnosis of exclusion, 49
 epithelioid cell, atypical, 43
 epithelioid cell with enlargement and
    binucleation, atypical, 43
 immunostains, 49
 microvacuolated cells, atypical, 44
 peritoneal fluid, paracentesis, 51
 pleural fluid, left, thoracentesis, 50
 pleural fluid, right, thoracentesis, 50
 rate and risk of malignancy, 51
 and SFM, 54

© Springer Nature Switzerland AG 2020
A. Chandra et al. (eds.), *The International System for Serous Fluid
Cytopathology*, https://doi.org/10.1007/978-3-030-53908-5

Atypia of undetermined significance (*cont.*)
    tight papillary clusters, atypical, 46
    two-step reporting approach, 49
Atypical cell clusters, 45, 48
Atypical epithelioid cell with enlargement and
        binucleation, 43
Atypical epithelioid cells, 43
Atypical mesothelial cells, 74
Atypical microvacuolated cells, 44
Atypical tight papillary clusters, 46

B
BAP1, 80, 88, 92, 142
BD Totalys™ multiprocessor, 247
BD Totalys® preparation, 248, 249
BD Totalys® SlidePrep instrument, 247, 248
Benign effusions, 20
Benign mesothelial cells, 69
Benign mesothelial cells with cytoplasmic
        pinching, 70
Benign ovarian epithelial tumors, 189
    Brenner/borderline Brenner tumors,
        190, 192
    endometrioid borderline tumors, 194
    endometrioid cystadenoma/
        adenofibroma, 190
    MBT, 193, 194
    mucinous cystadenoma/adenofibroma, 190
    ovarian borderline tumors, 192
    pelvic cavity, peritoneal lavage, 195
    pelvic cavity, peritoneal washings, 194
    seromucinous cystadenoma/
        adenofibroma, 190
    serous borderline tumors (SBT), 192
    serous cystadenoma, 190
Benign squamous cells, 108
Bile, 184, 185
    bile peritonitis, 185
    bile spillage, 185
Binucleated and multinucleated cells, 66
Binucleated mesothelial cell, 21
BRCA1, 169
BRCA2, 169
Breast adenocarcinoma, 224
Brenner/borderline Brenner tumors, 190, 192
Burkitt lymphoma, 115, 222

C
Calretinin, 83
Cancer-associated fibroblasts (CAFs), 289
Cannibalism, 25
Cannonballs, 102, 287

Carcinoembryonic antigen (CEA), 201
Carcinomatosis, 64
Carcinosarcoma, 221
Cell-based research, 154, 155
Cell block from peritoneal lavage, 26
Cell engulfing, 185
Cell free DNA, 154
Cellient® Automated Cell Block System®,
        240, 251, 259, 262, 264
Cell signaling D4D6 antibody on Ventana
        Benchmark, 136
Cellular clasping, 69
Cell wrapping, 25
Centrifugation (CF), 242, 243
Centrifugation sediment cell block
        technique, 252
Choriocarcinoma, 124
Chromogenic dual in situ hybridization
        (CISH), 146
Chronic lymphocytic leukemia/small
        lymphocytic lymphoma
        (CLL/SLL), 57, 113, 114
Ciliocytophthoria, 32, 176
Classical Hodgkin lymphoma, 118, 119
    cytological criteria, 118
Clear cell carcinoma (CCC), 208, 209
Clot cell block technique, 259
Collagen balls, 31, 32, 174, 175
Collodion bag method, 255, 257, 258
Colorectal adenocarcinoma, 230
Complementary DNA strand (cDNA), 152
Conditional reprogramming (CR), 155
Consistent with borderline tumor,
        46, 171
Curschmann's spirals, 34
Cytoblock™ cell block, 240
Cytocentrifugation, 242
Cytology, 169
Cytology-histology correlation (CHC), 273
CytoLyt®, 240
Cytopathology, 1
Cytopreparatory techniques, 239
    agar method, 255
    BD Totalys™ multiprocessor and BD
        Totalys™ SlidePrep, 247
    cell block preparations, 250, 251
    Cellient®cell block, 262, 264
    centrifugation, 242, 243
    centrifugation sediment, 251, 253
    collection and storage, 239, 240
    collodion bag method, 255, 257
    direct smear preparations, 241
    HistoGel™ (HG) method, 255
    molecular testing, 247, 248, 250

plasma thrombin/thrombin clot method, 253, 255
preparation methods, 240, 241
Shandon Cytoblock™ cell block, 257, 259
ThinPrep® liquid based preparation, 244, 245
CytoRich™, 240
CytoSpin®, 243, 244, 261

D
Daisy cells, 24
Death-associated protein kinase (DAPK), 151
Degenerating mesothelial cells in serous fluid, 10
Desmin, 82
Detached ciliary tufts, 33
Diffuse malignant mesothelioma (DMM), 64
Digital droplet polymerase chain reaction (ddPCR), 151
Digital polymerase chain reaction (dPCR), 151, 152
Digital solid polymerase chain reaction (dsPCR), 151
Disseminated peritoneal adenomucinosis (DPAM), 183
DNA testing
  methylation, 151
  next generation sequencing, 150, 151
  predictive DNA mutation analysis in effusions, 147
  Sanger sequencing, 150
  tumor cell enrichment, 148–150
Dysgerminoma, 217, 218

E
Early mesothelioma (EM), 73
Empyema, 30
Endocervical adenocarcinoma (ECA), 223, 227
Endocervical-type mucinous tumor, 190
Endodermal sinus tumor, *see* Yolk sac tumor (YST)
Endometrial serous carcinoma, 203
Endometrial stromal sarcoma, 221
Endometrioid adenocarcinoma, 198
Endometrioid borderline tumors (EBT), 194, 195
Endometrioid carcinoma (EC), 198, 199, 206, 207
Endometrioid cystadenoma/adenofibroma, 190
Endometriosis, 46, 179, 180

  cytologic criteria, 179, 180
Endosalpingiosis, 31, 46, 175, 176
EPICUP assay, 151
Epithelial membrane antigen (EMA), 81
Epithelial neoplasms, 227
Epithelial to mesenchymal transition (EMT), 280
Estrogen receptor (ER), 137
European Quality Assurance programs (EQA), 268
External quality assurance (EQA), 268

F
False keratinization and degeneration, 24
Favor benign, 47
Favor borderline tumor, 47
Favor reactive, 47
Ferruginous bodies, 33
Fistulas, 35
Fluorescent in situ hybridization (FISH) analysis, 57, 129, 134, 140, 142
  diagnostic testing
    in mesothelioma, 141–143
    in other tumor types, 143
  gene amplifications, 144, 146, 147
  gene rearrangements, 144
  malignant mesothelioma, 89, 90
  predictive testing, 143
  technical aspects, 140, 141
Follicular B-cell lymphoma, 143
Follicular lymphoma, 113

G
Gastrointestinal carcinomas, 228
GATA3, 87
Generalized hemolysis in a serous fluid, 13
Genomic biomarkers, 150
Germ cell tumors, 123, 124, 213
  dysgerminoma, 217, 218
  teratomas (benign and malignant), 214, 216
  yolk sac tumor (YST), 218, 219
Giant cells, 178
Goblet cells, 190
Granulosa cell tumor, 212–214

H
Hematolymphoid neoplasms, 129
Hemolysis in liquid based preparation, 14
Hemosiderin-laden macrophages, 178, 180
Hepatocellular carcinoma, 109

High-grade neoplastic cells, 200, 201, 211
  endometrioid carcinoma, 206
  HGSC, 201, 202
  malignant Brenner tumor/transitional cell
      carcinoma, 208, 210
  mucinous carcinoma, 202, 205, 206
  ovarian clear cell carcinoma, 207, 208
High-grade non-Hodgkin lymphoma, 114, 115
High-grade serous carcinoma (HGSC),
      201, 202
High-grade serous ovarian carcinoma
      (HGSOC), 201
High mobility group box 1 (HMGB1), 91
Histiocytes, 27, 28, 177
HistoGel™ (HG) method, 255, 256
Hodgkin lymphoma (HL), 112
Hodgkin/Reed-Sternberg (H/RS) cells, 119
Hologic ThinPrep® Processor, 246, 247
Homozygous deletion (HD), 89
Hyaluronan (hyaluronic acid), 90, 91
Hyperchromasia, 25

I
Immature teratoma, 214–216
Increased eosinophils, 29
Infectious organisms, 37
Inflammatory cells, 176–178
Inflammatory patterns, 29
International Organization of Standardization
      (ISO), 268
International System for Reporting Serous
      Fluid Cytopathology (TIS), 1
Intestinal contents, bowel rupture, 181
Ion AmpliSeq™ RNA Fusion Lung Cancer
      Panel, 153

K
Kirsten Rat Sarcoma Viral Oncogene
      Homolog (KRAS), 136

L
Laboratory information system, 269
Laboratory integration system, 247
Left pleural fluid, 38
Leiomyosarcoma, 220
Liquid based cytology (LBC), 132
Localized mesothelioma (LM), 64
Low-grade (appendiceal) mucinous
      neoplasm, 199
Low-grade mucinous neoplasm (with
      Pseudomyxoma peritonei), 199, 200

Low grade neoplastic cells, 189
Low-grade non-Hodgkin lymphoma, 113, 114
Low-grade serous carcinoma
      (LGSC), 196–199
Lung, right, thoracentesis, 38
Lupus erythematosus (LE) Cells, 34
Lymphocytic effusion, 57, 58
Lymphoma, 221
Lymphomatous, 112

M
Macrophages, 176–178
  cytologic criteria, 177
Malignant Brenner tumor, 208, 210
Malignant effusions, 155, 286, 287
Malignant low-grade epithelial tumors
  endometrioid carcinoma, 198, 199
  low-grade mucinous neoplasm (with
      Pseudomyxoma peritonei), 199, 200
  low-grade serous carcinoma (LGSC),
      196, 197
  micropapillary serous carcinoma
      (MPSC), 196
Malignant mesothelioma, 77
  asbestos exposure, 64
  benign vs. malignant mesothelial
      cells, 80–83
  benign mesothelial cells with cytoplasmic
      pinching, 70
  and carcinoma, 76, 83, 86, 87
  cellular effusion algorithm, 65
  cytological approach to fluids, 65–67
  cytologic criteria
      definitive criteria of malignancy, 70
      supportive criteria of malignancy, 71
  D2-40 stain, 86
  definition of, 67
  differential diagnosis, 75
  FISH, 89, 90
  frankly malignant with appropriate clinical
      presentation, 93
  frankly malignant with supportive
      immunochemistry, 92
  GATA-3 Stain, 87
  highly atypical mesothelial cells but
      insufficient material, 94
  highly cellular mesothelial sample with
      subtle atypia and supportive
      ancillary tests, 93
  highly cellular sample with atypia and
      inconclusive ancillary tests, 93
  highly cellular sample with atypia and no
      radiological abnormalities, 93

immunochemistry
  on cell block vs. smears, 79
  in work-up, 79
incidence of, 64
malignancy/clinical management, 91, 92
mesothelial cell brush border, 67
mesothelial cell glycogen expression, 67
mesothelial cells with calretinin stain, 84
mesothelioma with lipid, 68
moderately cellular sample with atypia and
      inconclusive ancillary tests, 94
prognostic and predictive markers for, 88
reactive mesothelial cells, 77, 79, 82
serous effusion, findings of, 69
soluble biomarkers, 90, 91
suspicious for mesothelioma, 72
versus carcinoma, 83, 86, 87
WT-1 stain, 85
Malignant Müllerian mixed tumor
      (MMMT), 221
Malignant pleural effusion, 149
Malignant-primary (MAL-P), *see* Malignant
      mesothelioma
Malignant-secondary (MAL-S), 99
ascitic fluid, 125
definition of, 100
diagnostic approach, 100
malignant effusions of epithelial origin
    adenocarcinoma, 101–104
    hepatocellular carcinoma, 109
    renal cell carcinoma, 109
    squamous cell carcinoma, 105–108
    urothelial carcinoma, 108
malignant effusions of germ cell and sex
      cord-stromal origin, 123, 124
malignant effusions of hematolymphoid
      origin, 112
    classical Hodgkin lymphoma, 118, 119
    non-Hodgkin lymphoma, 112–117
    plasma cell neoplasm, 119, 120
malignant effusions of melanocytic origin
    melanoma, 120, 121
    sarcomas, 122, 123
pleural fluid, 124, 125
rate and risk of malignancy/clinical
      management, 124
serous effusion specimens, 101
small cell neuroendocrine
      carcinoma, 109–111
squamous cell carcinoma, 108
Mantle cell lymphoma, 113
Marginal zone lymphoma, 113
Mature teratoma, 214–216
Melanoma, 120, 121

cytological criteria, 121
Merkel cell carcinoma, 111
Mesenchymal-epithelial-transition (*MET*)
      amplification, 146
Mesenchymal neoplasms, 220
Mesothelial cell, 18, 20, 21, 45, 66, 172, 173
  with calretinin stain, 84
  cytologic criteria, 174
  glycogen expression, 67
  reactive, 174
  with windows, 21
Mesothelial cell brush border, 67
Mesothelial-mesenchymal transition
      (MMT), 280
Mesothelial tumors, 64
Mesothelin, 90
Mesothelioma, 188
Mesothelioma in situ (MIS), 73
Metastatic adenocarcinoma, 101, 243, 251
Metastatic alveolar rhabdomyosarcoma, 122
Metastatic carcinoma, 223
  breast carcinoma, 103, 262
  endocervical adenocarcinoma, 223
  squamous cell carcinoma (SCC), 223, 226
Metastatic colorectal adenocarcinoma, 105
Metastatic gastric adenocarcinoma, 104, 205
Metastatic high grade serous carcinoma of
      ovary, 106
Metastatic lung adenocarcinoma, 260
Metastatic malignancy, 9
Metastatic melanoma, 121
Metastatic mucinous carcinoma, 204
Metastatic ovarian adenocarcinoma, 241,
      246, 253
Metastatic pulmonary adenocarcinoma, 107
Metastatic renal cell carcinoma, 110
Metastatic small cell carcinoma, 250
Metastatic small cell neuroendocrine
      carcinoma, 111
Metastatic squamous cell carcinoma, 108
Methylation, 151
Methylthioadenosine phosphorylase
      (MTAP), 81
Micropapillary serous carcinoma (MPSC), 196
MicroRNAs (miRNAs), 153, 154
Microsatellite instability (MSI), 139
Microsatellite stable (MSS), 139
Mixed acute and chronic inflammation, 177
Mixed epithelial and mesenchymal
      neoplasms, 220
Modified Giemsa or Papanicolaou methods, 20
Mucinous borderline tumors (MBT), 193, 194
Mucinous carcinoma, 202, 204–206
Mucinous cystadenoma, 190, 191

N

Necrotic material, 34
Negative for malignancy (NFM), 46, 51, 54,
        173, 271
    abdominal fluid, paracentesis, 38
    algorithmic approach to serous
            effusions, 19
    binucleated mesothelial cell, 21
    cell block from peritoneal lavage, 26
    cellular findings
        histiocytes, 27
        increased eosinophils, 29
        lymphocytes, 27
        mesothelial cells, 25
        neutrophils, 30
        without regard to volume/distribution,
            18, 20, 24
    ciliocytophthoria type change, 32
    criteria for, 18
    definition of, 17
    endosalpingiosis, 31
    false keratinization and degeneration, 24
    histiocytes, 28
    left pleural fluid, 38
    lung, right, thoracentesis, 38
    mesothelial cells, 20
    mesothelial cells with windows, 21
    peritoneal lavage, 24
    pleural effusion, 38
    psamomma body in peritoneal fluid, 30
    reactive mesothelial cells, 22
    right lung, pleural fluid, 38
    serous effusion, approach to, 18
    unexpected cellular and noncellular
            findings
        asbestos (ferruginous) bodies, 33
        collagen balls, 31
        Curschmann's spirals, 34
        detached ciliary tufts, 33
        fistulas, 35
        infectious organisms, 37
        lupus erythematosus cells, 34
        necrotic material, 34
        psammoma bodies, 31
        rate and risk of malignancy, 37
        unexpected benign cellular and non
            cellular findings, 31
        unexpected cell population (second cell
            population), 30
    various inflammatory patterns, 29
Neoplastic cells, 201
Neurotrophic receptor tyrosine kinase
        (NTRK), 137
    isoforms, 136

Next generation sequencing (NGS), 130, 134,
        150, 151
Nocardia in fluid, 36
Non-diagnostic (ND), 9, 11
    ascitic fluid, 13
    clinical management, 13
    definition of, 11
    degenerate sample, 12
    lung, right, thoracentesis, 15
    peritoneal cavity, paracentesis, 14
Non-hematolymphoid malignancies, 120
Non-Hodgkin lymphoma (NHL), 112, 113
    high-grade non-Hodgkin lymphoma,
            114, 115
    low-grade non-Hodgkin lymphoma,
            113, 114
    lymphocyte-rich serous fluid specimens,
            116, 117
    primary cavity-based malignant
            effusion, 117
Non-seminomatous germ cell tumors, 123
Non-small cell lung cancer (NSCLC),
        81, 132–134
Normal effusion, 18
Normal mesothelial cells, 173

O

Orangeophilia, 107
Organoids, 155
Organotypic spherical 3D ex vivo cancer
        models, 155
Osteopontin, 91
Ovarian borderline tumors, 192
Ovarian clear cell carcinoma (OCCC),
        207, 208
Ovarian sex cord stromal tumors, 211

P

Pancreatic adenocarcinoma, 224
Pancreaticobiliary, 205
Pan-TRK, 136, 137
Pap tests, 180
Para-malignant effusion, 286
Paucicellular specimens, 12
Periodic acid Schiff (PAS) stain, 66, 67
    PAS with diastase digestion
            (PASD), 83, 205
Peritoneal cavity, paracentesis, 14
Peritoneal inclusion cysts (PIC), 186
Peritoneal lavage, 24, 25
Peritoneal washings, 172
    benign background elements, 172

collagen balls, 174, 175
cytologic criteria, 174
endometriosis, 179, 180
endosalpingiosis, 175, 176
inflammatory Cells, 176–178
mesothelial cell, 173, 174
peritoneal fluid, lavage, 181
peritoneal fluid, washings, 180
cytopathologic approach, 170–172
differential diagnosis of bland epithelial/
low grade neoplastic cells, 189
endometrioid carcinoma, 207
high-grade neoplastic cells, 200, 201, 211
endometrioid carcinoma, 206
HGSC, 201, 202
malignant Brenner tumor/transitional
cell carcinoma, 208, 210
mucinous carcinoma, 202, 205, 206
ovarian clear cell carcinoma (OCCC),
207, 208
immunochemistry
for indeterminate cells in, 229–230
in peritoneal fluid, 227, 228
low grade neoplastic cells, 189
malignant low-grade epithelial tumors
abdominal cavity, peritoneal
lavage, 200
endometrioid carcinoma, 198, 199
low-grade mucinous neoplasm (with
Pseudomyxoma peritonei), 199, 200
low-grade serous carcinoma (LGSC),
196, 197
micropapillary serous carcinoma
(MPSC), 196
mesothelial proliferations, 186
right pelvis, peritoneal washings, 187
well differentiated papillary
mesothelioma (WDPM), 187
nonepithelial elements, 181, 182
abdominal cavity, peritoneal
lavage, 186
acellular mucin, 183
bile, 184, 185
peritoneal lavage, 186
Psammoma bodies, 182, 183
serous benign/borderline ovarian tumors
from malignant tumors, 228
staging and clinical relevance, 168–170
staging of carcinoma by tumor origin, 168
unusual and uncommon
gynecologic tumors
germ cell tumors, 213, 214, 216–219
granulosa cell tumor, 212, 213
lymphoma, 221

mesenchymal neoplasms, 220
metastatic carcinoma, 223, 226
mixed epithelial and mesenchymal
neoplasms, 220
ovarian sex cord stromal tumors, 211
pelvis, left gutter, washing, 219
Pigmented macrophages, 185
Plasma cell myeloma, 120
Plasma cell neoplasm, 119, 222
CD138 expression, 120
cytologic alcriteria, 119
Plasma thrombin cell block technique, 254
Plasma thrombin (PT) method, 253, 255
Pleomorphism, 78
Pleural effusion, 38, 60
Pleural malignant effusion (ME), 148
Pleural metastasis of breast cancer, 138
Pleural rind, 64
Poorly differentiated/non-keratinizing
squamous cell carcinoma, 106, 107
PreservCyt™, 244, 262
Primary cavity-based malignant effusion, 117
Primary effusion lymphoma (PEL), 117, 118
Progesterone receptor (PR), 137
Programmed cell death ligand 1 (PD-L1),
88, 131–133
Prostate adenocarcinoma, 224
Psammoma bodies, 31, 176, 182, 183
in peritoneal fluid, 30
Pseudokeratotic cells, 74
Pseudomyxoma peritonei (PMP), 58, 103,
172, 183, 190, 193, 199, 206
Pulmonary adenocarcinomas, 135

Q
Quality assurance (QA), 268
elements of, 270
Quality control (QC), 268
Quality improvement (QI), 268
Quality management (QM)
analytic phase, 269
analytic phase monitors, 271–274
component of, 268
post-analytic phase, 269, 274, 275
pre-analytic phase, 269, 271
quality assurance, elements of, 270
for serous fluid cytopathology, 270

R
Rapid on-site assessment (ROSE), 248
Reactive mesothelial cells, 22, 23, 77,
79, 82, 174

Reactive mesothelium (RM), 75, 76
Rearranged during transfection (RET), 144
Receptor tyrosine kinase (ROS1), 134, 135
Renal cell carcinoma, 109
Retinoic acid receptor β (RARβ), 151
Rheumatoid changes, 35
Rheumatoid disease, 35
Rheumatoid serositis, 35
Richard-Allan Scientific™ HistoGel™
          Specimen Processing Gel, 255
Right lung, pleural fluid, 38
Risk of malignancy (ROM), 5, 6, 37, 41
    AUS, 51
    MAL-S, 124
    SFM, 58, 59
RNA quantity and quality evaluation, 152
ROS1, 136

S
Sanger sequencing, 150
Sarcomas, 122, 123
Sarcomatoid component, 64
Secondary malignant effusions,
          sources of, 101
Seminoma/dysgerminoma, 123
Sequencing by synthesis approach, 150
Seromucinous cystadenoma/
          adenofibroma, 190
Serosal cavity anatomy and fluid dynamics
    pericardium, 284
    peritoneum, 282, 283
    pleurae, 283, 284
Serosal fluid formation and
          resorption, 284–286
Serosal membranes, pathophysiology of
          metastases, 287–290
Serous borderline tumors (SBT), 192, 193
Serous carcinoma, 192
Serous cystadenoma, 190, 191
Serous effusions
    algorithmic approach, 19
    cytology, 4, 5, 239
    cytopathology, reporting format, 4
    negative for malignancy (NFM), 18
Serous endometrial carcinoma (SEC), 201
Serous fluid
    cytology, 37
    degenerating mesothelial cells in, 10
    generalized hemolysis in, 13
    terminology, 1
Serous fluid cytopathology
    rate and risk of malignancy, 5, 6
    report format, 3, 4

Serous membranes, 279–282
Serous neoplasms, 227
Sex cord-stromal tumor, 123, 124
Shandon Cytoblock™ cell block, 257, 259
Signet-ring cells, 205
Small cell neuroendocrine carcinoma,
          109, 111
    cytological criteria, 110
Small cluster of mesothelial cells, 177
Soluble biomarkers, malignant
          mesothelioma, 90, 91
Soluble mesothelin-related protein
          (SMRP), 90
Spherical organoids, 156
Squamous cell carcinoma (SCC), 78, 87, 105,
          107, 108, 223, 225, 226
    cytological criteria, 106, 107
Starling equation, 285
Starling forces, 285
SurePath™, 240, 250
Suspicious for malignancy (SFM), 44, 51,
          56–58, 74
    algorithm for, 55
    ascitic fluid, paracentesis, 59
    and AUS, 54
    cytologic criteria, 54, 55
    definition, 54
    immunochemistry, 55–57
    lung, left pleura, thoracentesis, 59, 60
    pleural effusion, 60
    rate and risk of malignancy/clinical
          management, 58, 59
Suspicious for mesothelioma, 72
Systemic lupus erythematosus (SLE), 34

T
Talcum powder crystal in pelvic washing
          fluid, 181
T-cell acute lymphoblastic leukemia/
          lymphoma (T-cell ALL/LBL),
          115, 116
Tenascin, 91
Teratomas (benign and malignant), 214, 216
Testicular germ cell tumors, 201
The Bethesda System (TBS), 1
The International System (TIS), 2
The International System for Reporting Serous
          Fluid Cytopathology (TIS), 2, 5
ThermoScientific Cytoblock® cell block
          preparation system, 257, 261
ThermoScientific CytoSpin® Processor, 243
Thermo Scientific™ Shandon™ Cytoblock™ cell
          block, 240

Thick mucin with atypical cells, 184
ThinPrep®, 240, 244–246
Thoracentesis, 148
Thrombin clot method, 253, 255
Transitional cell carcinoma, 208, 210
Tumor proportion score (TPS), 132
Two-toned cytoplasm, 20

U
Unexpected cell population (second cell
        population), 30, 31
United Kingdom National External Quality
        Assessment Service (UK
        NEQAS), 268
Urothelial carcinoma, 78, 108
UroVysion® multi-probe FISH assay, 142

V
Vascular endothelial growth factor
        (VEGF), 290
Ventana ALK (D5F3) assay, 134

W
Walthard's rest, 172, 192
Well differentiated/keratinizing squamous cell
        carcinoma, 106
Well-differentiated mucinous carcinoma, 184
Well differentiated papillary mesothelioma
        (WDPM), 64, 187

Y
Yolk sac tumor (YST), 218, 219